CIRCULATING NOW, FULL CIRCLE

CIRCULATING NOW, FULL CIRCLE

From the Historical Collections of the National Library of Medicine

Edited by

Elizabeth A. Mullen and Jeffrey S. Reznick

VIRGINIA TECH™
PUBLISHING

CIRCULATING NOW
From the Historical Collections of the National Library of Medicine

First published 2024 by Virginia Tech Publishing

This open access book was realized in part by staff of the National Library of Medicine (NLM), with support from the NLM.

Virginia Tech Publishing
University Libraries at Virginia Tech
560 Drillfield Drive
Blacksburg, VA, 24061

Cataloging in Publication Data

Name: Elizabeth A. Mullen | Jeffrey S. Reznick—editors.

Title: Circulating Now, Full Circle: From the Historical Collections of the National Library of Medicine

Description: Blacksburg, VA: Virginia Tech Publishing, 2024.

Identifiers: ISBN: 978-1-962841-96-2 (PDF) • ISBN: 978-1-962841-97-9 (EPUB) •
ISBN: 978-1-962841-98-6 (PRINT)
DOI: https://doi.org/10.21061/circulating-now

Subjects: History | Blogs | Libraries and Archives

To all who contributed to the creation of this book,
all who have contributed to its foundation, *Circulating Now*,
and all who value the historical collections of the
National Library of Medicine, today and tomorrow.

CONTENTS

ACKNOWLEDGMENTS

This open access book, like *Circulating Now*, the blog upon which it is based, was a highly collaborative initiative made possible by the time and talent of many individuals. We thank the authors of the chapter introductions for their insightful framing of the selected blog posts that follow their work. We thank the original contributors to *Circulating Now* for their enthusiastic support to include their posts in this book, and especially those who generously agreed to offer reflections on their original contributions, which provide enlightening interludes in each chapter. We also thank the leadership of the National Library of Medicine (NLM) for supporting *Circulating Now* from its inception, the founding and former blog editorial board members for their guidance and leadership, the current board for their support, and the leadership of the NLM History of Medicine Division who reviewed and supported the original project proposal. Additionally, we thank Peter Potter of Virginia Tech Publishing for his willingness to take on this project; Mary Culler for her work in tracking all the details of the project and preparing the files and metadata; Caitlin Bean, Robert Browder, Corinne Guimont, and Emily Hills for their experience and expertise; and Kristina Dunne, NLM Pathways Intern, for her careful proofreading of the penultimate manuscript. We also thank Allison Cao, NLM Pathways Intern, for her careful review of the hyperlinks. We also extend our thanks to E. Thomas Ewing for his enthusiasm and generous support, and to the three anonymous peer reviewers who offered outstanding feedback on our original manuscript and many ideas to improve it.

We have made every effort to trace and acquire permissions from the copyright holders of material reproduced here, which was originally published on *Circulating Now* according to the Association for Research Libraries' Code of Best Practices in Fair Use and which does not otherwise fall into the public domain. With regard to our copyright research, we are especially grateful to our colleagues Douglas Atkins, Nicole Baker, Sarah Eilers, Lindsay Franz, Margaret Kaiser, Jiwon Kim, Christie Moffatt, Jill L. Newmark, John Rees, Ginny A. Roth, Susan L. Speaker, and Rebecca Warlow, and, for their own valuable time and thoughtful support, Joyce Backus, Eric Gallinek, Todd Gallinek, Becky Lyon, Jan Schultz, Marti Spiegelman, and James Wanner. We also thank our many colleagues in archives, libraries, and other institutions who kindly responded to our copyright inquires and offered their experience and expertise, including Claire Bassett and JoAnn Pospisil, Library and Archives, Baylor College of Medicine; Ros Bidmead, Michelle Cunliffe, Caroline Gilchrist, and Jake Stayt, Anna Freud Centre; Dawn Bonner, George Washington's Mount Vernon, Mount Vernon Ladies' Association; Ruth Bryan, Jason Flahardy, and Megan Mummey, Special Collections Research Center, University of Kentucky Libraries; Michelle Chiles and Hilary Gunnels, Phillips Memorial Library, Providence College; Mary Catherine DeNoble, Queens University; Stephanie Desmon, The Johns Hopkins Center for Communication Programs; Christie Hartmann and Fiona Maynard, Playboy Archives; Christy Henshaw, Wellcome Collection; Sharon Knecht, Oblate Sisters of Providence Archives; Sarah Lepinski, The Metropolitan Museum of Art; Sharon Li-shiuan Yang and Xiao-He Ma, Harvard-Yenching Library; Patrick Maxton, Chris Schoenherr, Emily Simkin, and Kimberley Washington, Abbott Historical Archives; Sammi Merritt, Jameatris Yvette Rimkus, and Linda S. Stepp, University Archives, University of Illinois at Urbana-Champaign; Patrick O'Dowd, The University Press of Kentucky; Stephanie Plunkett, Norman Rockwell Museum; Matthew Richardson, Texas Medical Center Library; Margaret Rockwell, Norman Rockwell Family Agency; Barbara Ryan, Association for Computing Machinery; Patrick Spero, American Philosophical Society; and Samuel Thrope, The National Library of Israel.

Any errors in this book are our own, and we would appreciate hearing from anyone who would contact us with corrections. Should any copyright holders step forward after publication, due acknowledgement will gladly be made.

ELIZABETH A. MULLEN AND JEFFREY S. REZNICK
July 2024

HOW TO READ THIS BOOK

NOTE ABOUT ITS ONLINE AND PRINT EDITIONS

To achieve the widest possible distribution, this volume is available in both online and print editions. The online edition can be found, free of charge, on the Virginia Tech Publishing website at https://doi.org/10.21061/circulating-now. The print edition can be purchased through Amazon.

Much of the content of this book consists of blog posts reprinted from their original born-digital publication *Circulating Now*, a blog dedicated to the historical collections of the National Library of Medicine (NLM). In their original format, these posts include a significant layer of context and content intrinsic to online publication platforms in the form of hyperlinks. These hyperlinks provide access to full text, digitized documents, resources, and further information from a wide network of sources. We encourage readers of the print edition to explore the online edition, which retains the hyperlinks included in the original text. We also encourage readers to follow the URLs provided in the text to the original posts in order to experience them in context and encounter the full content of *Circulating Now*.

The print and online versions of this book bring the project full circle as they become part of the NLM's historical collections, preserved for future generations. As such, they are available in the NLM reading room and online in the NLM Digital Collections at https://collections.nlm.nih.gov/CirculatingNowFullCircle. The online publication *Circulating Now* is also being preserved in the collections as part of the NLM Web Collecting initiative via the Internet Archive at https://wayback.archive-it.org/3758/*/https://circulatingnow.nlm.nih.gov/.

PREFACE

MARY CULLER AND E. THOMAS EWING

Circulating Now, the blog of the National Library of Medicine (NLM), sustains and grows the commitment of the NLM "to provide knowledge and expertise freely and to inspire people and enrich lives." As this collection illustrates, *Circulating Now* has become a virtual space that brings the rich and world-renowned historical collections and related resources of the NLM into public dialogue with medical experts, librarians, historians, and the thoughtful public. This open-access book underscores the value of *Circulating Now* by introducing its dynamic content into the twenty-first-century scholarly publishing ecosystem as a resource to be even more widely appreciated, referenced, and shared by interested readers and preserved for the future.

The chapter introductions of this book, along with the selected posts that appear in each chapter, demonstrate the remarkable range of chronological, thematic, and geographical content provided by *Circulating Now*: from sixteenth-century European medical books to mid twentieth-century Chinese pamphlets detailing proper public health behaviors to twenty-first-century digital collections of websites, and much, much more. These various collections have inspired writers from a variety of backgrounds to explore a plethora of themes related to medicine such as race, gender, war, and many other aspects of the human condition. Along the way, many of these writers address broader themes of collaboration, clear communication with the public, and highlighting underrepresented stories. The depth and breadth of these posts represent the richness of the historical collections and related resources of the NLM. This book will inspire you to delve deep into *Circulating Now*, and, by extension, the collections of the world's largest biomedical library, which have been acquired, organized, and made freely available by generations of civil servants and valued by generations of researchers, teachers, and many others.

As an open access platform, *Circulating Now* provides its posts freely to the public, scholars, educators, and students at a time when so much content, especially academic journals in specialized medical fields, has been placed behind paywalls or requires subscriptions. Given that accessing a single article from a medical journal can cost close to fifty dollars, and annual subscriptions run into thousands of dollars, *Circulating Now* is an outstanding public service and public history initiative. Moreover, publishing with *Circulating Now* offers scholars and students the opportunity to share their research openly and with a wide audience.

Circulating Now is part of an emerging information ecosystem that connects academic writing, public audiences, and important contemporary issues. While academics have historically found a public voice by writing newspaper op-eds, speaking at public venues, and being interviewed on radio or television, the expansion of public discourse through blogs, newsletters, and social media has created remarkable new opportunities for engaging public audiences with relevant issues. While *Circulating Now* is managed by the staff of a federal agency, other blogs serving a similar purpose of bringing academic writing to public audiences are associated with media organizations (*Made by History* from *The Washington Post*), professional associations (the American Historical Association or Medical Heritage Library), or autonomous collaborations of academics (*Nursing Clio*). Together, these scholarly and publicly accessible blogs contribute to the democratization of knowledge—carrying on this important commitment and tradition of libraries—as their curated content creates and sustains an open dialogue among readers as well as authors, regardless of institutional affiliation or personal resources. Within higher education, these writings for public audiences are increasingly valued along with more traditional forms of scholarship such as monographs, chapters in edited volumes, and peer-reviewed journal articles. In fact, these publicly engaged forms of scholarship often complement, reinforce, and augment more traditional forms of scholarship, as authors or editors of books, for example, use the format of the academic blog to make their original research more accessible to the public—and thus build an audience for their scholarly works as well.

Circulating Now therefore responds to and advances this important shift in scholarship in the humanities, and especially medical history, toward engaging broad audiences and enhancing public understanding of important issues. The remarkable scope of *Circulating Now* posts on the COVID-19 pandemic is just the most recent example of how this platform contributes and responds to urgent public health questions. In higher education, increasing value is being placed on scholarship that addresses important social issues, engages diverse perspectives, and contributes to public understanding of important topics. While traditional scholarly platforms such as peer-reviewed journals or academic books remain important for academics, faculty have come to appreciate that publicly engaged scholarship should also be part of their academic trajectory. In addition to broadening the audience for original scholarly works, academic blogs like *Circulating Now* require a different approach to scholarly writing that should also be part of the portfolio of any academic—and the training of undergraduate and graduate students.

Circulating Now also provides an important public service by providing reliable, trusted, and verified medical information for all readers. Its numerous posts on vaccines, for example, provide reliable information about a topic that has broad implications for community health as well as public discourse. These posts recognize that vaccines have a complicated history, including public resistance, unsuccessful outcomes, and differential impacts, yet each post clearly distinguishes between contested meanings and deliberate misinformation, while providing links directly to trusted medical sources that confirm the efficacy of vaccines. By building posts around primary sources available from the historical collections and related resources of the NLM, *Circulating Now* ensures that readers can track this analysis back to original archival or published sources. "NLM Collections Tour: Vaccines" provides readers and viewers with access to information about the history of vaccines in the form of posters, movies, books, and journals. The early history of vaccines is explored in "Edward Jenner and 'The Happy Immunity'," which directly addresses the controversial origins of many vaccines: "The public has often had trouble putting their trust into something as counter intuitive as giving yourself the germs you're trying to protect yourself from." By tracing the history of the smallpox vaccine from discovery to testing to vaccination, however, this post provides substantive evidence for a vital conclusion: "When you get vaccinated and develop immunity to certain, sometimes deadly, diseases, the entire population benefits from it." "Rashes to Research" acquaints readers with the eponymous NLM exhibition on the 1964 rubella epidemic, during which public health officials communicated a message especially relevant during the COVID-19 pandemic that "vaccination is something we do for others as much as we do for ourselves." The commitment of *Circulating Now* to public engagement is clearly evident in "Don't Hesitate. Vaccinate." Here is a poster featuring characters from the 1977 film *Star Wars*, which offers the humorous, yet vital, question: "Parents of Earth, are your children fully immunized?" Once again, a historical review, in this case, of the remarkable advance in vaccine discovery in the 1970s, lends support to a conclusion urgent for our COVID times during which this book was conceived and produced—and for inevitable future pandemics—the fact that a standard regimen of vaccines is needed for all age groups as part of a commitment to improving the health of society.

Circulating Now posts are particularly well suited for use in educational settings to advance students' appreciation for the complex history of medicine. *Circulating Now* has provided opportunities for students—including interns, graduate students, and undergraduates completing academic projects—to present their research as emerging scholars, or as part of a research team. For students in the humanities, this opportunity to take part in research projects that produce outcomes for evaluation according to set standards has some similarities to the laboratory experiences of students in Science, Technology, Engineering, and Mathematics (STEM), yet also requires the analytical skills appropriate for interpreting complex materials and engaging with important questions. The timeline of academic blogs, with efficient reviews and steps toward publication, in combination with rigorous scholarly review and guidance on reaching broad public audiences, make this format ideal for early-stage researchers. Additionally, *Circulating Now* posts can be assigned as reading material for courses, since the platform allows access by students and instructors regardless of institutional affiliation. By connecting to primary sources in digital form, many of these posts make it possible for students to "do history" on their own, as they can examine the source materials while preparing the steps toward writing an original analytical post accessible to all readers.

As an interpretative resource, *Circulating Now* serves as a portal to the collections of the NLM while expanding public recognition of the Library, fostering interest in the history of medicine and biomedical sciences and allowing people to "visit" the Library virtually and experience the work that happens there. Now this book—as its title conveys—brings *Circulating Now* full circle in a discrete publication that re-introduces and augments this valuable public resource. As a part of the very collections it aims to enhance, this book itself will now circulate widely, helping these collections reach new audiences and, in doing so, advance public understanding of the history of medicine.

INTRODUCTION

ELIZABETH A. MULLEN AND JEFFREY S. REZNICK

"Free things like air,
Vital things like blood,
Living things like ideas . . .
Circulate"

With this introduction, we launched *Circulating Now* in 2013. The idea was—and remains—a simple yet meaningful one:

> For over 175 years the National Library of Medicine's historical collections have circulated to generations within the reading rooms of its current and previous locations in and around Washington, DC. Today, these collections—as part of the trillions of bytes of data produced and delivered by the world's largest biomedical library—circulate daily to millions of people around the world, including scientists, health professionals, scholars, educators, students, and the general public.

Ten years on and stretching into the COVID-19 pandemic, many dozens of individuals of varied backgrounds have published hundreds of stories on *Circulating Now* about their appreciation and use of the vast historical collections of the National Library of Medicine (NLM) to advance research, teaching, and learning about the human condition. Each in their own way, through their attention, interest, engagement, and perspectives, these individuals have become a community contributing to a shared and open knowledge base that consistently enriches our understanding of medical history. This community also reinforces the intellectual and cultural connections between the NLM and other archives, libraries, federal agencies, professional associations, and non-profit organizations, and, by extension, the stewardship of their related collections and resources. Each post authored, co-authored, and read; each link followed; each connection made; and each collaboration surfaced and celebrated further defines and expands this network, shaping it and growing its multitude of access points to the collections and to the authors and the work they are doing. Such individual and collective engagement with and support of the NLM—a federal institution long dedicated to openness, public access, and the surfacing of meaningful stories at the intersection of medicine, science, and society—makes a difference in the ongoing public service of our institution as a national library and a key component of the National Institutes of Health (NIH).

This book marries newly written material with selected posts from the archives of *Circulating Now*, which we have organized thematically to examine, annotate, and enhance what Erin Blakemore of the *Washington Post* called the "varied, lively and sometimes surprising" content of its original source. Throughout, readers will also find a dozen reflections on selected posts written by their original authors—interludes that convey the persistent meaning in the lives of their authors of their contributions and the subjects they address. The resulting volume expands and realizes anew the original mission of *Circulating Now* while joining an increasing number and variety of scholarly and popular books born from and inspired by blogs: from historical fiction and nonfiction to web-based comics and travel guides, Twitter handbooks and best practices in business to animal-welfare advocacy initiatives and advice columns. By extension, as Mary Culler and E. Thomas Ewing explain in their preface, this book contributes to evolving conversations about and guidelines informing how blogs, blogging, and collections born from blogs reflect not only the convergence of our digital age with new ways of writing and longstanding appreciation of "the book" and traditional book culture, but also the diverse and changing ways in which academics undertake research, teach, and talk with their colleagues and the public; students learn and engage with technology and contemporary events; authors and editors conceive, reconceive, and share their work; and readers and publishers receive this work and engage with it.

We conceived this project first and foremost as an open access ebook. While it is available as a physical edition, we hope readers will embrace the virtual version and circulate it widely among colleagues and friends to yield even more points of access, more connections, more research, and even greater use and appreciation of the historical collections and related programs of the NLM. There is no limit to the stories these public resources can reveal, today and tomorrow.

CHAPTER 1

COMMUNICATING COLLECTIONS

INTRODUCTION • JAMES LABOSIER

While the historical collections of the National Library of Medicine (NLM) are preserved for posterity, seemingly unchanging, they are, in fact, ever dynamic as they are studied by one generation after another. Prior to widespread online exposure of these collections, much of what was said about them was confined to articles in print publications. These articles appeared mainly in journals devoted to various fields of medical historical research, written for specific and often academic audiences. With wider access to the collections through the internet came the impetus to connect them to a wider audience. In the midst of this change came "the blog," a common, flexible, informal, and immediately accessible communication platform adaptable to virtually any topic or idea. Enter *Circulating Now,* an ideal project to reach new and broader audiences and engage them in the value and relevance of the historical collections of the NLM. With *Circulating*

Now, curious readers of a variety of backgrounds and located anywhere could connect with and articulate their appreciation of these collections.

In a sense, a blog joins its readers along a common path and leads them to destinations previously undiscovered. Contributors to *Circulating Now* have taken this approach by connecting collections to subjects that are attractive and widely relatable. The authors of these posts, a selection of which appear in this chapter, connected their subjects to the interests of readers through general conventions such as familiar objects, aspects of daily life, anniversaries, and current events. Each in their own way, these authors believed that if an equation could be made between something familiar and an aspect of the historical collections of the NLM, a reader would be more likely to continue reading and therefore exploring down the path created by the blog and its many contributors.

To most people, there is not much novel or exciting about a microscope, but it is a familiar object. They may have used it in school. They understand that it symbolizes science. Likewise, everyone is aware of cancer in one context or another. From these points of general reference and through the expertise of historian Michael Sappol, readers can make connections to, and therefore better appreciate, unique and intriguing collection items. In "How to See . . . With the Microscope," Sappol begins with such familiarity, engaging his readers through a unique book in the historical collections of the NLM to teach them that a microscope is a relatively recent invention. The book itself is special because, in addition to being signed by its author, it was one of the first written to instruct professionals in how to use a microscope. Through Sappol's creative narrative, readers can imagine being one of these early users. Similarly, in "Global Healing," by Ginny A. Roth, readers feel the connections and commonalities we all have as humans as we view the photographs of Patricia Gallinek, a registered nurse who volunteered as a photographer for years with organizations involved in international healthcare. Through Gallinek's generous donation of more than 500 of her photographs, the Library continues to preserve the lived experiences of health and healing around the globe for public access and future research. These posts by Sappol and Roth represent how contributors to the blog have drawn effectively upon common knowledge to convey and enrich the meaning and importance of the historical collections of the NLM. Moreover, through these posts and many others, readers can see that the NLM preserves much more than books.

Anniversaries hold almost universal attraction. For most people, anniversaries represent major milestones and invest objects with meaning that can become more significant with the passage of time. *Circulating Now* has focused on a variety of anniversaries, some going as far back as 500 years, as in the case of the pioneer anatomist Andreas Vesalius. In "Andreas Vesalius at 500," Michael J. North encourages readers to view his foundational works, but also to learn more about Vesalius as a person. "America's National Parks: Preserved for Public Health," authored by Anne Rothfeld, focuses on the more recent centenary of the National Park Service through the lens of photographs that document the public health facilities of many parks. "MCCR Was There" and "Smoking in America: 50 Years On" mark fifty-year anniversaries through photographs of healthcare professionals who took part in the 1963 March on Washington and the collected reports of the Surgeon General on the health effects of smoking produced annually since 1964. These posts by Elizabeth A. Mullen and Christie Moffatt highlight the range of time represented in the collections.

Annual and monthly recognitions of widespread diseases and conditions offer opportunities to reflect on past awareness and address current and future challenges to individual and community health. Here, too, contributors to *Circulating Now* have made contributions to remembering these causes. Readers learn from "Alzheimer's Disease Collection Received," authored by Margaret Kaiser, that the month of November has been dedicated to Alzheimer's disease awareness, and through this lens she highlights the NLM's acquisition of the Alzheimer's Disease Education and Referral (ADEAR) Center's collection of public health education publications from the National Institute on Aging since 1983. Kaiser's post shares details of a collection of books, pamphlets, and flyers produced to educate the general public and makes the reader aware that the NLM still actively acquires related individual items and collections, both ancient and modern.

Even global events seemingly unrelated to the history of medicine, such as the World Cup soccer championship, have served to introduce facets of the historical collections of the NLM. "Kick Polio Out of Nigeria," authored by Erika Mills, describes public health posters produced in Nigeria in 1998 that use soccer as a theme to encourage polio vaccinations. Although this article did not appear on a specific anniversary, the 2014 entry appeared in a World Cup championship year, as did the 1998 posters.

The series that helped to introduce *Circulating Now* to the world, "'The President Is Somewhat Restless...,'" by Jeffrey S. Reznick and Lenore Barbian demonstrates that general interest in American history can be a gateway to learning about a fascinating collection. Presidential assassinations are both historically noteworthy and necessarily relevant to medicine. President James Garfield's death in 1881 followed months of protracted suffering. During this period, the president's physicians issued regular bulletins about his condition, sometimes up to three such notices daily. More than a hundred years later, *Circulating Now* recounted this harrowing national event by publishing the text of these bulletins in a series of posts aligned with the actual timing of the original events, allowing readers to engage with them in real time. Periodic posts focused on Garfield's doctors, deterioration, and eventual autopsy, revealing the disparity between the public pronouncements and the true progression of the president's decline.

Taken together, the posts featured in this chapter demonstrate how, from the very beginning of *Circulating Now*, its diverse contributors drew on their own expertise to showcase collections of the Library in ways that could entice and engage readers and teach them that "historical collections" encompass materials of recent vintage, not simply antique books. Moreover, readers learn that important and relevant histories of medicine reside in video recordings as well as ephemeral objects such as posters, pamphlets, and flyers. While outwardly appearing to be a brief and innocent diversion, *Circulating Now* from its earliest posts had higher ambitions to inform, engage, and reveal to a wide audience as never before the vast collections of the world's largest biomedical library.

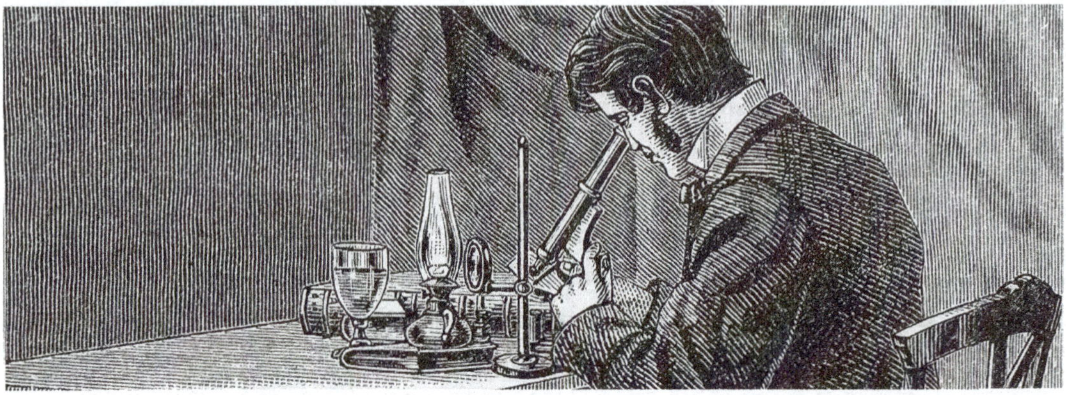

HOW TO . . . SEE WITH THE MICROSCOPE

https://circulatingnow.nlm.nih.gov/2014/06/04/how-to-see-with-the-microscope/

June 4, 2014 • Rare Books & Journals

MICHAEL SAPPOL

Microscopy was the coming thing in late nineteenth-century medicine. If you were an ambitious doctor, no matter what your field of interest, you probably wanted to own a good microscope, and apply it to the questions at hand. What do the structures of human and non-human bodies look like? How does that help us learn what these structures do? What happens in the human body when disease occurs? What do diseased tissues look like? And, really exciting, what microorganisms are present in diseased tissue? To find the answers to all these questions, you could consult Dr. J. Edwards Smith's book *How to See with the Microscope*.

But before you could do any of that, you had to obtain a fine quality instrument (which could be pricy). Then you could begin to learn how to see with it. Which was not an obvious or easy thing to do. If you didn't know how, you might just end up confusing optical effects and distortions with the object you wanted to see or missing the fine details that distinguish

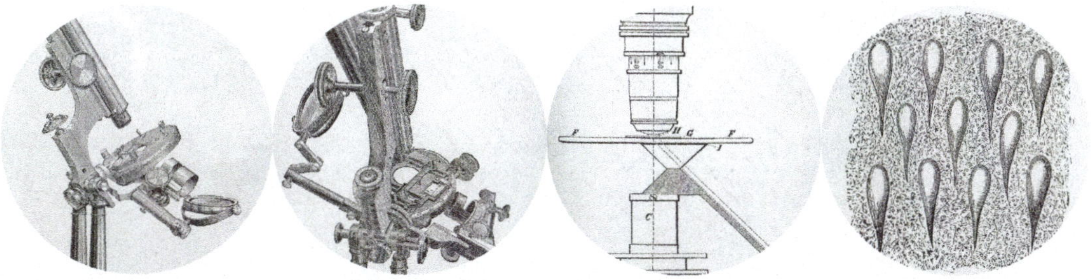

LEFT TO RIGHT **(1)** Zentmayer's American Centennial Stand, constructed especially for the Centennial Exhibition **(2)** Bulloch's First Class Microscope, a binocular model **(3)** An accessory for illumination developed by Col. J. J. Woodward, of the U.S. Army **(4)** The scales of 'Podura' (Collembola, springtail) insects are one of the earliest subjects reported as a test subject for the microscope. Edwards uses them here to demonstrate the light and shade that should be seen.

one microorganism or tissue sample from another. Historians like Jutta Schickore and Jonathan Crary have shown that seeing with microscopes was something that had to be learned and practiced, and that the practice of seeing with microscopes changed how doctors, patients, and the general public saw things and saw themselves. There were, Jonathan Crary tells us, "techniques of the observer," and many technologies of viewing.

How to See with the Microscope is a book for beginners, containing "useful hints connected with the selection and use of the instrument," and advice on monocular, binocular, and "duplex" microscopes, stands, apertures, lenses, lighting, high and low magnification, preparation of slides, "the uses and abuses of the microscope," and even the positioning of the person looking *through* the scope (a whole chapter on that). And "also some discussion of the claims and capacity of the modern high-angled objectives, as compared with those of medium aperture; with instructions as to the selection and use of American object-glasses of wide aperture." All of which, at the time, were matters of disagreement and even some controversy. There was even a "war of the apertures" conducted in the medical press. Obviously you had a lot to learn, and the book's author, Dr. J. Edwards Smith, was a vocal advocate of "eye training."

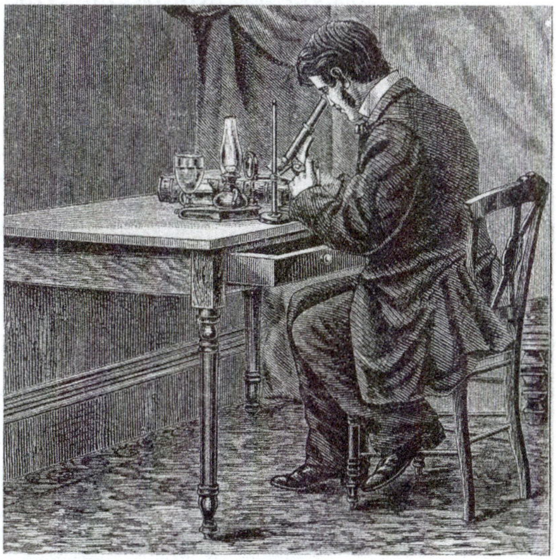

Position of the observer

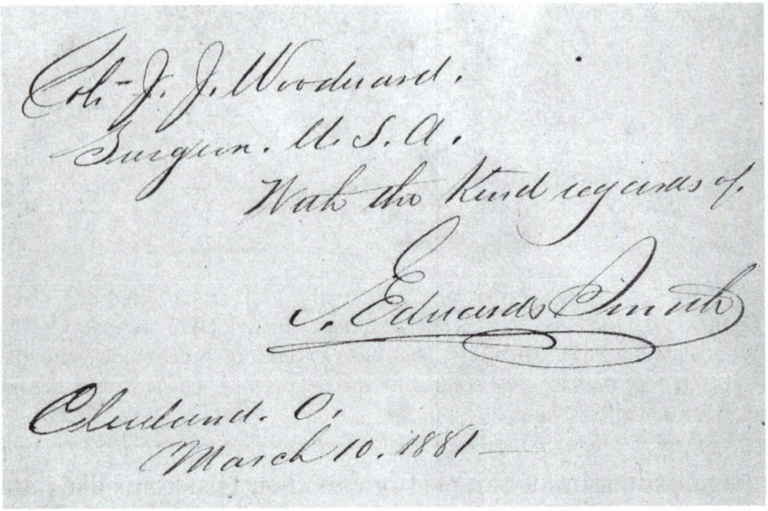
Col. J. J. Woodward,
Surgeon. U.S.A.
With the kind regards of,
Edwards Smith
Cleveland. O.
March 10. 1881

Inscription to J.J. Woodward

Interestingly, Dr. Smith was a "Professor of Histology and Microscopy in the Cleveland (O.) Homœopathic Hospital"—homeopathists were as much interested in microscopy as regular physicians—and he consorted with regular physicians as a member of the Illinois State Microscopical Association and the American Association for the Advancement of Science.

The National Library of Medicine's copy of the book was touched by Smith's hand. He autographed it and presented it to Joseph Janvier Woodward, MD, then a prestigious surgeon and curator at the Army Medical Museum and Army Medical Library (the ancestor of the National Library of Medicine). Sixteen years earlier, Woodward had performed autopsies on both Abraham Lincoln and John Wilkes Booth. In 1881 he served as one of the attending physicians to President James Garfield, following Garfield being shot by Charles Guiteau, and during this period Woodward was well-known in microscopical circles for his work in developing photomicrography.

• • •

Edwards Smith, MD, How to See with the Microscope *(Chicago: Duncan Brothers, 1880). 410 pp. illustrated.*

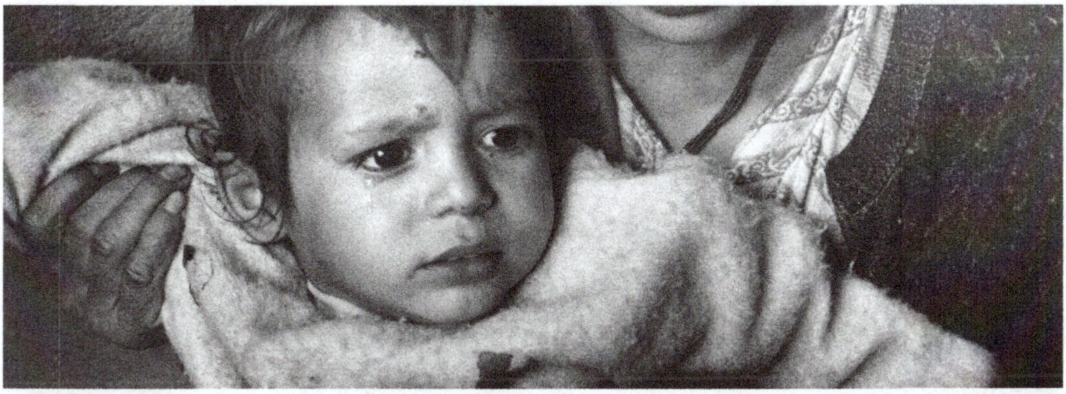

GLOBAL HEALING

https://circulatingnow.nlm.nih.gov/2015/02/11/global-healing/

February 11, 2015 • Prints & Photographs

GINNY A. ROTH

> "I have always been drawn to people and have sought to see them compassionately and with understanding through the lens of my eyes, my heart and soul as well as the lens of my camera."
>
> —Patricia Gallinek

Serving in many roles such as caregiver, decision maker, patient advocate, and teacher, nurses are pivotal players in the healthcare profession. Patricia Gallinek, RN, took her duties a step further, deeply immersing herself into the lives of hundreds of men, women, and children in need of healthcare and compassion. Ms. Gallinek has always had a love for photography, and through it she found a way to enrich her life, and those of others.

In 1990, after retiring from thirty years in the nursing profession, Ms. Gallinek returned to college to study photojournalism, documentary

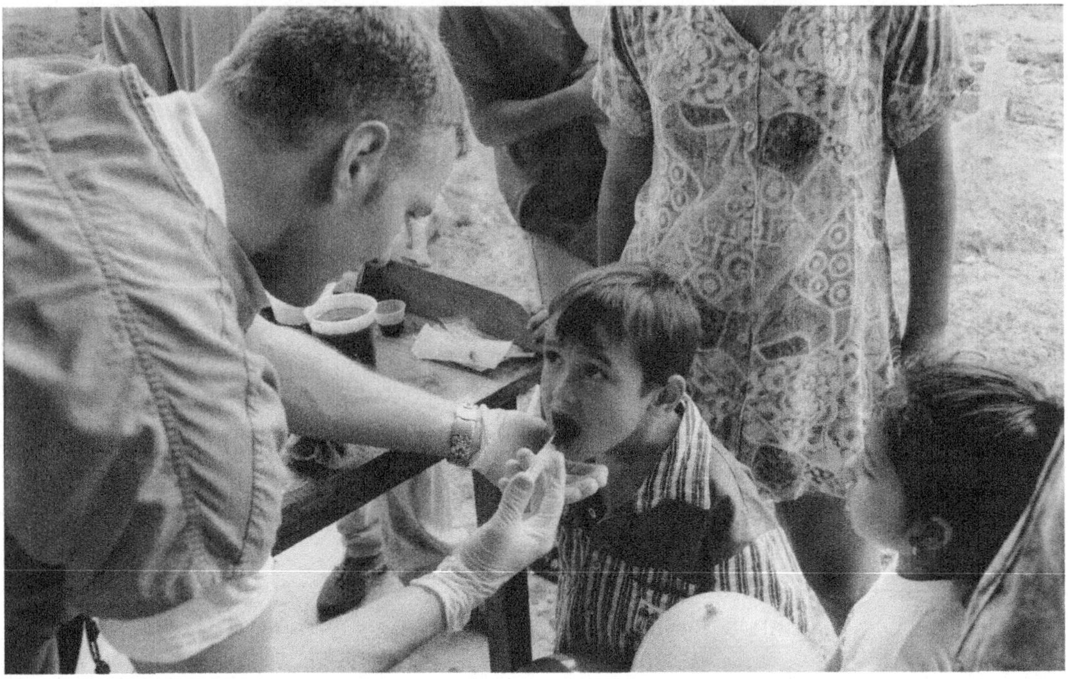

Volunteer Medical School student Clinton Keilman administers oral medication to children for parasitic infestation while on mission in Honduras in 1999.

photography, and communications. Her goal was clear: it was her calling to document healthcare around the world on film and, in her own words, "bring awareness to the heart-wrenching healthcare problems and those extraordinary volunteers whose selfless devotion relieves suffering and improves medical care around our world."

Born through her love of photography and the most genuine concern for humankind, she embarked on a new vocation to volunteer as a photographer for organizations involved in international healthcare. Despite language barriers, rough terrain, and challenging climates, and even through intensely emotional scenes of despair, her images thoughtfully and respectfully evoke the sense of humanity, perseverance, and friendship that she found in the communities she visited.

Ms. Gallinek has generously donated to the National Library of Medicine (NLM) over 500 photographs that she herself printed from her journeys around the globe, each carefully described and documented when the photograph was made. Below is a small selection of images from the collection.

All images are copyright Patricia Gallinek and used with permission.

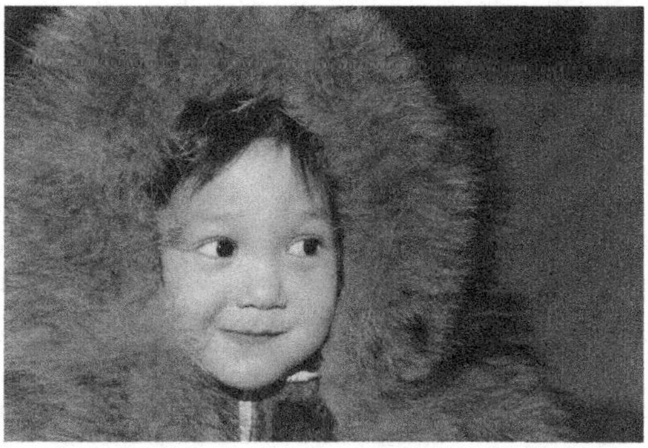

All smiles today, a young boy arrives at dental clinic for consultation. Maniilaq Health Center—Kotzebue, Northwest Alaska, USA, 2004.

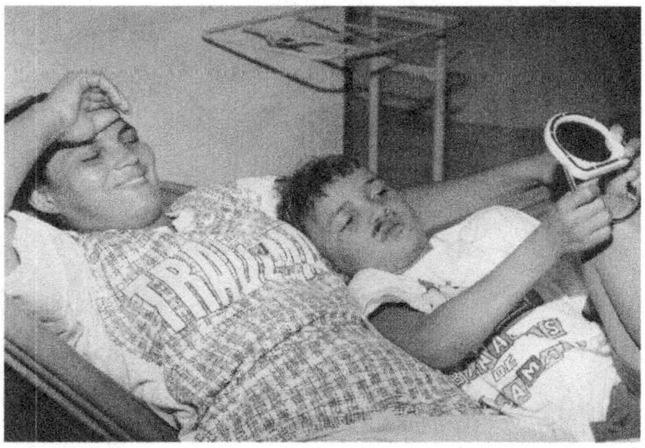

Following reconstructive surgery for a cleft lip performed by Esperança volunteer Dr. John Gibney, a little boy and his mother rest in their clinic hammock. The little boy studies his face in the mirror. His mother looks on with pride, relief, and happiness. Brazil, 1998.

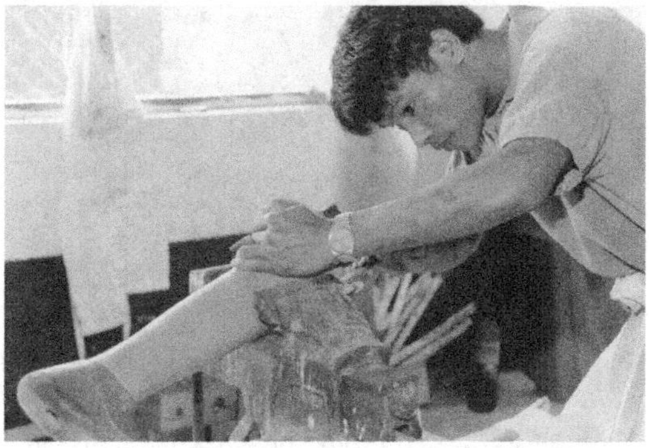

In 2001 Mae Tao Clinic inaugurated a prosthetics fabrication facility for landmine victims and other amputees. Border of Burma, 2004.

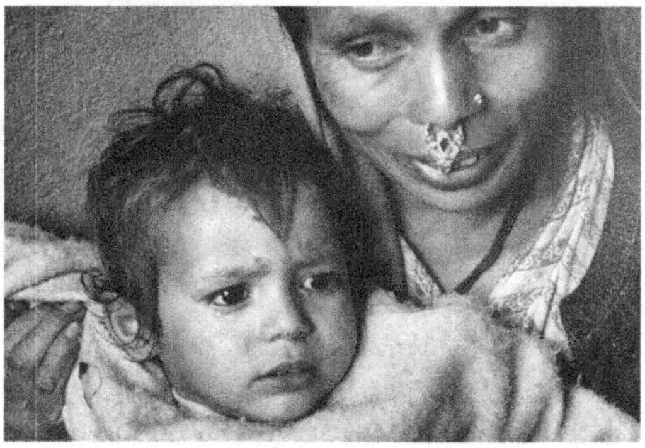

This forlorn mother and child are part of an endless line of people in Ilam, Nepal, waiting patiently, pain in their eyes, and their feet sore and bleeding from walking for days on rocky roads. 1994.

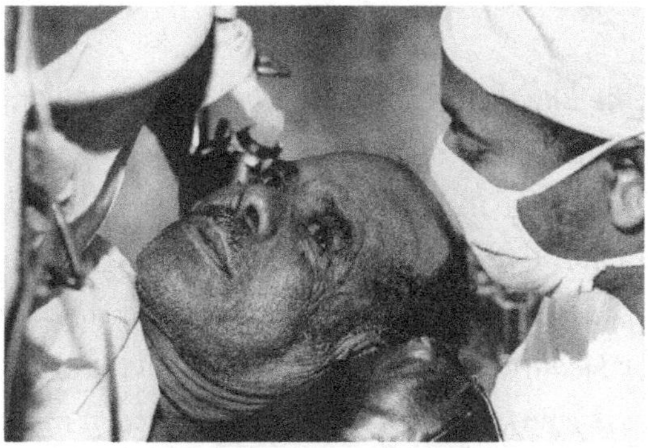

An anesthesiologist monitors a patient moments before knee surgery. Health Volunteers Overseas, Black Lion Hospital, Addis Ababa, Ethiopia, 1955.

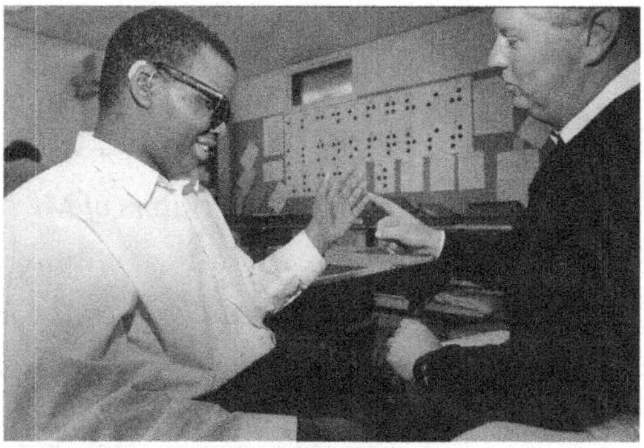

A teacher and student at the Dorton House School for the Blind, United Kingdom, 2003.

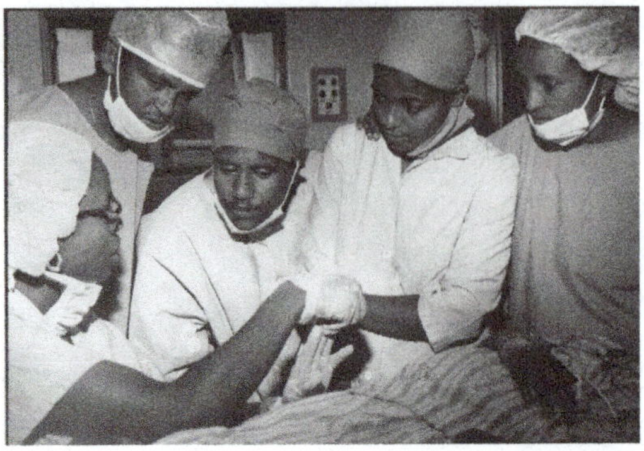

Yale University hospital volunteer anesthesiologist Dr. Adelle Williams (left) shares medical experiences with Ethiopian student nurse anesthetists. These students attend anesthesia school in Ethiopia. Ethiopia, 1995.

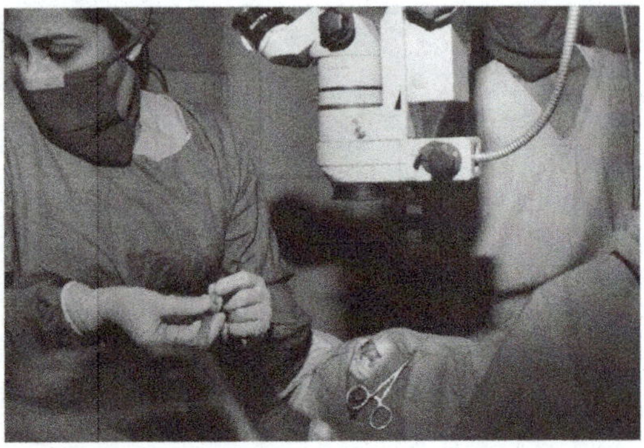

Dr. Reena Sethi, wife of Dr. Arun Sethi and volunteer eye surgeon performs cataract surgery and intraocular lens implantation on a 50-year-old patient. "We welcome more volunteers," Dr. Sethi says. Eye Care Project, India, 1997.

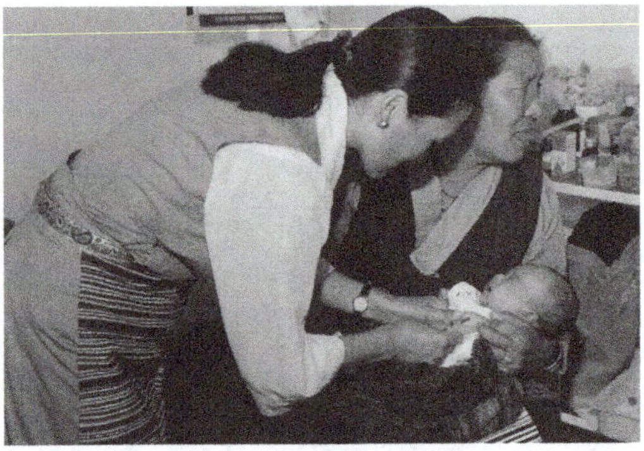

Looking away as Delek Hospital staff nurse gives immunization to one month old infant in the outpatient clinic at Delek Hospital. Tibetans living in exile, Dharamsala, India, 2002.

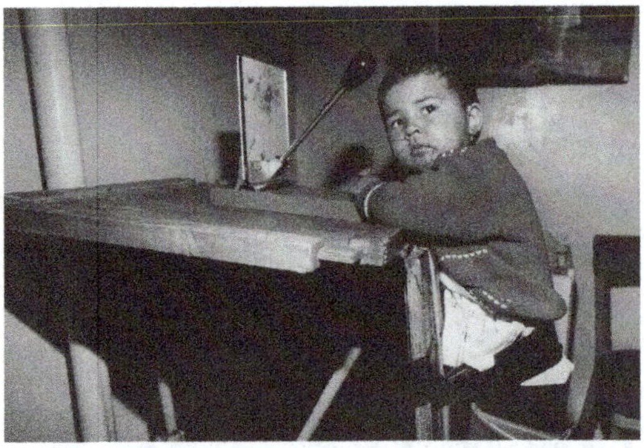

A young boy is physically challenged. He sits in a harness chair. This chair enables him to sit upright and to be more comfortable during his acupuncture treatment. UMID Medical Rehabilitation Center, Uzbekistan, 1997.

• • •

Ms. Gallinek was the recipient of the Elizabeth Lobkowicz Photography Award for Academic Honors in the Arts and Humanities, presented by the faculty and administrators of Mt. Vernon College in Washington, DC. Ms. Gallinek also received the International Civil Golden Award by the Distinguished Civil Forum of Nepal for her outstanding contribution in the field of photography. Her photo essays for HealthCare Traveler can be found at http://healthcaretraveler.modernmedicine.com/authorDetails/19461. To learn more about donating to the NLM please visit our Donations to the National Library of Medicine page.

Reflection

The "caregiver" is a well-known archetype, one into which nurses fall seamlessly for their compassionate, protective, and nurturing dispositions. Patricia Gallinek, RN, maintained these traits throughout her thirty-year career as a nurse and subsequent career as an international documentary photographer of healthcare concerns.

I met Patricia in January 2015 when picking up her donation to the NLM of over 500 photographs. She showed me her expansive darkroom where she printed the photographs after returning from Ethiopia, Burma, India, Honduras, and countless other regions where she used her camera as a tool to raise public awareness of individuals and communities suffering the effects of healthcare disparities caused largely by socio-economic, geographic, and language barriers. She also documented the selfless volunteers who dedicated their lives to easing distress in these communities through medical assistance.

Patricia passed away on March 19, 2022. A wave of sadness flowed through me when I learned this. Seven years after writing "Global Healing," I look at her photographs and see the power that just a few dedicated individuals can possess to make a difference. Patricia's photographs are a revelation not only because she traveled as a volunteer to the far reaches of the world to "vocalize" in images the desperation of those whose voices remain unheard but also because she simultaneously captured in their faces the human spirit, hope, bravery, and resolve.

Patricia truly was "the caregiver." I feel blessed to have known her and comforted that her life and work will endure in the historical archives of the NLM. —Ginny A. Roth, 2023

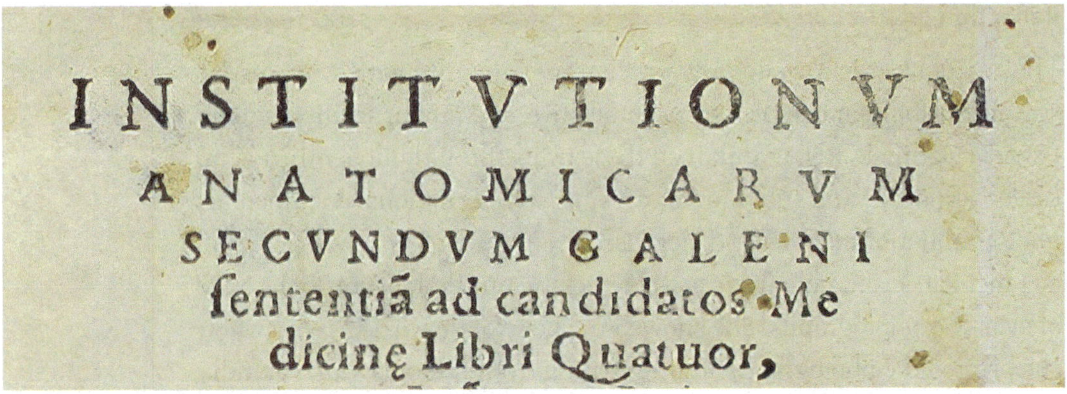

ANDREAS VESALIUS AT 500

https://circulatingnow.nlm.nih.gov/2013/12/31/andreas-vesalius-at-500/

December 31, 2013 • Rare Books & Journals

MICHAEL J. NORTH

Today marks the 499th birthday of the great, sixteenth-century anatomist Andreas Vesalius, born on December 31, 1514. Throughout 2014 *Circulating Now* will be joining many others in celebrating this 500-year landmark in the history of medicine.

Very fortuitously, the Library has recently acquired a rare copy of a dissection manual edited by Vesalius: Johann Guenther's *Institutionum Anatomicarum Secundum Galeni Sententiam ad Candidatos Medicinae Libri Quatuor* (*Four books on anatomical dissection for medical students following the method of Galen*), published in Venice in about 1540.

Johann Guenther von Andernach (1505–1574) was a medical humanist and professor at the Universities of Paris and Louvain. He was especially well-known for his Latin translation of, and commentary on, the newly discovered text of Galen's *De Anatomicis Administrationibus* (*On Anatomic

Procedures) in 1531, which was the ancient physician's own guide to dissection. The world of anatomists was jolted by the text and the new method of dissection took medical schools by storm. In 1536, Guenther published this pocket-sized dissection manual based on Galen's text especially for medical students, the *Institutionum Anatomicarum*, in which he made reference to the talents of his young pupil Andreas Vesalius, who probably assisted in editing it.

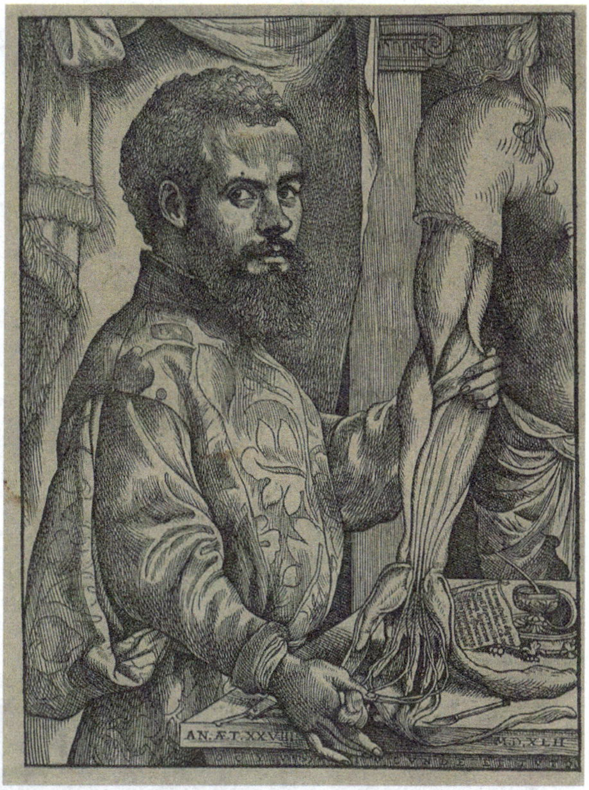

Andreas Vesalius, 1543 • Woodcut portrait of Andreas Vesalius from his *De Humani Corporis Fabrica Libri Septem*, 1543

Andreas Vesalius (1514–1564) was descended from a long line of medical men and was the son of the Flemish apothecary to the Holy Roman Emperor Maximilian. Born in Brabant in what is now Belgium, he began attending the University of Louvain at a young age and was a keen student of Greek, Latin, and eventually anatomy under Guenther; it was quite likely he was present when the scholar performed his famed translation of Galen's dissection manual.

After graduating from medical school in 1537 (having written a thesis on the work of tenth-century Persian physician Rhazes), Vesalius went to Venice, where he soon received an appointment from the Senate of the Republic of Venice to teach anatomy at the prestigious University of Padua. The following year he published his famous *Tabulae Anatomicae Sex*, which contained six anatomical plates with detailed explanations that would foreshadow his more important anatomical work five years later.

Only a month after the publication of *Tabulae*, Vesalius issued his own revised edition of Guenther's *Institutionum Anatomicarum*, without Guenther's permission. With high praise for his former instructor throughout the preface, Vesalius claimed that there were merely some

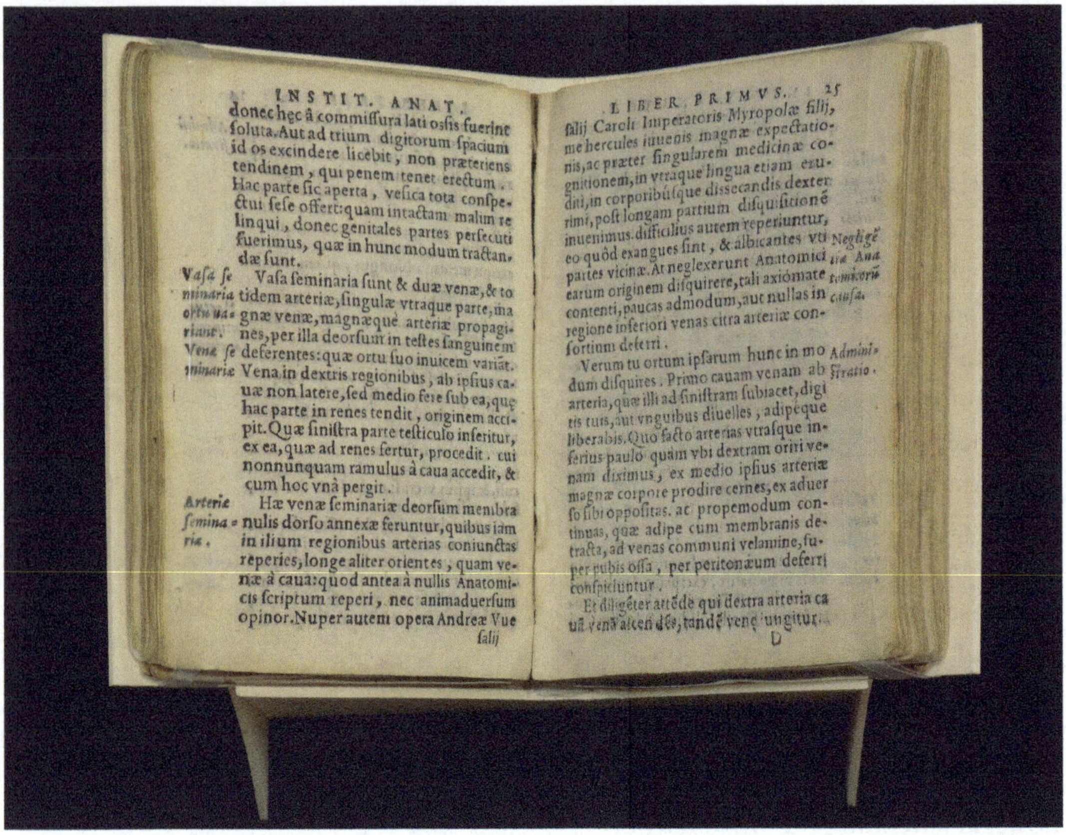

Institutionum Anatomicarum, 1540 • *National Library of Medicine #101594641*

printing errors that needed correction, however, he made numerous changes following his own experience with dissections; he was careful to leave untouched the praise that Guenther had written about him on pages 46 and 47. In about 1540, this undated second edition of Vesalius' revised edition of the *Institutionum Anatomicarum* came out. The Library has long owned a first edition of this revised work, but the acquisition of this second edition makes our collection of materials by and about Vesalius nearly complete.

The book itself is tiny, less than four-and-a-half inches tall and bound in limp vellum, which was usually a sign that the volume was cheaply sewn together to go into circulation immediately. Surviving copies of these manuals are rare; most likely they were carried in students' pockets and passed around the dissection theater while instruction was taking place.

Only three years later, Andreas Vesalius wrote his important De Humani Corporis Fabrica Libri Septem (Seven Books on the Fabric of the Human Body), published in Basel in 1543. This beautifully illustrated book has frequently been cited as the first modern anatomical work, as it examined the body in such great detail and compared it to the works of Galen.

To learn more about Vesalius and his achievement in creating *De Fabrica,* visit the National Library of Medicine's Turning the Pages project featuring this important work. To view selections from the Library's collection of anatomical atlases, visit Historical Anatomies on the Web.

•••

This article is the first in a series to commemorate the 500th anniversary of the birth of the great anatomist Andreas Vesalius, born on December 31, 1514.

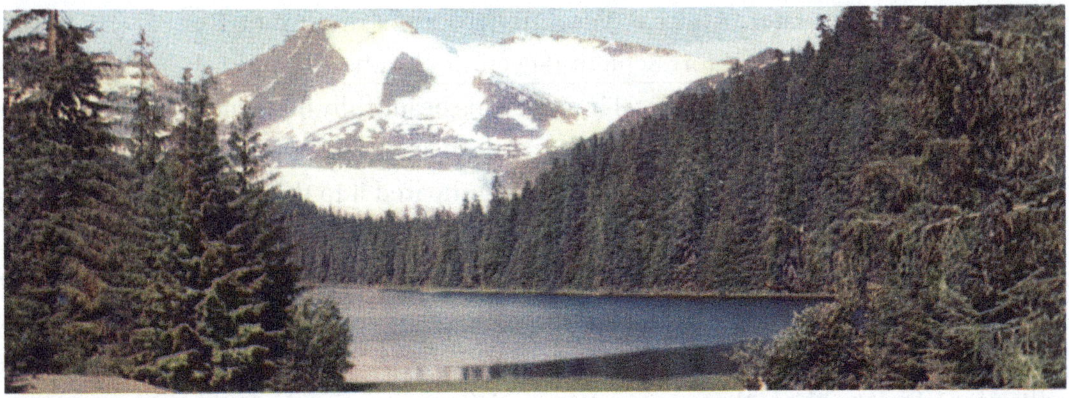

AMERICA'S NATIONAL PARKS: PRESERVED FOR PUBLIC HEALTH

https://circulatingnow.nlm.nih.gov/2016/08/25/americas-national-parks-recreation-for-public-health/

August 25, 2016 • Prints & Photographs

ANNE ROTHFELD

The National Park Service (NPS) celebrates its centennial on August 25, 2016. From Maine to Hawaii, the breadth of NPS includes parks, seashores, monuments, Indian reservations, and historic sites. America's parks are filled with an abundance of natural wonders: glaciers and rivers, flora and fauna, animals and insects, canyons and sand dunes, stargazing and camping.

Yellowstone became the first national park in 1872, and later, through the Forest Reserve Act, Congress enacted the protection of "forest reserves." Over a period of sixteen years, three presidents added more than 150 million acres of forest and parkland, including Sequoia, Yosemite, Mt. Rainier, Crater Lake, and Glacier. Beginning in 1901, Congress enacted multiple

ABOVE A Postcard from Alaska • Mendenhall Glacier, Alaska, early twentieth century • *Courtesy Abbott Historical Archives. National Library of Medicine #101460855*

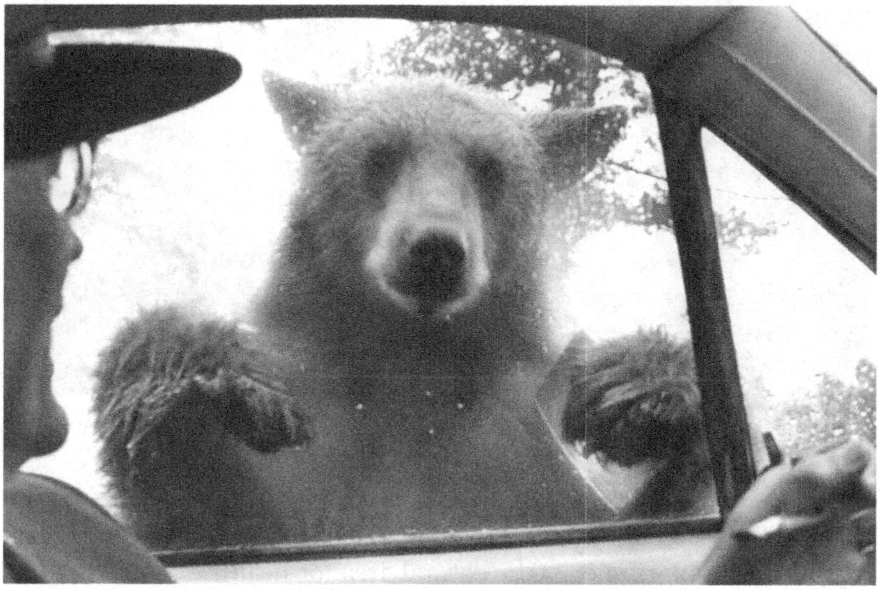

A Fauna Encounter • A bear "greets" a visitor in a national park. Public Health Service at work in the national parks, 1960s • *National Library of Medicine #101547480*

pieces of legislation to protect the country's parks and monuments, the foundation of today's NPS. President Woodrow Wilson signed the Organic Act of 1916, which created the NPS, to establish the conservation of nature and wildlife, and the preservation of historical landmarks and structures. In 1935, the Historic Sites Act broadened NPS's responsibilities of historic preservation, including presidential homes, Civil War battlefields and cemeteries, and the C&O Canal. By the late twentieth century, the scope of NPS expanded to include the Land and Water Conservation Fund, National Wilderness Preservation System, National Historic Preservation, National Trails System, and National Wild and Scenic Rivers System. Excursions from urban areas to the national parks continue to offer public health benefits to Americans: fresh air and water, sunshine, and cooler temperatures in summer; visiting the parks helps restore physical and psychological health to those who languish.

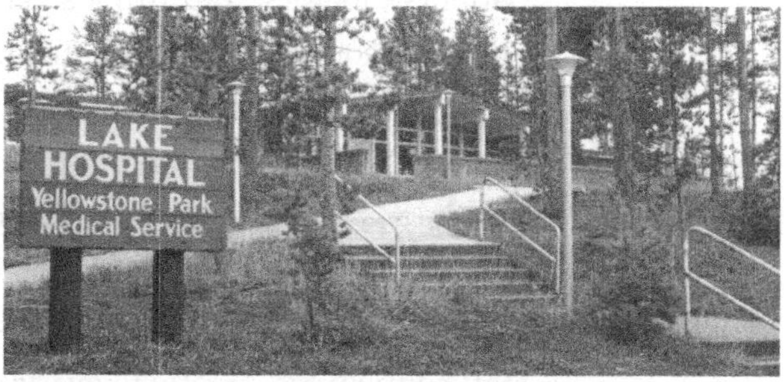

A Hospital in the Woods • Medical facility in Yellowstone National Park. Public Health Service at work in the national parks, 1960s • *National Library of Medicine #101547480*

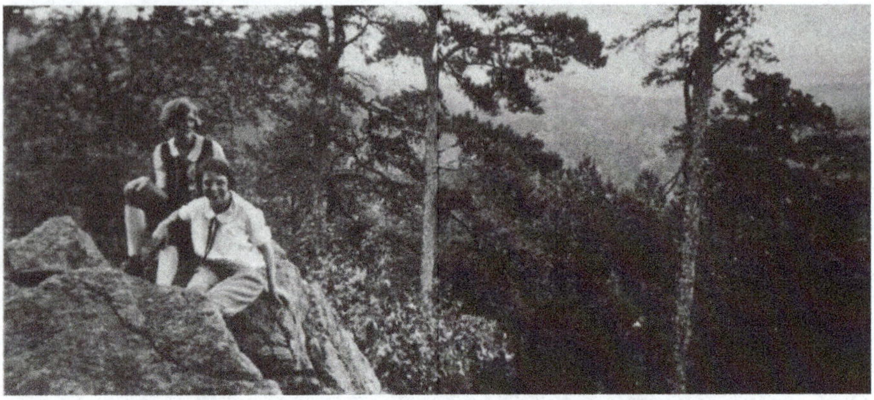

Recreation for Nurses • Nurses hiking in Hot Springs National Park, Arkansas, Army and Navy General Hospital, 1940s • *National Library of Medicine #101400633*

In twentieth-century Europe, "taking the cure," a phrase meaning to visit a mineral spring or other natural area for health reasons, became highly fashionable. In the United States, following the American Civil War, bathhouses and hotels near natural areas grew in number as hot springs became popular resort attractions. The U.S. military had the same idea. Hot Springs, Arkansas, for example, where over forty springs rise from the mountain's base, became the site of the first joint Army-Navy military hospital. In 1882, President Chester A. Arthur signed a bill authorizing the hospital, which became the army's primary facility for patients afflicted with arthritis and paralysis. In 1921, Congress designated the Hot Springs area a national park. Returning military personnel who suffered from severe wounds and/or loss of limbs in World War II took advantage of the hydro-therapy treatments available at the facility.

During World War II, national parks offered nature's healing to military patients, doctors, and nurses. The Navy and Army departments built rehabilitation hospitals in Sequoia, Carlsbad Caverns, Grand Canyon, and Yosemite. Under the direction of the Navy Department, the Ahwahnee Hotel in Yosemite offered injured military personnel a place to convalesce. Similarly, the Army built a rehabilitation camp in Denali National Park where nearby military personnel soldiers could fish, hike, skate, and relax. Cabins built near these hospitals for the families of patients and staff contributed greatly to everyone's morale.

For many people today, the outdoors' tranquility and expansiveness serve as a tonic to calm nerves and revive energy. Areas for healthy

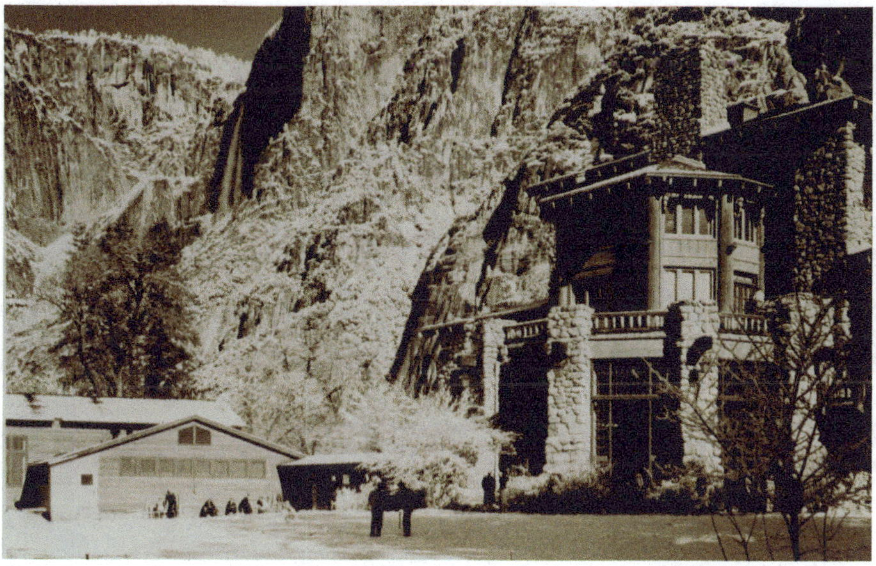

An Inland Naval Hospital • U.S. Naval Convalescent Hospital, Yosemite National Park, CA, 1944 • *National Library of Medicine #101403068*

recreational activities, observing nature, and learning about cultural heritage are preserved all over the country by the National Park Service and support the health and well-being of people today and for future generations.

Each national park offers unique environments and educational opportunities. You can experience: biodiversity of shorelines and woodlands in Acadia (Maine), conservation of 2,000 stone bridges in Utah's Arches National Park, aurora borealis over Denali (Alaska), endangered marine life in the barrier islands of the Gulf Islands National Seashore (Florida and Mississippi), and fossil formations in Zion (Utah). Natural wonders call to us to pause and renew our senses.

• • •

As we celebrate the NPS, we welcome you to share your experiences of a national park or historic landmark.

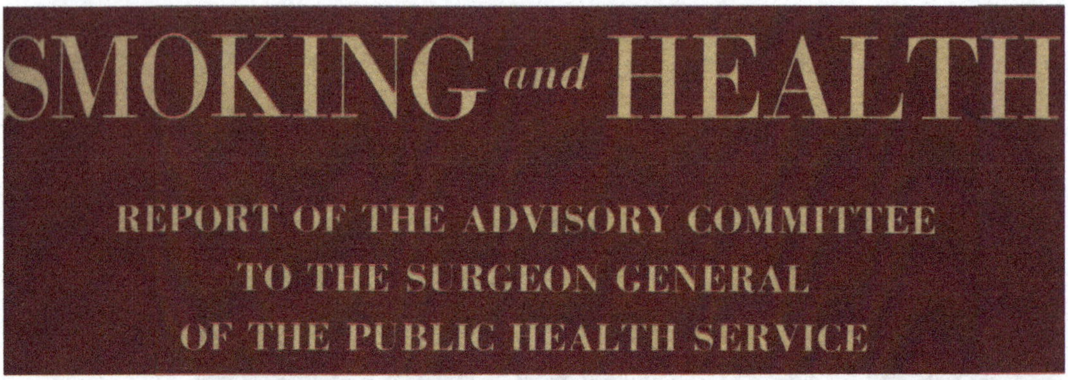

SMOKING IN AMERICA: 50 YEARS ON

https://circulatingnow.nlm.nih.gov/2014/01/10/smoking-in-america-50-years-on/

January 10, 2014 • Archives & Manuscripts

CHRISTIE MOFFATT

Fifty years ago, on January 11, 1964, the Surgeon General of the United States, Luther L. Terry, issued Smoking and Health: Report of the Advisory Committee to the Surgeon General. *In recognition of this landmark document in the history of medicine and the United States, let's recall its history through the National Library of Medicine (NLM)'s* Profiles in Science*:*

• • •

No single issue has preoccupied the Surgeons General of the past four decades more than smoking. The reports of the Surgeon General have alerted the nation to the health risk of smoking and have transformed the issue from one of individual and consumer choice to one of epidemiology, public health, and risk for smokers and non-smokers alike.

Debate over the hazards and benefits of smoking has divided physicians, scientists, governments, smokers, and non-smokers since *Tobacco*

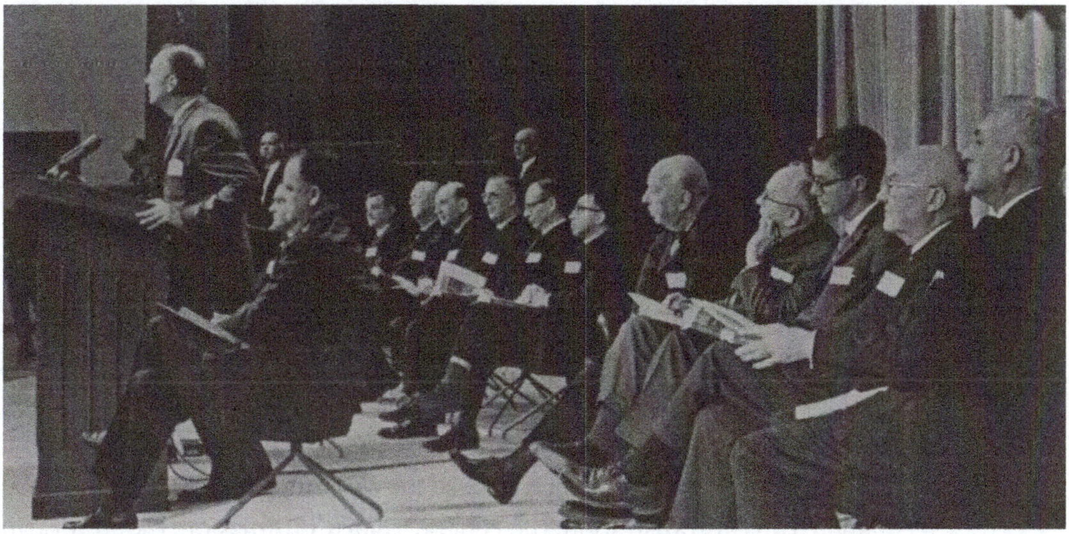

U.S. Surgeon General Luther Terry addressing a press conference at the release of the 1964 report on *Smoking and Health*, 1964 • *NLM's* Profiles in Science *#101584932*

nicotiana was first imported to Europe from its native soil in the Americas in the sixteenth century. A dramatic increase in cigarette smoking in the United States in the twentieth century called forth anti-smoking movements. Reformers, hygienists, and public health officials argued that smoking brought about general malaise, physiological malfunction, and a decline in mental and physical efficiency. Evidence of the ill effects of smoking accumulated during the 1930s, 1940s, and 1950s. Epidemiologists used statistics and large-scale, long-term, case-control surveys to link the increase in lung cancer mortality to smoking. Pathologists and laboratory scientists confirmed the statistical relationship of smoking to lung cancer as well as to other serious diseases, such as bronchitis, emphysema, and coronary heart disease. Smoking, these studies suggested, and not air pollution, asbestos contamination, or radioactive materials, was the chief cause of the epidemic rise of lung cancer in the twentieth century. On June 12, 1957, Surgeon General Leroy E. Burney declared it the official position of the U.S. Public Health Service that the evidence pointed to a causal relationship between smoking and lung cancer.

The impulse for an official report on smoking and health, however, came from an alliance of prominent private health organizations. In June 1961, the American Cancer Society, the American Heart Association, the National Tuberculosis Association, and the American Public Health Association addressed a letter to President John F. Kennedy, in which they called for a national commission on smoking, dedicated to "seeking a solution to this health problem that would interfere least with the freedom of industry or the happiness of individuals." The Kennedy administration responded the following year, after prompting from a widely circulated critical study on cigarette smoking by the Royal College of Physicians of London. On June 7, 1962, recently appointed Surgeon General Luther L. Terry announced that he would convene a committee of experts to conduct a comprehensive review of the scientific literature on the smoking question. Terry invited representatives of the four voluntary medical organizations who had first proposed the commission, as well as the Food and Drug Administration, the Federal Trade Commission, the American Medical Association, and the Tobacco Institute (the lobbying arm of the tobacco industry) to nominate commission members. Ten were finally chosen, representing a wide swath of disciplines in medicine, surgery, pharmacology, and statistics, though none in psychology or the social sciences. Candidates qualified only if they had taken no previous stand on tobacco use.

Meeting at the National Library of Medicine on the campus of the National Institutes of Health (NIH) in Bethesda, Maryland, from November 1962 through January 1964, the committee reviewed more than 7,000 scientific articles with the help of over 150 consultants. Terry issued the commission's report on January 11, 1964, choosing a Saturday to minimize the effect on the stock market and to maximize coverage in the Sunday papers. As Terry remembered the event, two decades later, the report "hit the country like a bombshell. It was front page news and a lead story on every radio and television station in the United States and many abroad."

The report highlighted the deleterious health consequences of tobacco use. *Smoking and Health: Report of the Advisory Committee to the Surgeon General* held cigarette smoking responsible for a 70 percent increase in the mortality rate of smokers over non-smokers. The report estimated that average smokers had a nine- to ten-fold risk of developing lung cancer compared to non-smokers; heavy smokers had at least a twenty-fold risk. The risk rose with the duration of smoking and diminished with

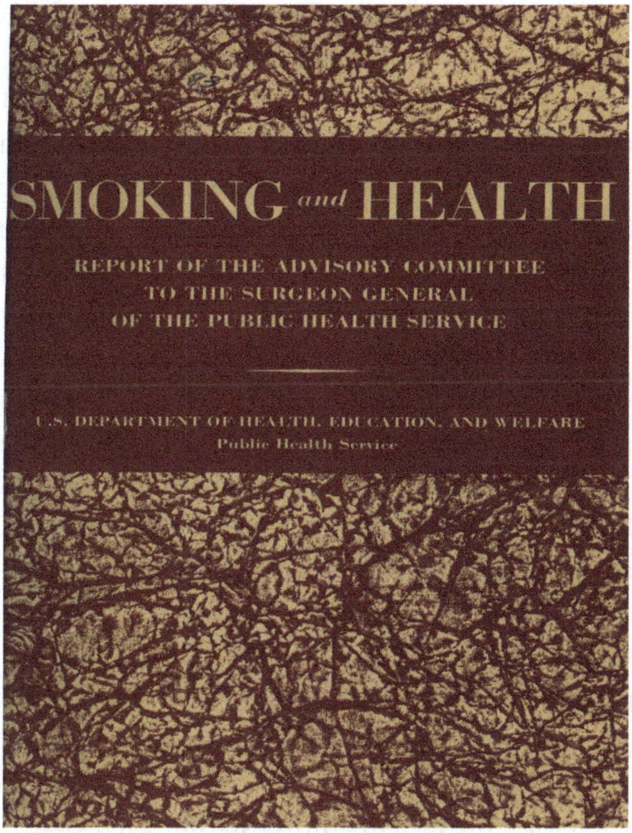

Smoking and Health: Report of the Advisory Committee to the Surgeon General of the Public Health Service, 1964 • *NLM's* Profiles in Science #101584932

the cessation of smoking. The report also named smoking as the most important cause of chronic bronchitis and pointed to a correlation between smoking and emphysema, and smoking and coronary heart disease. It noted that smoking during pregnancy reduced the average weight of newborns. On one issue the committee hedged: nicotine addiction. It insisted that the "tobacco habit should be characterized as an habituation rather than an addiction," in part because the addictive properties of nicotine were not yet fully understood, in part because of differences over the meaning of addiction.

The 1964 report on smoking and health had an impact on public attitudes and policy. A Gallup survey conducted in 1958 found that only 44 percent of Americans believed smoking caused cancer, while 78 percent believed so by 1968. In the course of a decade, it had become common knowledge that smoking damaged health, and mounting evidence of health risks gave Terry's 1964 report public resonance. Yet, while the report proclaimed that "cigarette smoking is a health hazard of sufficient importance in the United States to warrant appropriate remedial action," it remained silent on concrete remedies. That challenge fell to politicians. In 1965, Congress required all cigarette packages distributed in the United States to carry a health warning, and since 1970 this warning is made in the name of the Surgeon General. In 1969, cigarette advertising on television and radio was banned, effective September 1970. The Public Health Cigarette Smoking Act of 1969 requires that the Surgeon General produce an annual report reviewing the latest scientific findings on the effects of smoking on health. As a result, more than half of all reports published under the auspices of the Surgeon General during the past forty years have dealt with this issue.

Fifty years after the release of the first Surgeon General's report on smoking and health, remarkable progress has been made. Since 1964, smoking prevalence among U.S. adults has been reduced by half. Unfortunately, tobacco use remains the leading preventable cause of disease, disability, and death in the United States. In January 2014, the Surgeon General will release the fiftieth anniversary Surgeon General's Report on smoking and health. The report will highlight fifty years of progress in tobacco control and prevention, present new data on the health consequences of tobacco use, and detail initiatives that can end the tobacco use epidemic in the U.S.

• • •

The Reports of the Surgeon General *through the year 2000, including those on smoking and health, have been digitized and made available on NLM's* Profiles in Science. *Reports and other publications of the Surgeon General from 2001 to the present are available as full text in NLM's HSTAT (Health Services/Technology Assessment Texts) system.* Reports of the Surgeon General *on* Profiles in Science *was launched in 2002. This post features text written by Dr. K. Walter Hickel, a historian in the Digital Manuscript Program.*

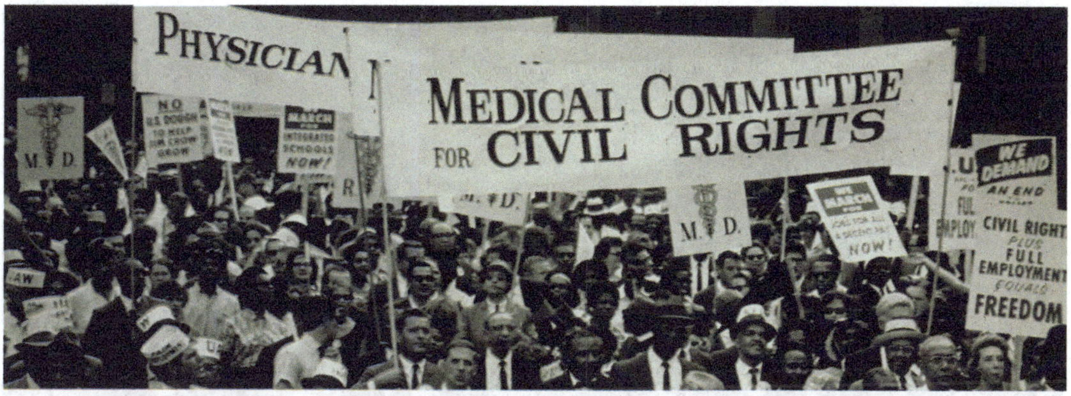

MCCR WAS THERE

https://circulatingnow.nlm.nih.gov/2013/08/28/mccr-was-there/

August 28, 2013 • Prints & Photographs

ELIZABETH A. MULLEN

As crowds gather today on the Mall in Washington, DC—on the occasion of the fiftieth anniversary of the March on Washington for Jobs and Freedom—we remember that participants in the March came from all parts of society. In this photograph a contingent of medical workers, doctors, nurses, and others march under the banner of the Medical Committee for Civil Rights (MCCR). The MCCR was a short-lived organization, initially formed by physician Walter Lear to protest the AMA's policy of non-integration at its annual convention in Atlantic City in 1963. Following that protest, Dr. Lear brought together over 200 healthcare workers to join the March on Washington. While the MCCR disbanded shortly afterward, it gave rise to the Medical Committee for Human Rights, which formed in 1964 to support volunteer medical workers providing care to civil rights workers, activists, and volunteers working on the Mississippi Summer Project, known as Freedom Summer, a volunteer project organized by

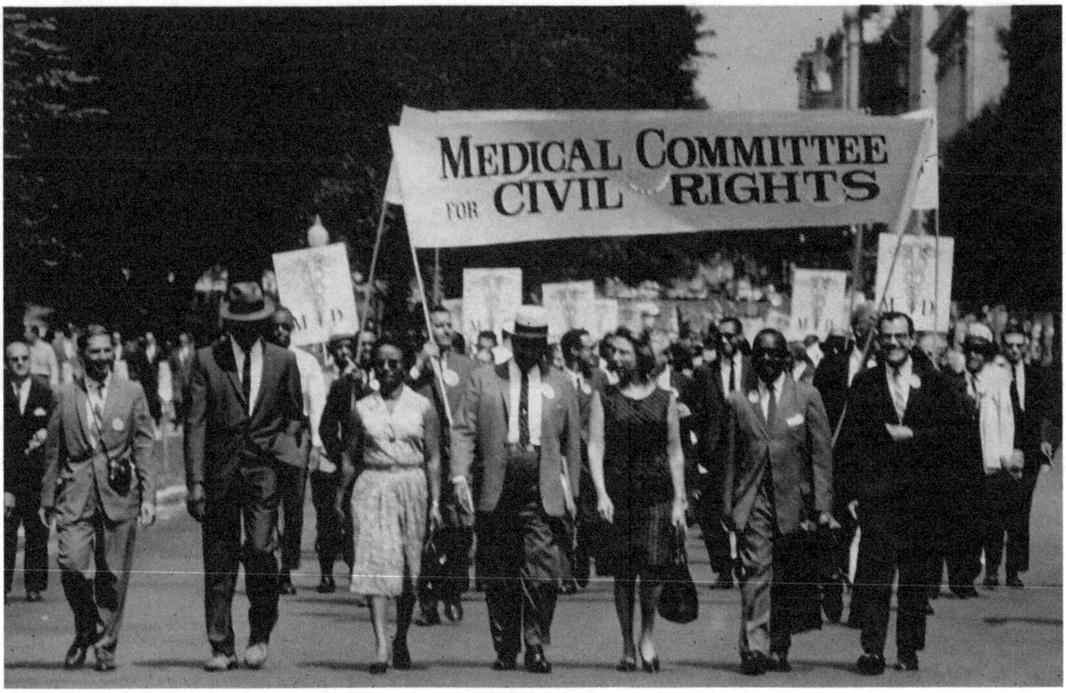

Members of the Medical Committee for Civil Rights at the March on Washington for Jobs and Freedom, 1963 • *National Library of Medicine #101455945*

the Council of Federated Organizations, a coalition of the Mississippi branches of the four major civil rights organizations (SNCC, CORE, NAACP, and SCLC) to register African American voters in Mississippi.

The March of 1963 touched hundreds of thousands of lives that day in Washington, DC, transforming a generation. Today we recall the March, the generation that experienced it directly, and the legacy of Dr. Martin Luther King Jr.'s "I Have a Dream" speech, in which he described the event as "the greatest demonstration for freedom in the history of our nation."

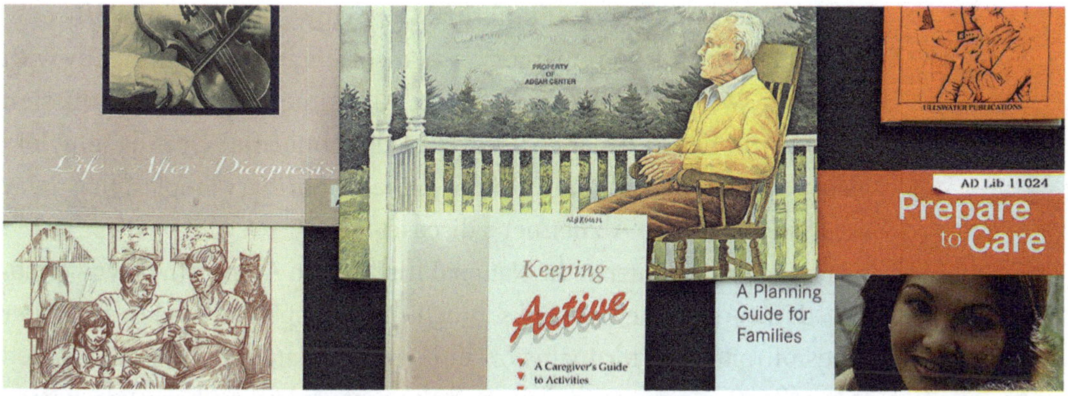

ALZHEIMER'S DISEASE COLLECTION RECEIVED

https://circulatingnow.nlm.nih.gov/2013/11/15/alzheimers-disease-collection-received/

November 15, 2013 • Rare Books & Journals

MARGARET KAISER

Recently, the Library received from the National Institute on Aging (NIA)'s Alzheimer's Disease Education and Referral (ADEAR) Center an excellent collection of public health education materials dealing with Alzheimer's disease. Caring for a person with Alzheimer's disease is demanding and can present many challenges, and this collection is particularly strong in the areas of caregiver guidance and training.

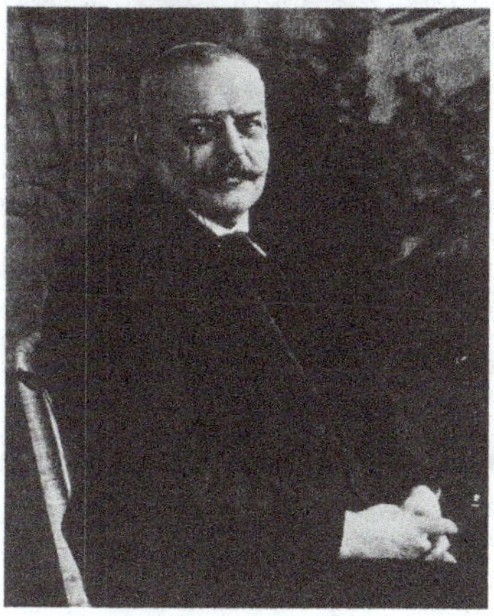

Portrait of Alois Alzheimer, ca. 1900 • *National Library of Medicine #101448035*

Alzheimer's disease is a progressive and irreversible brain disease. The disease is named after Bavarian physician, Dr. Alois Alzheimer (1864–1915), who, in 1901 began following the case of Auguste

Deter, a mental patient in Frankfurt, Germany. Although only fifty-one, she was suffering from memory loss, disorientation, and difficulty with language. When she died in 1906, Dr. Alzheimer requested permission to examine her brain and discovered the abnormal clumps (amyloid plaques) and tangled bundles of fibers (neurofibrillary tangles) that today are associated with Alzheimer's disease.

The ADEAR Center at the National Institute on Aging, which was established in 1990, reviewed books, brochures, pamphlets, guides, and other types of materials for inclusion in its online database. The NIA ended this collection activity in 2012 and the materials have been transferred to the Library. The collection consists of materials published between the 1980s and 2012 and documents the research in Alzheimer's disease as well as its assessment, diagnosis, and management. The collection includes brochures, pamphlets, workbooks, and fact sheets that provide information on a wide range of topics pertaining to both patient care and

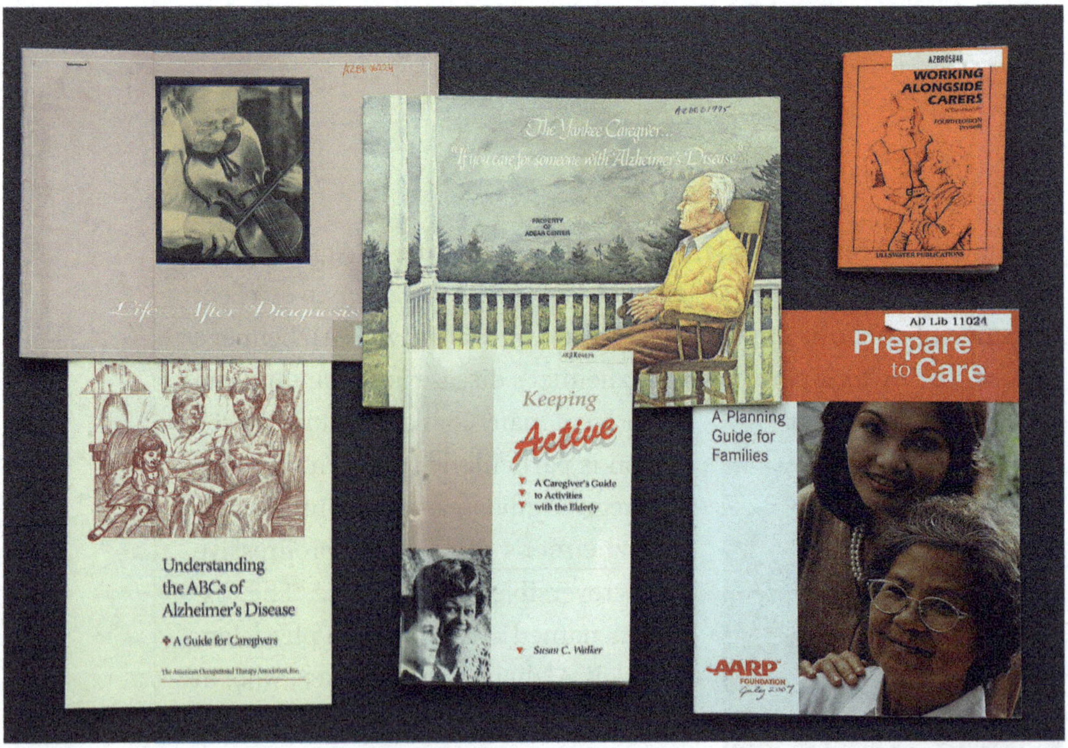

Titles include: *Life after Diagnosis*, *Understanding the ABCs of Alzheimer's Disease*, *The Yankee Caregiver*, *Keeping Active*, *Working Alongside Carers*, and *Prepare to Care*

caregiver needs. Subjects include coping with behaviors, financial and legal issues, and choosing a care facility.

November is National Alzheimer's Disease Awareness Month and National Caregiver Month. For current health information visit the National Institute on Aging's Alzheimer's Disease Education and Referral (ADEAR) Center, the government's leading resource on Alzheimer's disease. The ADEAR Center staff answers telephone, email, and written requests from families, caregivers, and professionals.

• • •

As of the date of this post, this recently acquired collection is currently being processed for inclusion in the collections of the Library. For questions about any of these titles, including how to consult them, please contact the History of Medicine Division reference staff via NLM Customer Support.

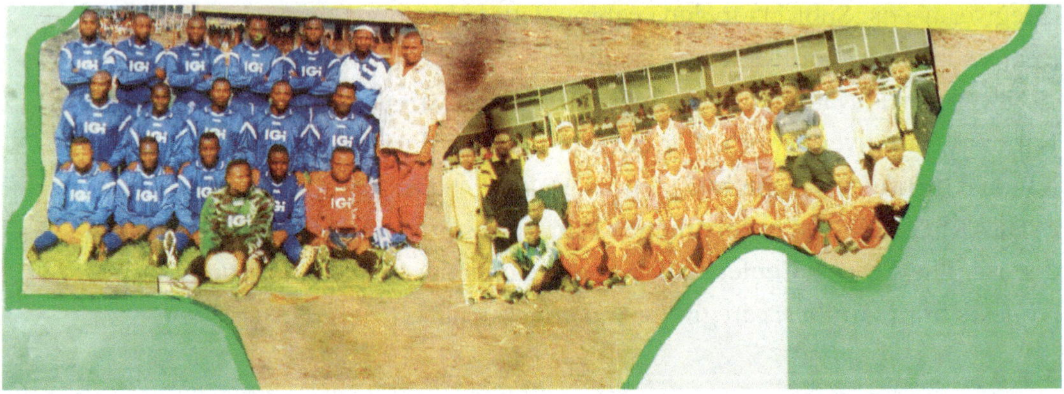

KICK POLIO OUT OF NIGERIA

https://circulatingnow.nlm.nih.gov/2014/06/25/kick-polio-out-of-nigeria/

June 25, 2014 • Prints & Photographs

ERIKA MILLS

During the World Cup, the globe is consumed by The Beautiful Game. Soccer is everywhere—even in public health messages! This poster encouraged parents to have their small children vaccinated against poliomyelitis during the 1998 National Immunisation Days in Nigeria. It points out that a healthy child may grow up to play on the national soccer team, a topical twist on an important message, as Nigeria competed in the World Cup that year. "Kick polio out of Nigeria" is the slogan at the bottom of the poster, and in subsequent World Cup tournament years, polio eradication efforts have used similar, soccer-based mantras.

National Immunization Days have been a vital part of polio eradication programs around the world. All children who are five years old or younger are taken to designated immunization centers where they receive the oral vaccine, regardless of whether they've already had doses in their routine immunizations. A month later, they return for another dose.

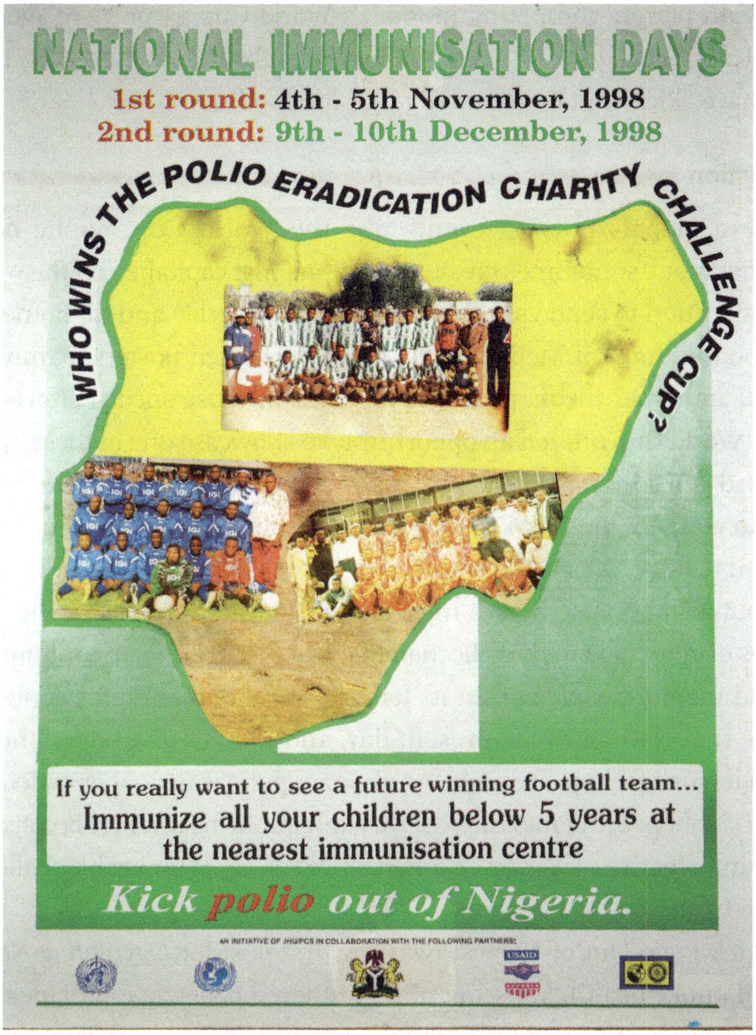

National Immunisation Days, ca. 1998 • *National Library of Medicine #101455309*

These large-scale efforts must mobilize communities en masse to be effective. According to UNICEF, in 2005, forty-five million doses of vaccine were given in Nigeria by 138,220 vaccinators. National Immunization Days, along with routine immunization, surveillance, and targeted "mop up" campaigns to contain outbreaks, have cleared the disease from most areas of the world. Today, polio remains endemic in only three countries: Nigeria, Afghanistan, and Pakistan.

As the poster suggests, perhaps some of the children who received the vaccine in 1998 grew up to become the soccer stars of today. A few of the

Nigerian players competing in today's World Cup game were aged five or younger back in 1998. Here's hoping that by the next World Cup, we will have "kicked polio out of Nigeria" for good!

Reflection

During global sporting events like the World Cup, public health organizations sometimes create campaigns that capitalize on the world's rapt attention to send vital messages that reach wide and hit home. The National Library of Medicine (NLM) has collected posters, pamphlets, films, and other media produced for some of those special efforts. The 2014 World Cup offered an opportunity to showcase one of these sports-themed items from the NLM's extensive collection of public health posters and to connect the NLM's historical collection to current events. I was excited to write "Kick Polio Out of Nigeria," not only because I am a soccer fan but also because it gave me a chance to highlight one of the many pieces of ephemera in the collection that had the potential to communicate to and inspire people within its temporal and demographic context, to relate that context to the present day, and to help us understand and learn lessons from past events. As of 2020, polio is no longer endemic in Nigeria, but peering into the past through public health media continues to be informative as we search for effective solutions for health challenges of the future.

"Kick Polio Out of Nigeria" was my first post for *Circulating Now* on global public health. Subsequently, I authored posts on topics including malaria eradication and Olympics-themed public health posters. In 2019, I co-curated an exhibition called *World Health Organization: Picturing Health for All* with my colleague and fellow *Circulating Now* editorial board member Ginny A. Roth. Curatorial work, like writing blog posts and developing exhibitions, allows me to connect patrons to the NLM's vital health information and our vast collection and promote public health, which is part of the NLM's mission, but also to foster an understanding of how biomedical science has been both shaped by and has helped shape society. —Erika Mills, 2023

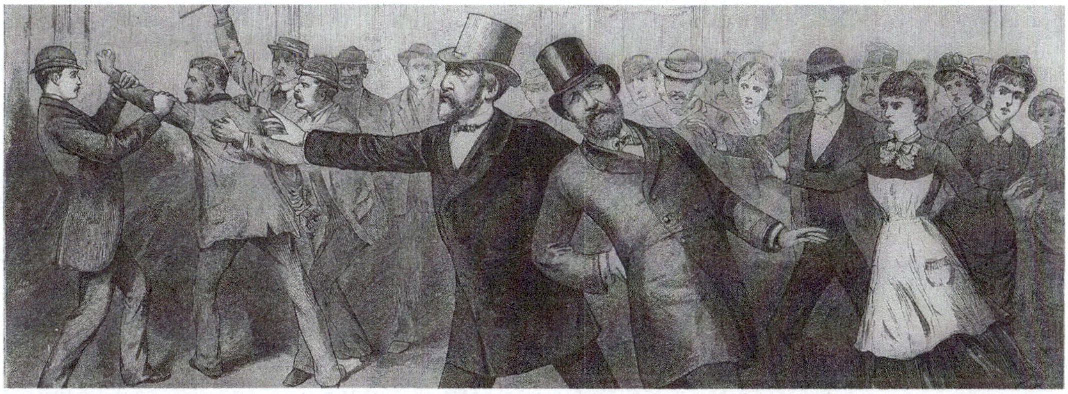

"THE PRESIDENT IS SOMEWHAT RESTLESS . . ."

https://circulatingnow.nlm.nih.gov/2013/07/02/the-president-is-somewhat-restless-reenacting-the-summer-of-1881-and-the-days-following-the-assassination-of-president-james-a-garfield/

July 2, 2013 • Garfield Assassination

JEFFREY S. REZNICK AND LENORE BARBIAN

Reenacting the Summer of 1881, and the Days Following the Assassination of President James A. Garfield

• • •

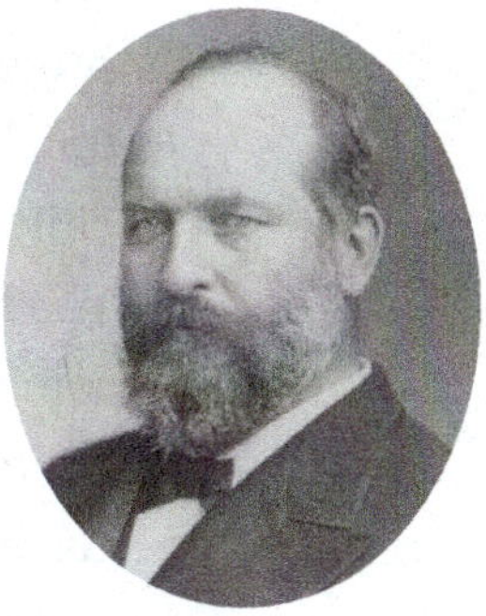

One-hundred-and-thirty-two years ago today—on July 2, 1881—the 20th president of the United States, James A. Garfield, entered the Baltimore and Potomac Railroad Station in Washington, DC, to board a train bound for Williamstown, Massachusetts. Charles Guiteau, who was angry that Garfield failed to appoint him to a diplomatic post and believing that God was instructing him to

TOP A detail of "The attack on the President's life—Scene in the ladies' room of the Baltimore and Ohio Railroad depot—The arrest of the assassin," *Frank Leslie's Illustrated Newspaper*, July 16, 1881, pp. 332–333. • *Courtesy Library of Congress*

RIGHT President James A. Garfield (1831–1881) • *Courtesy Library of Congress*

kill the President, stepped toward Garfield from a station door and fired two shots. One bullet grazed the President's right arm. The second bullet entered his lower right back. As bystanders seized Guiteau, Garfield collapsed onto the floor, mortally wounded.

Within an hour after the shooting, a group of notable physicians assembled to take over the President's case. Their prime concern was the bullet still lodged in Garfield's abdomen. It was this bullet and the path that it took through Garfield's internal organs that would haunt the doctors that attended him. Garfield received the very best in medical care of the time, but in 1881 the germ theory of disease was not yet established in America. There were no CT scans, PET scans, or even x-rays. There was no blood typing, and blood transfusions were rarely successful. Abdominal surgery was seldom attempted since it was almost always fatal. The best that doctors could do for the President was to probe his wound to determine the path of the bullet and, therefore, the extent of his injures, dress his wounds, provide him with nourishment, and make him comfortable. Many did not expect the President to live for more than a few hours, but Garfield surprised them all by surviving throughout the night and waking cheerful and rested. Now despite the seriousness of Garfield's wound, there was hope. The doctors' medical experience during the Civil War had shown them that some could survive wounds similar to Garfield's, and Garfield was a relatively young and athletic man who was always playful with his children.

America—and eventually the world—reacted to Garfield's attempted assassination with deep despair. The President's physicians issued daily progress reports, which the public eagerly awaited and newspapers quickly reprinted for their readers. Letters by the bushel basket came daily to the White House offering advice on various forms of treatment. The famous American inventor, Alexander Graham Bell, volunteered to come to Washington and help with Garfield's case. Yet, despite the care of prominent doctors and the heartfelt concern of the American people, Garfield would fail to recover from his injuries.

This series of blog posts is based in part on research completed for a 2006 temporary exhibition at the National Museum of Health and Medicine commemorating the 125th anniversary of the assassination of President Garfield. However, this summer, we invite you to experience the aftermath of the Garfield assassination in a way that was not part of that exhibition: through the series of bulletins that appeared regularly in newspapers across the country in the summer of 1881. Millions of Americans read these bulletins in newspapers large and small, following the drama involving Garfield and the medical care he received from his doctors. Beginning today they will appear here—in real historical time—for the first time since they were originally issued 132 years ago this summer.

Many of these original bulletins, in manuscript and printed form, are held in the archival collections of the National Library of Medicine (NLM), specifically within the papers of Joseph Janvier Woodward (1833–1884), one of President Garfield's attending physicians.

The entire set of the published bulletins are in the NLM's copy of Charles A. Wimer's Complete Medical Record of President Garfield's Case (Washington, DC, 1881), which also contains a rare set of photographs of the President's spine, taken following his death. All of this material, combined with sources held by the Library of Congress and the National Museum of Health and Medicine, opens a new window into the aftermath of Garfield's assassination.

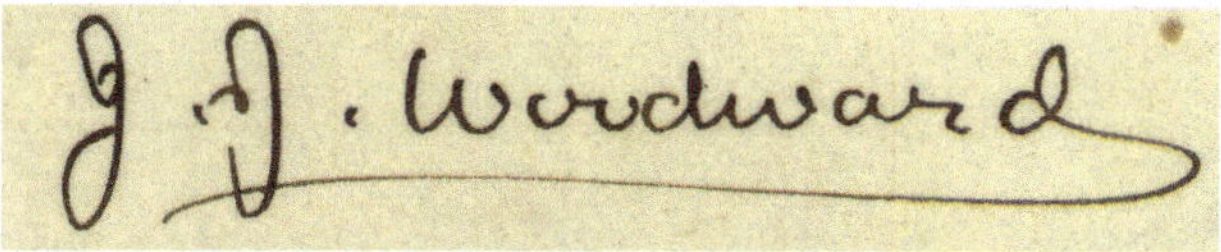

Signature of J. J. Woodward, a physician to President Garfield • *National Library of Medicine*

• • •

This post is one of a series reenacting the official bulletins released to the public by the physicians to President Garfield during his illness after the shooting on July 2, 1881.

CHAPTER 2
HISTORY IN HAND

INTRODUCTION • LAURA HARTMAN

To hold a piece of history in your hand can be a very profound sensory experience. The weight, the texture, the materials, the technique, the color, even the smell and sound, transport you to another time. A close look reveals the character and personality of the item. A long perusal triggers memories and emotions; a sense of nostalgia; or, perhaps, in the presence of a truly old or pioneering work, a sense of awe. Historical materials intrinsically connect and resonate with the (be)holder.

In the twenty-first-century world of print-on-demand, audiobooks, and digitized images and texts, the focus is on providing information. Researchers never need to leave the comfort of their own home to read or view the content of a collection item. In this context, format often means downloadable formats such as PDFs, JPEGs, or MOVs. The original physical format is at worst cropped out or at best simulated through the digital format or relegated to a footnote or piece of metadata. In this digital environment, *Circulating Now* provides a critical bridge between the intellectual content and physical context.

With tens of millions of items in the historical collections of the National Library of Medicine (NLM), there is ample opportunity for NLM staff, volunteers, and interns to engage with the materials that pass through their hands as part of their daily work. The blog posts in this chapter, written by catalogers, conservators, and curators, spotlight the physical nature of the materials that have resonated with their holders. Each in their own way, these authors share their detailed knowledge about the craftsmanship of the collection items with readers, while pointing out historical significance and unique features.

Circulating Now allows virtual visitors an up close and personal inspection of materials, an experience that simply is not possible even for those lucky enough to visit the Library and participate in a tour. Few people, including historians of medicine, get a chance to hold early modern manuscripts or rare books. Pre-dating the Industrial Revolution, they are artifacts from a time when absolutely everything was made by hand.

Krista Stracka's celebration of National Handwriting Day is less about penmanship and more about the scribal craft. Vivid language transports one to the scriptorium where the vellum is stretched, scraped, pricked, and ruled. You can almost see the pricking wheel marking the sheet and the correcting knife scraping away the errors. The manuscript is beautifully written, illuminated and rubricated in fifteenth-century style. The important practical text, that of Avicenna's *Canon,* a medical work in use for nine centuries, takes a back seat to evidence of craftmanship and construction.

Similarly, Stephen J. Greenberg's description of the 1610 edition of the *Prognosticatio* by Paracelsus is a study of book production in the hand-press period. The dizzying complexities of page imposition, folding, and nesting seem like a master class in origami. Given the frequent chance for human error in this process, it is no wonder that every copy of a hand-press period book has the potential to be completely unique. And yet this inspection of the sheets, how they are composed and folded, is not normally possible for researchers once the sheets have been bound—librarians frown when researchers pick at bindings to see how they are sewn together.

Some of the rare volumes patiently sitting on the shelves conceal illustrations that make them unique, extraordinary copies of a text. Homira Pashai's post on the curiously illustrated Mughal period manuscript is one such case. Painted over the text of Rhazes' medical work are images from a well-known Persian love story. It is as if someone took a copy of *Gray's Anatomy* and painted scenes from *Romeo and Juliet* over the text. Pashai speculates that the paintings were added to increase the manuscript's value. Perhaps the subterfuge was an attempt to sell the item to an unsuspecting purchaser who did not read Persian. Certainly, these beautiful imperfections have value to the art historian. They also firmly wed the medical side of Persian culture with the literary culture of the time.

Posts about visual materials highlight special characteristics that need to be seen to be understood. One advantage *Circulating Now* has over traditional two-dimensional digital repositories is the ability to showcase collection materials as objects, from new angles, in new settings, even in video. Like digital collections, this gives staff the ability to display, and the online audience an opportunity to examine, items while limiting the wear and tear on physical books and scrapbooks that might be increased by repeated openings and view fragile film without damaging the original.

The co-authored post by Kenneth M. Koyle, Ginny A. Roth, and Krista Stracka, on the *Memorials of Captain Hedley Vicars*, describes how an added illustration, specifically a fore-edge painting, elevates a popular biography to a piece of art. The short video demonstrating how one must hold the physical volume at just the right angle and fan the pages of the text block to reveal the painting mesmerizes and begs to be replayed, over and over again. As a closed volume there appears to be nothing but gilt on the fore-edge. Then suddenly a highly detailed hospital scene appears. The digital capture is in some ways superior to an in-person experience—you can view it at home, you can see it very close, you can repeat it infinitely. This charming, almost magical, feature infuses the volume with personality as it reflects the anecdotes within.

The concept of added value is not limited to textual works. Sarah Eilers featured the historical film, *The Medical Service of the Finnish Armed Forces in Winter* in the post, "Winter Wounds, Paper Dressing." In between the description of the subject matter—the military medical practice of using paper dressings to staunch war wounds—lie many references to the physical film and its embellishments—the whiteness, the poor resolution, the lost footage, the poor splicing, the editing, the translations, and the orchestration. The reader can both view the subject of the film and see the film as an object. The multiplicity of language tracks, music tracks, and footage exemplify the complexities of preserving such cultural artifacts. The film has passed through many hands, each person added to either its content or its physical nature. The unknown provenance of the film, as well as the mystery of who transformed it into what it is today, is as interesting as the medical knowledge captured in its footage. Breaking the theatrical fourth wall, this post directly solicits the audience to help solve the unanswered questions about this film.

Ephemeral and tiny, postage stamps feature beautiful artwork and have their own intrinsic preservation needs. Ginny A. Roth's post, simply titled "Dr. Schwartz's Stamp Collection," is a visual feast for the eyes, a kaleidoscope of color. The post focuses on a single-page miniature exhibition on the millennia-old practice of medical astrology. Colorful stamps depicting the twelve zodiac signs are artfully arranged in a circular "clock-face" design. Other stamps, many reflecting the international nature of the collection, honor famous physicians and commemorate significant medical discoveries. All, however, are acidic and in need of rehousing. Remounting them on acid-free paper ensures that the once ephemeral will become historical artifacts saved for future generations.

Computer technology is often short-lived. It serves its purpose and is then discarded in favor of the next state-of-the-art program. Although the NLM does not normally collect objects, it does collect pioneering technology related to medical data and research. John Rees's interview with Jan Schultz, the creator of PROMIS (Problem-Oriented Medical Information System), an early computer-based system of medical records, provides a rare opportunity to understand the intent or psychology of one such pioneering work. Schultz laments that he hoped medical procedure codes would help physicians characterize diagnoses; he never intended for them to be used by insurance companies to decide what was medically necessary or covered under individual policies. From the physical point of view, what may be most striking about this early computer program is that it was built with a touchscreen. Suddenly this 1970s pioneering medical records system becomes all too familiar to those of us in the twenty-first century. Just like a smartphone, it needs a person to interact with it. What was first perceived as an empty shell suddenly whirrs to life in the reader's mind.

Conservators are the physicians of the special collections world. They examine the physiopathology of historical materials, make a diagnosis, and treat the patient. Sometimes the patient is a celebrity, like the Nirenberg Genetic Code Chart. This Nobel Prize winning research is arguably one of the most awe-inspiring items in the historical collections of the NLM. The protein sequences and results of protein synthesis are handwritten in several different colors, with a successful experiment circled in red. As striking as these colors are, the acid in the ink is detrimental to its own preservation. In "Preserving Nirenberg's Genetic Code Chart," Kristi Wright and Holly Herro chronicle the struggle of the conservator to preserve this seminal award-winning research for posterity. Their work highlights the use of chemical analysis and Photoshop Assisted Spectroscopy to identify appropriate housing to slow the degradation caused by the ballpoint ink. They show how scientific techniques are applied to help save the research, while respecting its construction.

Circulating Now encourages posts from interns experiencing historical collections at the very beginning of their career journeys. In "Doctoring the Art of Medicine Series," conservation intern Laura McNulty reflects on her experience rehousing May Lesser's series of prints. McNulty writes that "by focusing on the people rather than the tools and techniques, [Lesser] made doctors and their work more human." Conversely, it is McNulty's focus on conservation tools and techniques that bring her internship experience to life. One can picture McNulty wielding her micro-spatula and jar of methylcellulose, spitting on a cotton swab, and applying heat to remove the offending adhesives. Few consider what is involved with cleaning and rehousing artwork. The pride in McNulty's sense of accomplishment and her personal connection to the collection shine through.

Collectively, *Circulating Now* enables readers to see the diverse breadth and depth of the NLM's physical collections and understand how the staff engage and care for them. The entire object is brought into focus and these historical materials are given a platform to speak for themselves.

The posts tease out their secrets, reveal their imperfections, and show off their individual personalities. These historical materials revel in both their intellectual significance and their physical context. Artifact, image, text, and video thrive in situ; when they cannot, conservators find ways to preserve them for future generations to experience.

Now, come get acquainted with the myriad physical formats in the historical collections of the NLM. Learn about their craftsmanship and their character. See the miniscule magnified. View the artistic and visual splendor. Be transported to the medieval scriptorium. Visit the NLM Conservation Lab where modern technology and traditional handiwork combine to preserve materials. Puzzle over the mysteries of provenance. Reflect on the intent of the creator and the created work, as you experience that profound sense of holding a piece of history in your hand.

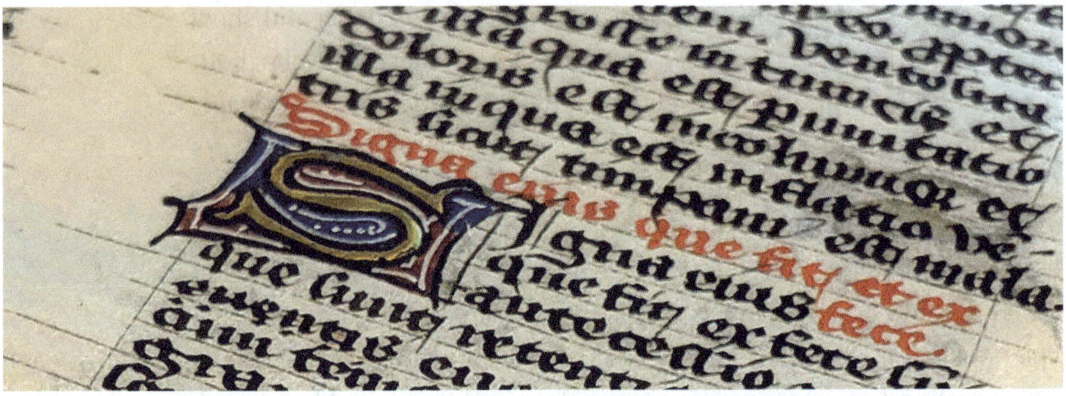

PEN TO PARCHMENT: NATIONAL HANDWRITING DAY

https://circulatingnow.nlm.nih.gov/2020/01/23/pen-to-parchment-national-handwriting-day/

January 23, 2020 • Rare Books & Journals

KRISTA STRACKA

In honor of National Handwriting Day, we recognize the craft of the highly skilled medieval scribes and artists who meticulously copied and illuminated the fifteenth-century *Liber medicinalis* (or *The Book of Medicine*), a Latin translation of selected portions of *al-Qānūn fī al-tibb* [*The Canon of Medicine*] by Ibn Sīnā held at the National Library of Medicine.

Ibn Sīnā, also known as Avicenna, was a Persian physician and polymath who first wrote the *Canon* in 1025, an encyclopedic work that is revered as one of the most influential books on medicine. Used for centuries as the standard textbook for physicians, the *Canon* was described by William Osler as "a medical bible." Within the five extensive books are important contributions to fields like neuroscience and drug research.

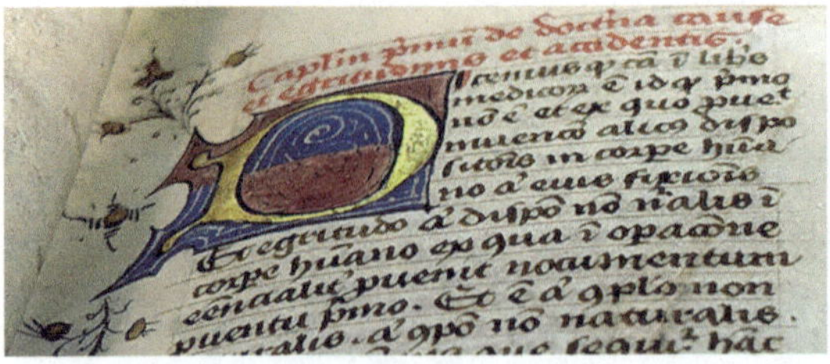

Detail of lettering in *Liber medicinalis*, 1450 • *National Library of Medicine #101141493*

No matter how often this early manuscript is pulled to display for tours, it never ceases to amaze all who gaze upon it, not only for the significance of its content but for its physical features. After the original clasps are released from the edge of the sixteenth-century brown calf binding, the cover is opened to reveal the beautiful gold leaf of the ornamental initial and the tiniest script in Gothic book-hand on the vellum page, often mistaken at first for printed text. How could lettering so small and consistent possibly have been handwritten? In short, the answer is a lot of preparation and teamwork.

Scribes

As demand for books increased in the later medieval period, scribal work expanded outside of the monastery to include secular, professional scribes. For any scribe of this period, the first step was the completion of a lengthy apprenticeship to gain mastery of this often grueling and tedious work. Production of just one book could take months or even years. To speed up the process, the work was often distributed among multiple scribes who worked concurrently on different sections. At least three different "hands" (another term for scribes) wrote the five sections of the *Liber medicinalis*. The first scribe (leaves 1–78) was a calligrapher active in Bruges during the 1450s named Willelmus de Predio, who is identified on leaf 78. Based on unique variations in the writing of the individuals, he and a second scribe (leaves 379–388) are likely to have written later sections as well. For instance, the second scribe chose to pen flourish letters in the top lines with heads in profile, decorations that were also added in the fourth section (leaves 389–460).

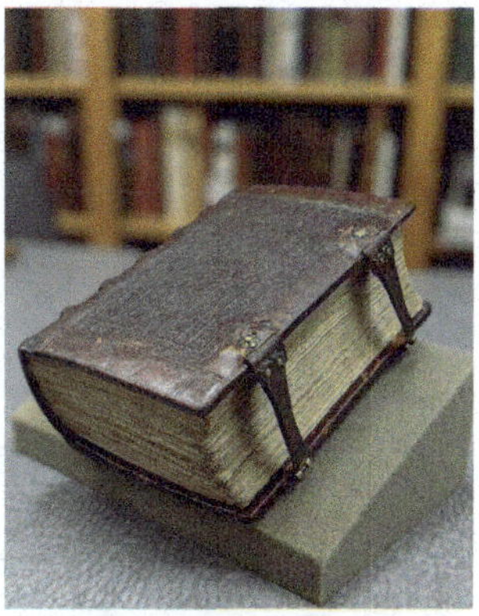

Liber medicinalis, 1450 • *National Library of Medicine #101141493*

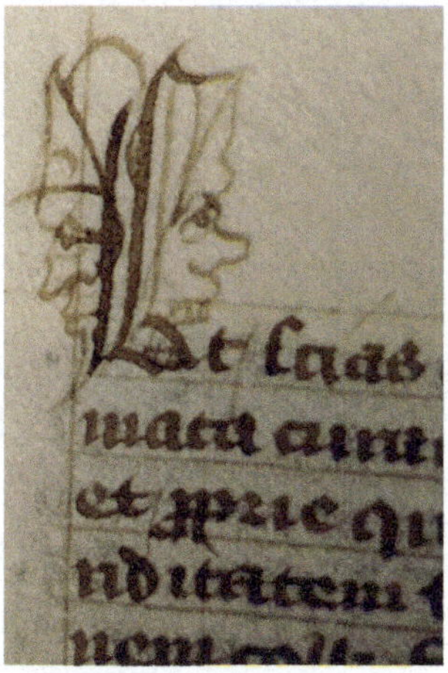

Flourishes in *Liber medicinalis*, 1450

Preparing the Parchment

Before these scribes put a pen to the page, the design and layout was planned and the writing surface was prepared, a process based on the book's intended purpose. Although the use of paper in bookmaking had increased by the 1450s, this manuscript was written on softened, untanned

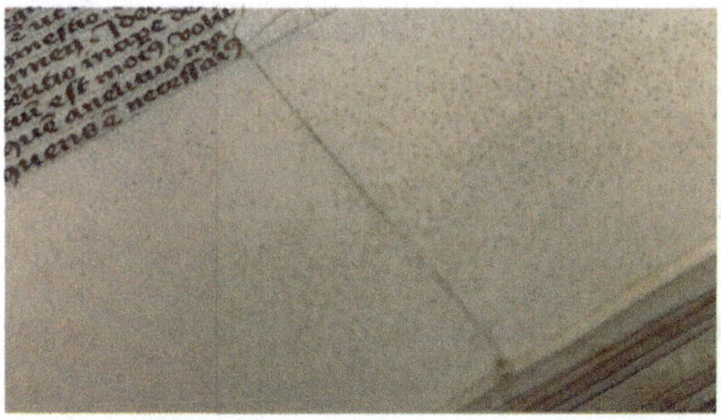

Detail showing follicles in the parchment of *Liber medicinalis*, 1450

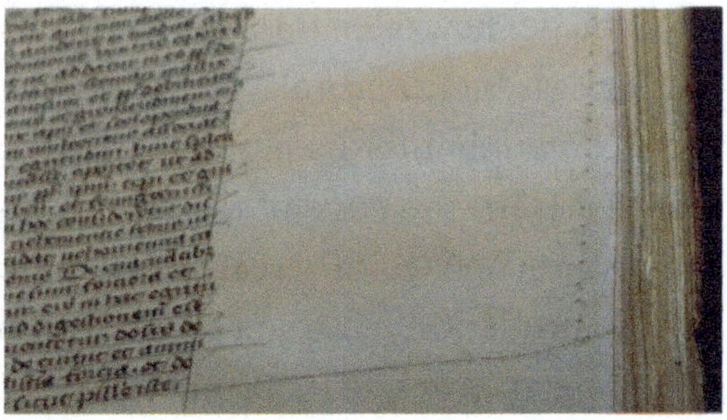

Pricked edge in *Liber medicinalis*, 1450

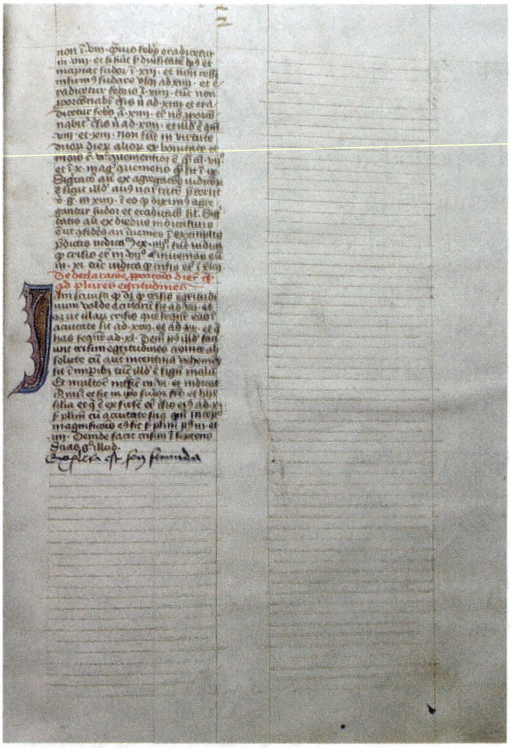

Unfilled ruling in *Liber medicinalis*, 1450

calfskin known as vellum, or more broadly as parchment—a term that also includes the skin of goat and sheep. To create a thin smooth surface for writing, the laborious work of parchment-making included steps to stretch, scrape, clean, and treat the skin before cutting it to size and sending to the scribes as sheets.

With the parchment in hand, the scribe or the apprentice prepared it for writing by first "pricking" and then "ruling" the page to create a template for that precise script. Pricking the parchment involved the use of an instrument like a spiked wheel to add puncture marks (or "prickings") at designated intervals. These prickings served to guide the drawing of the horizontal and vertical ruling pattern for the columns and rows. The ruling layout of this manuscript is most visible on the final leaf as most of the inked lines were left unfilled. The design called for two columns of sixty lines each, which measures to about twelve handwritten lines per inch!

Script and Scribal Tools

To fill these lines, the scribes used one of the most important tools in their kit—knowledge and skill of the script planned in the design. Each scribe used a formal Gothic book-hand to write this book—a script characterized by upright, unjoined letters made with sharp strokes that required frequent lifting of the pen. To fit the selected portions of the *Canon* in one book as opposed to multiple bound volumes, it required use of a small font.

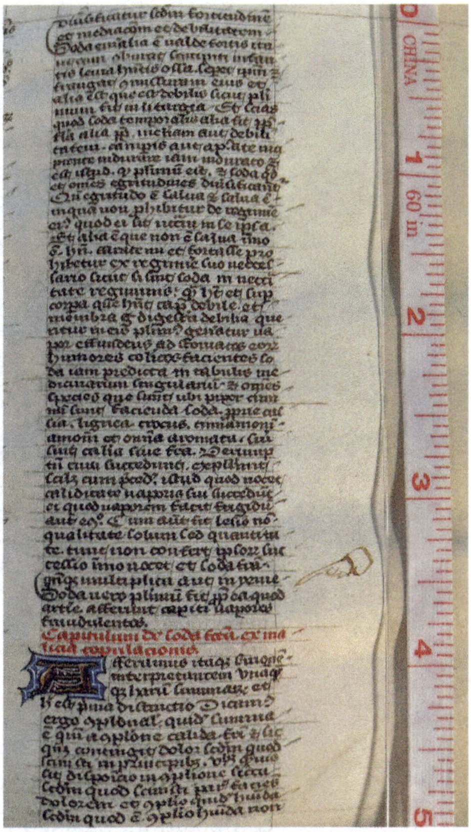

Very small writing in *Liber medicinalis*, 1450

So, with the parchment prepped and tools at hand, the scribes copied word for word from an existing book (the "exemplar"). The *Canon* was first translated from Arabic into Latin by Gerard of Cremona in the late twelfth century, a copy likely serving as the exemplar for this book. Seated at an angled desk with the exemplar placed in a reading frame and a filled ink pot readily at hand, the scribe held a quill pen in his right hand and a knife in the other to sharpen the pen and scrape mistakes from the page. Though beautifully executed, this manuscript is not entirely error-free. The second scribe mistakenly called the section beginning on leaf 79 the second book, but correctly calls it "liber tertius" in the explicit on leaf 423. A knife was not taken to the page to correct this error.

Process of Illumination

Finally, during the process of writing, the scribes left spaces for the highly skilled illuminators to illustrate, paint, and apply gold leaf to create the decorated initials found throughout the book. At the beginning of Book III, space for a 25-line initial was left blank, unintentionally offering the opportunity for us to view this step in the process. The largest initials can be found at the beginnings of Books I and IV with smaller 2-line and 3-line initials at beginning of paragraphs throughout, all beautifully illuminated in gold, blue, pink, and white.

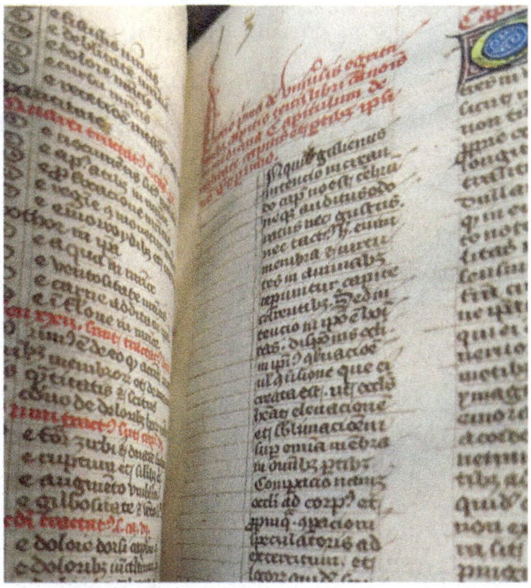

Space for an illustration in *Liber medicinalis*, 1450

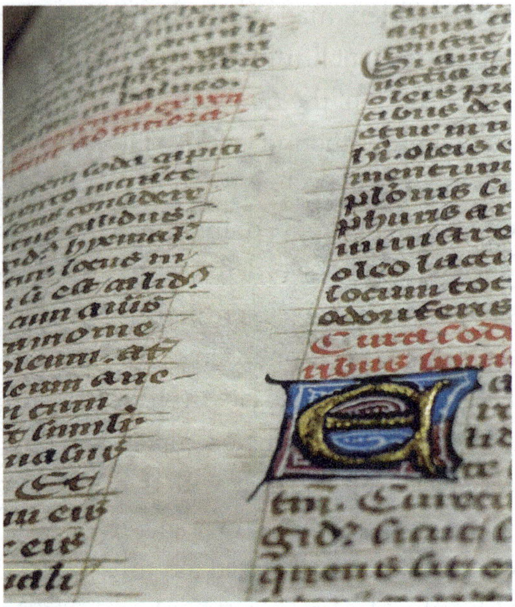

An illuminated letter in *Liber medicinalis*, 1450

Conclusion

Each manuscript book is unique and reveals clues about the story of its composition. Based on the high quality of the vellum, its decorated letters, the clean margins, and the selection of a font size that is not exactly reader-friendly, it is likely the *Liber medicinalis* was intended as a gift, once belonging to the Benedictines of Saint-Amand near Valenciennes. Due to its condition, we are currently unable to digitize the book but invite you to appreciate the penmanship of these scribes in person throughout the year, not only on National Handwriting Day.

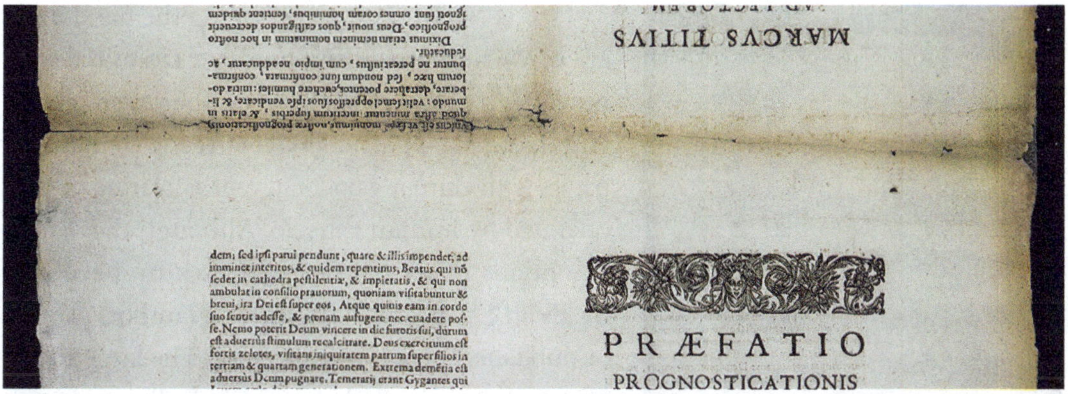

A BOOK UNFINISHED: PARACELSUS IN HAND-PRESS SHEETS

https://circulatingnow.nlm.nih.gov/2016/11/29/a-book-unfinished-paracelsus-in-hand-press-sheets/

November 29, 2016 • Rare Books & Journals

STEPHEN J. GREENBERG

Books today, as physical objects, have reached a very odd place in our consciousness. Readers are increasingly offered books (or at least texts—there is a difference: books are physical objects; texts are their intellectual contents) in a bewildering array of electronic alternatives. Print (on paper) is dead, we are told, at the same time that the latest Harry Potter story sold two million print copies in the United States and Canada in its first two days of availability.

Moreover, at no time in the history of printing has it been easier to produce a physical book. Websites such as Blurb.com and Lulu.com allow authors to self-publish books in a variety of formats, with drag-and-drop interfaces, fast turnover times, and remarkably good results. Self-publishing is hardly new, but modern technology allows for extremely small pressruns; even as small as a single copy.

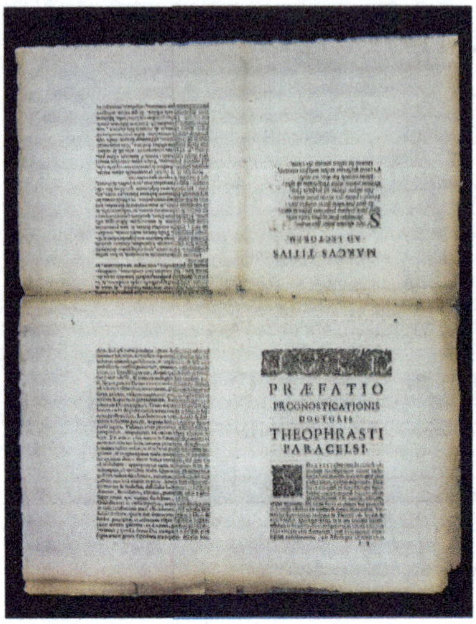

A full sheet of the *Prognosticatio* from a hand-press showing the preface and three other pages of text, 1610

This is NOT how it was. During the hand-press era of Western printing (roughly 1450 to the early nineteenth century), books were laboriously created with hand-set type, on single sheets of handmade paper, with clumsy wooden (eventually iron) presses operated by human muscle. Although there were exceptions in special cases, a pressrun needed to be about 1,500 copies for anyone (author, printer, or publisher) to make any money. The large sheets of paper were printed on one side, allowed to dry, printed on the other side (the technical term was "perfecting"), allowed to dry again, folded, gathered, stitched, and (possibly) bound for sale. None of this work was mechanized until well into the nineteenth century.

It is exceedingly rare to see an original hand-press book in an intermediate stage of production. But in the collections of the National Library of Medicine, there exists just such a book: printed sheets from 1610, never folded, never bound, never quite finished. It is entitled *Prognosticatio Eximii Doctoris Theophrasti Paracelsi*, which translates (roughly) from the Latin as predictions or prophecies from the famous doctor, pharmacologist, alchemist, astrologer, and much else, Philippus Aureolus Theophrastus Bombastus von Hohenheim (1493–1541), normally just known as Paracelsus. His work in toxicology, particularly involving the medical uses of mercury, was groundbreaking. His philosophical and mystical work, particularly as shown in this book, which was reprinted many times, simply demonstrates how flexible the boundaries were between science and medicine at the time.

The *Prognosticatio* consists of ten sheets, roughly 47 × 38 centimeters (18.5 × 15 inches) each, of handmade paper just as it would have emerged from the press after the second side was printed. Four pages of text and illustrations are visible on each side of the sheet; their orientation depending on how the sheet was to be folded. In this case, the sheet was to be folded twice, to provide a quarto-format gathering of eight pages. Had the sheet shown two pages per side, designed to be folded once, it would have been a folio; had it been printed with eight pages showing,

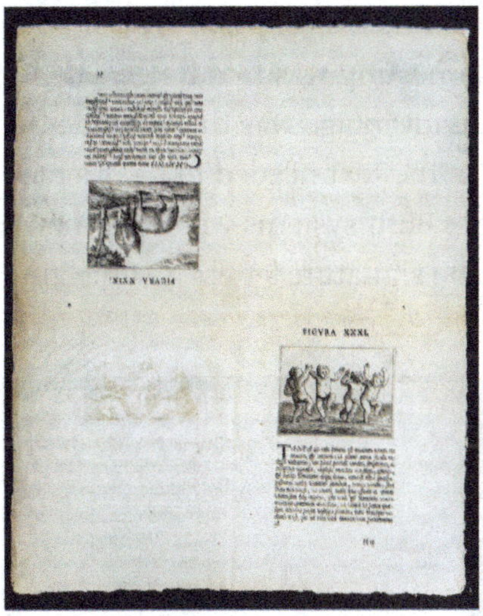

A full sheet showing letterpress text and engraved illustrations

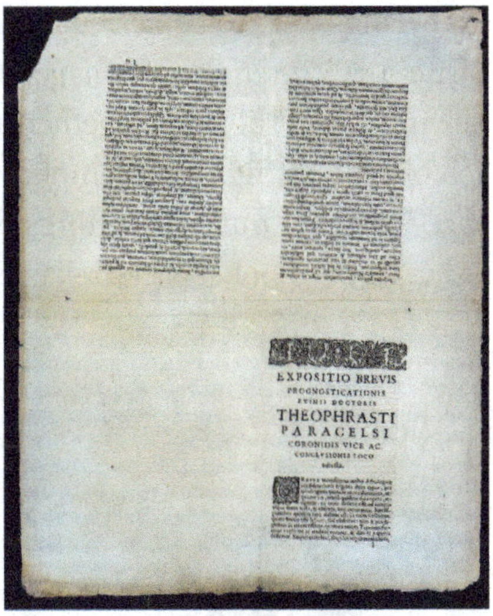

In another full sheet, carelessly printed, the paper was not well secured in the printing press.

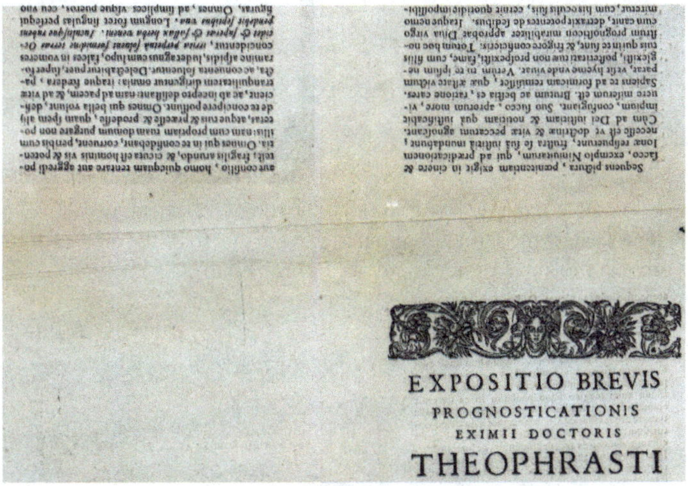

A close-up of the preceding sheet shows how the text needed to be oriented to give the proper order once the sheet was folded.

designed to be folded three times, it would have been an octavo. It's worth remembering that the terms folio, quarto, octavo, and so on refer to how the sheet was to be folded after printing. They have no direct bearing on the size of the book itself in the hand-press era.

Often, printed sheets would have additional letters called "signatures" in the lower margins to help the bookbinder place the gatherings in the correct order for sewing. This would be especially important when gatherings were to be nested inside each other, a common type of book structure. The main advantage of such nesting was that it needed less sewing to put the book together; the disadvantage was that it made the job of typesetting more complicated, as the text needed to be oriented just right over multiple settings of type. Both systems were commonly used. In this book it is clear, based on the signature letters, that nesting

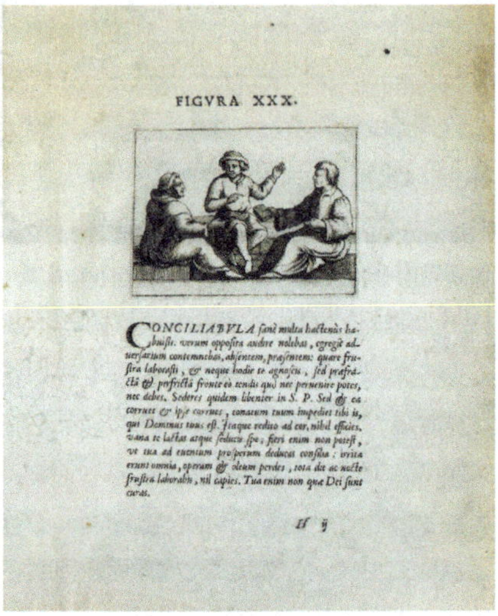

A close-up of a single page with text and illustration shows where the signature letter is clearly visible in the lower right corner.

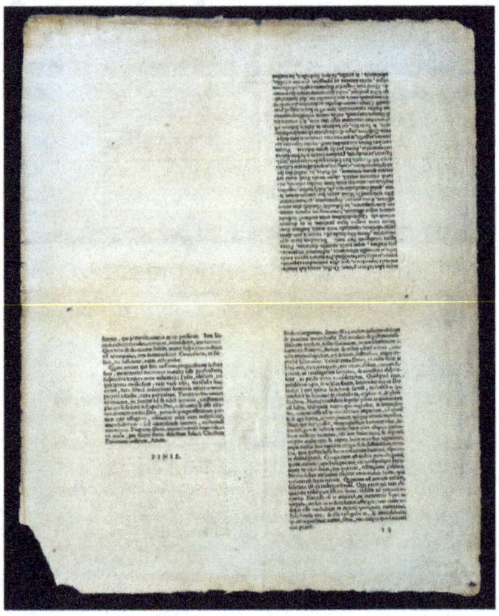

The final full sheet, with the work "Finis," confirms that the set of ten sheets is complete.

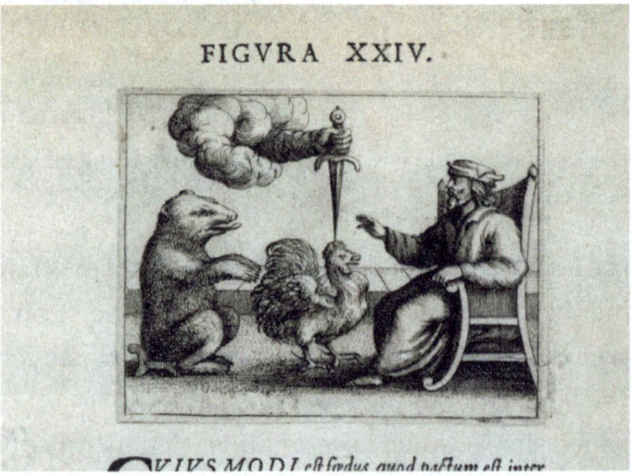

A close-up of an engraved illustration shows the plate mark (the slightly darker rim around the picture), which is the tell-tale evidence of the use of a rolling press to print the engraving.

was not used. The letters also indicate that the book is complete, as there are no gaps in the letter order.

The *Prognosticatio* does, however, present one additional complication. It is profusely illustrated with obscure, if interesting, mystical pictures. In this edition, they are copperplate engravings. The engravings are beautifully done, and clearly added meaning to the text (for those in the know), but for the printer, they added another layer of complexity to the production. For technical reasons, the copperplates needed to go through a different sort of press for printing. Earlier editions were illustrated with woodcuts, which did not present this problem, but were also inferior in quality to the engravings. For the printer, including engravings meant that each sheet of paper went through presses four times: once on each side for the image, and once on each side for the text.

It will never be known why this copy was left uncompleted. Presumably, it simply didn't sell. Sheets could be bound at the time of sale, or folded and stitched without binding, or even sold loose and unfolded, with the purchaser taking responsibility for the finishing. However, someone must have thought the sheets worth keeping. There were many other uses to which waste sheets could be put by either the printer or the bookbinder.

• • •

For more information about this book and other collections, please contact the History of Medicine Division via NLM Customer Support.

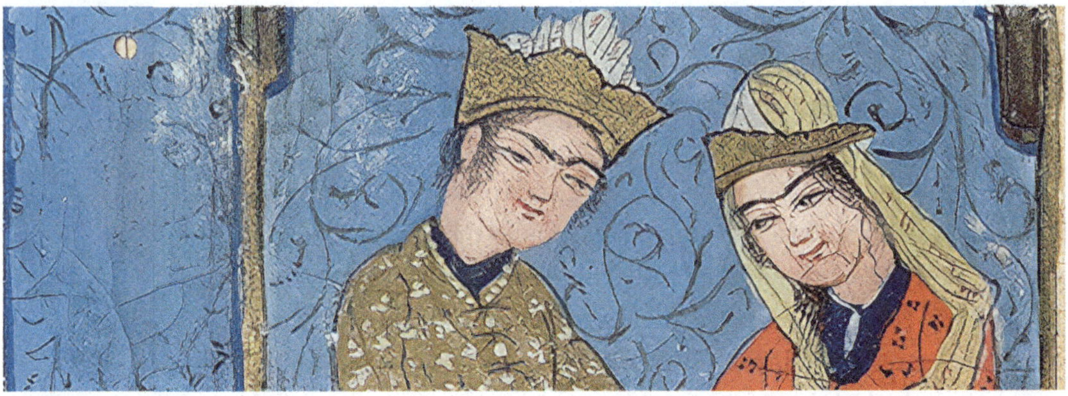

A MUGHAL ERA MANUSCRIPT CURIOUSLY ILLUSTRATED

https://circulatingnow.nlm.nih.gov/2016/05/05/a-mughal-era-manuscript-curiously-illustrated/

May 5, 2016 • Rare Books & Journals

HOMIRA PASHAI

The National Library of Medicine is the home of many precious manuscripts belonging to the Indian Mughal era (sixteenth- to eighteenth-century). Among these manuscripts, there is a unique copy of *Kitab-i fi al-tibb al-mansuri* (*Book on Medicine Dedicated to al-Mansur*) by Muhammad Zakariya al-Razi (died 925 AD). Al-Razi's text on the subject of therapeutics, diet, hygiene, anatomy, physiology, general pathology, and practical surgery was extremely influential and extensively copied into the seventeenth century. This copy from the early sixteenth century is unique because it includes six illustrations—not related to the text—that were painted onto the manuscript covering some of the text maybe

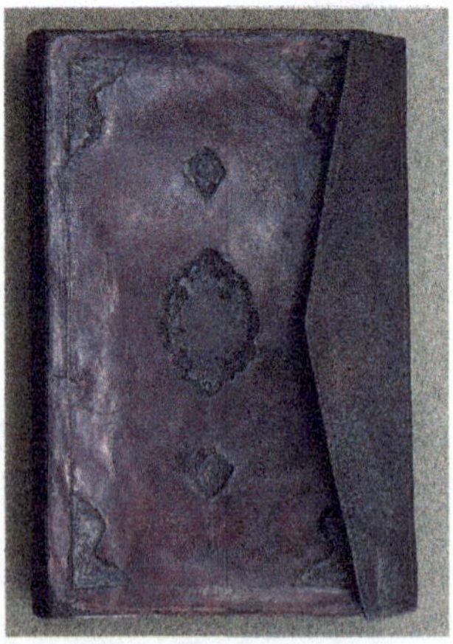

Kitab-i fi al-tibb al-mansuri by Muhammad Zakariya al-Razi, early sixteenth century • *National Library of Medicine*

well over a century ago. The reason is not known, but it was likely done in order to make the manuscript appear more valuable. As a result, this medical manuscript has been infused with illustrations from the genre of poetry and the product is a most precious work that is worth studying.

The inscriptions and seals that appear on the two flyleaves of this *Kitab-i fi al-tibb al-mansuri* attest to the long history of ownership of the manuscript. The twelve seals of the manuscript vary from the name of God, *Ya Karim*, to the name of individuals–evidently librarians–with the most notable one the seal of Shah Jahan *'Inayat Khan* AH 1068 (CE 1657). The inscriptions are written in Persian, the language of the Mughal court, and are written at slight but varied angles, which distinguish them from the neatly aligned text. The inscriptions and seals elaborate on the notion of distinct levels of authority in the imperial library. Inspector librarians, like Muhammad Hossein identified from the flyleaf AH 1002 (CE 1594), used inscriptions to sign the flyleaf with their name, date, and other information, while superintendents, designated officials, who held the greater positions of *nazim* and *darugha* (head library officials) used seals designed with their names on inscribed manuscripts.

Thus, Mughal librarians, like modern curators, used the codified system of inscriptions and seals to record the transfer of custody of the manuscripts. The common phrase *"vared arz shud,"* which means

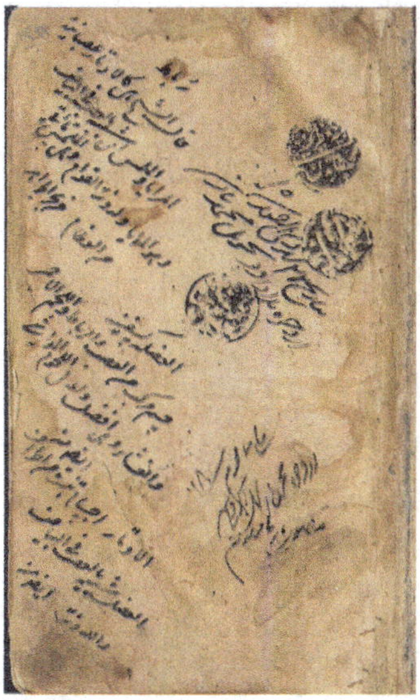

Flyleaf

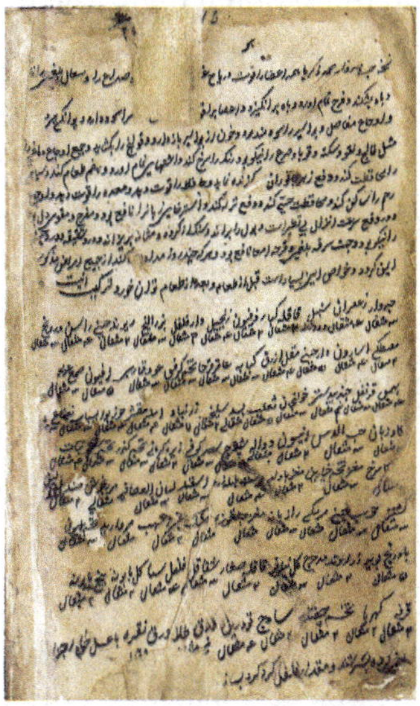

Endleaf

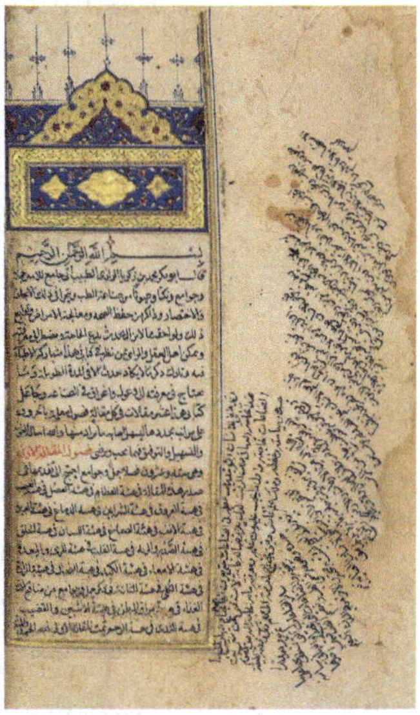

Saelawh

the manuscript "entered the library," usually appears, followed by the respective dates of accessions and the name of the librarian who supervised the task of manuscript transference. Also, the most ubiquitous type of inspection included the word *"arzdida"* meaning "received by" with the name, date, and month provided. The inspection note *"tahwil"* meaning "entrusted" was also used in conjunction with the name of the librarian and the date of transfer. Thus, during Shah Jahan's rule (CE 1628–1658), in the Mughal libraries, a chain of individuals practiced the codified transfer of custody to make sure the manuscripts were not lost.

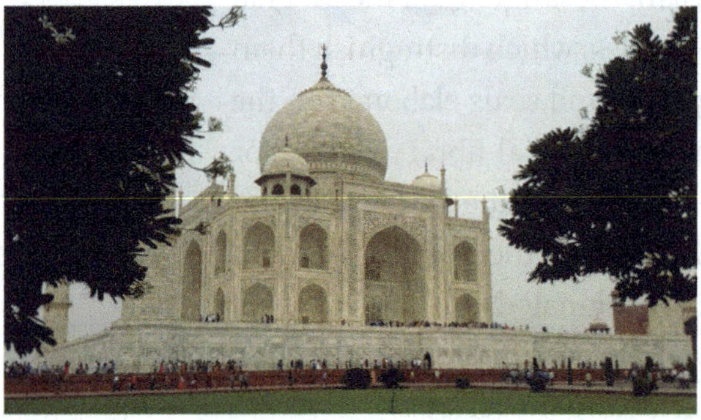
The Taj Mahal ca. 2016 • *Courtesy Joyce Backus*

'Inayat Khan, whose seal appears on the flyleaf of this manuscript, according to the *Shah Jahannama* (*History of Shah Jahan*), was appointed as the overall superintendent of the royal library (*darugha-yi kitabkhana*) most likely in Agra or Delhi, on AH 1068 (CE 1657) during the reign of Shah Jahan. *'Inayat Khan*, meaning 'the blessed lord' is a title bestowed upon Mirza Muhammad Tahir Ashena (died 1670 CE) who was one of the high-ranking civil officers (*sahib mansab*) of the Mughal court. His father Zafar Khan Ahsan Turbati was the governor (*wali*) of Kabul and Kashmir during the Mughal reign and his mother was Buzurg Khanum, the sister of Mumtaz Mahal, the beloved Persian wife of Shah Jahan, in whose commemoration the Taj Mahal was commissioned in 1632 CE. A great patron of literature and art, *'Inayat Khan* compiled *Kitab-i Mulkhas Tavarikh Shah Jahan* (*Extracts from the History of Shah Jahan*) based on the writings of Abdulhamid Lahuri and other historical accounts. His work on literature also includes a Divan of Poetry. *'Inayat Khan's* seal began to appear on manuscripts held in the royal library immediately after his appointment. Unfortunately, his seal was only in use for a short period due to the termination of Shah Jahan's reign less than twelve months later. Afterward, beginning the reign of Aurangzeb in 1658, he began a life of solitude in Kashmir.

The illustrations, added to the original centuries after it was created, are unrelated to medicine. They are in the Persian style of the fifteenth- to the beginning of the seventeenth-century paintings based on illustrations most likely from the Persian story of tragic romance *Khosrow va Shirin* by the poet Nizami Ganjavi (died 1209 CE). In this famous story the Sasanian King Khosrow Parviz II, the King of Persia, falls in love with the Armenian Princess Shirin. Farhad, the rival of Khosrow for the love of Shirin, is

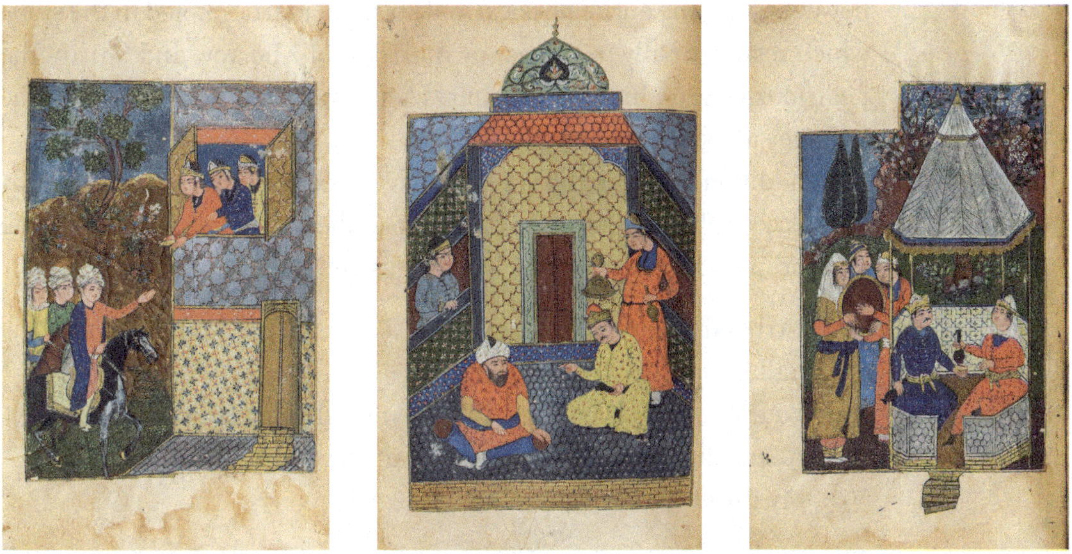

FROM LEFT TO RIGHT (1) Most likely Khosrow visiting Shirin's palace **(2)** Most likely Khosrow conversing with Shapur **(3)** Most likely Khosrow and Shirin feasting

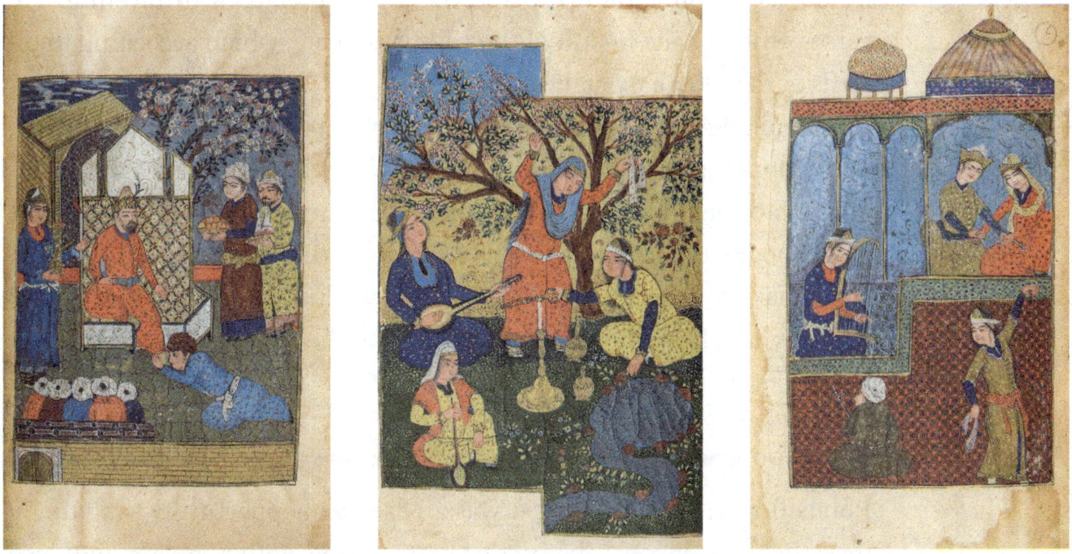

FROM LEFT TO RIGHT (1) Most likely Farhad summoned by Khosrow **(2)** Most likely celebration of the nuptial of Khosrow and Shirin **(3)** Most likely celebration of the nuptial of Khosrow and Shirin

the symbol of the selfless warrior who undertakes the task of cutting a canal through the rocks of the Bisotun Mountain for transportation of milk to Shirin's palace. Although in this circle of love Farhad's concept of love is heroic and Khosrow's sensual, Khosrow's lack of reasoning in a debate with Farhad results in betraying Farhad by sending him the false news of Shirin's death that leads to Farhad's demise. Typical of romances, however, after the entire physical and spiritual journey noted in the story, which results finally in the happy marriage of Khosrow and Shirin, the nefarious villain Shirviyeh conspires later against the couple, and in the end they are separated by death.

In addition to the images, verses have been inserted in the flyleaf by an unknown librarian, connoisseur, or scribe on the wisdom of reading and companionship of books. The verses are:

> "Art O'thou the one whose qualification is my faculty of speech (talking) capital
> Your occupation puts a bridle on my willfulness
> As the dust of your road became my place of worship
> My unsettled thought turned blemish"

These verses come to the aid of any historian to examine the manuscript through a social justice lens that elaborates on the respect of the time for books as companionship and the joy for metaphor unraveling. The verses embrace the breath of the compassionate, which according to the Sufis is the root of existence.

Overall, the manuscript is a unique artifact that takes us on a journey to the Imperial Mughal Library (1526–1707) where groups of artists and artisans copied, painted, and embellished the texts and the guardians of the books undertook the task of transferring and cataloging them. Papermakers, leatherworkers, bookbinders, illuminators, scribes, gilders, painters, and librarians used their skills on the refinement of the library institution in the Mughal court.

Reflection

Publishing in *Circulating Now* was an excellent opportunity to share my investigations of some distinctive manuscripts with a greater audience. I often noticed the annotation on the margins and their lucidity, from a sherbet recipe for sleep for the Ottoman Sultan Bayezid to instruction for making hair dyes during the Middle Ages.

Close companionship with the manuscripts familiarized me with the scribes and the thought processes of their authors. In the introduction of one "manual for eyes," for instance, the author explained his own life experience, noting that, since he had lost all his children to diseases, he decided to heal himself and raise awareness of his healing by writing the very manuscript I held in my hand.

Examining these manuscripts reveals how our predecessors were actively engaged in acquiring knowledge and refining it for their posterity. At the same time, this examination itself creates a human connection between us and people of the past. Such proximity establishes an incredible bond between the author and the reader, one which transcends time and space. The bond then results in the oneness, the unity, of the author and the reader of the manuscript. As a result, the reader, intellectually acquainted with the author, away from the cultural assumptions and conceptual differences of our modern time, perceives humanity as a whole. The privilege and pleasure of examining these manuscripts first-hand led to an expansion of my own self-awareness, becoming open to others, and being open to the world. —Homira Pashai, 2023

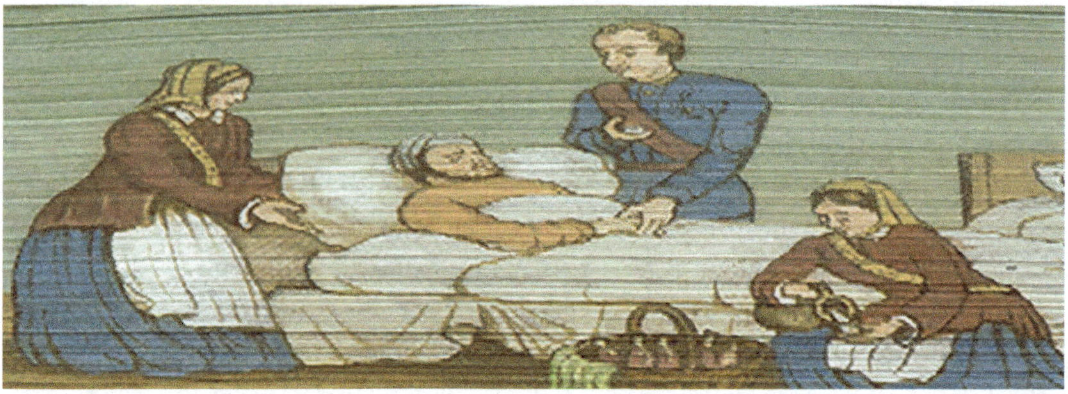

ART ON THE EDGE

https://circulatingnow.nlm.nih.gov/2017/03/22/art-on-the-edge/

March 22, 2017 • Rare Books & Journals

KENNETH M. KOYLE, GINNY A. ROTH, AND KRISTA STRACKA

Hedley Vicars was not a war hero. He was not a renowned strategist or tactician; his presence on the battlefield did not strike fear in the hearts of his enemies. In fact, Captain Hedley Vicars was killed by a Russian musket ball during his first direct combat engagement on the hills in front of Sebastopol on March 22, 1855. If not for his friendship with the biographer Catherine Marsh, Hedley Vicars' legacy would likely have been little more than a forgotten grave on a Crimean War battlefield. Catherine Marsh did count Hedley as a close friend, however, so when he died she was moved to immortalize him as a veritable Christian saint in a book that would eventually be translated into no fewer than eight languages, with hundreds of thousands of copies (plus a few plagiarized variants) printed and sold around the world from 1855 until the early twentieth century.

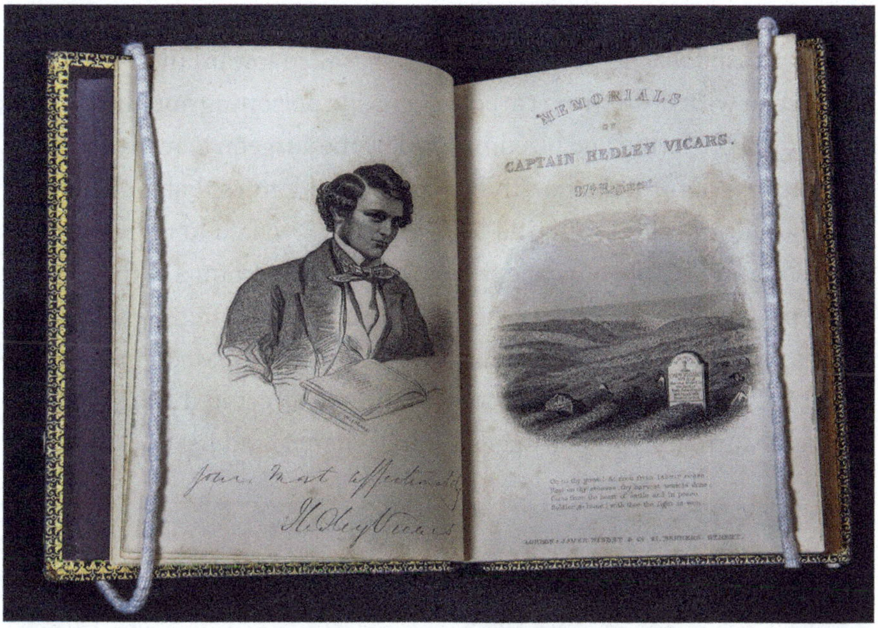

Memorials of Captain Hedley Vicars, Ninety-Seventh Regiment, 1870

The book *Memorials of Captain Hedley Vicars, Ninety-Seventh Regiment* belongs to a literary genre known as "evangelical biography." The main purpose of the book seems to be as much to convince readers of the piety, humility, and Christian faithfulness of its subject as to recount the events of his life. The book opens with a few entertaining stories from Vicars' youth and his early experiences as a British army officer, but the author is obviously eager to transition to her real focus—his Christian "awakening" and subsequent devotion to Bible study, prayer, and proselytizing. The book quotes liberally from Vicars' diary entries and letters he wrote to family and friends, incorporating dozens of complete letters transcribed directly into the text. These letters almost universally—if somewhat redundantly—proclaim his faith and rejoice in his zealous adherence to his gospel principles. In one passage he describes his daily routine, which included equal time dedicated to religious pursuits as to his work as an officer.

Interspersed among the pages of evangelical prose are several first-hand accounts of nineteenth-century military medicine, including the mournful tale of a friend dying of an unnamed disease while they were stationed in Jamaica, the "sickening feeling" of seeing the infamous military hospital at Scutari as his regiment sailed toward the Crimea, his own brush with death from carbon monoxide poisoning and the "severe" methods of blistering and bleeding used by the surgeon to revive him, and vivid descriptions of the horrifying cholera epidemics that took the lives of hundreds of soldiers around him while they waited to march against the Russian forces at Alma and Sebastopol. These accounts of the medical care and medical challenges Vicars encountered during his travels are the reason this book resides in the National Library of Medicine (NLM)'s historical collections, but our copy of the book, printed in 1870, has a unique feature that gives it special value, charm, and beauty.

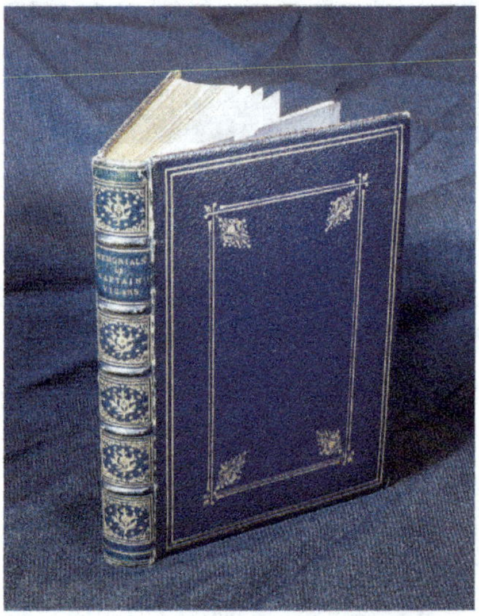

Beautifully bound, about 7 inches high

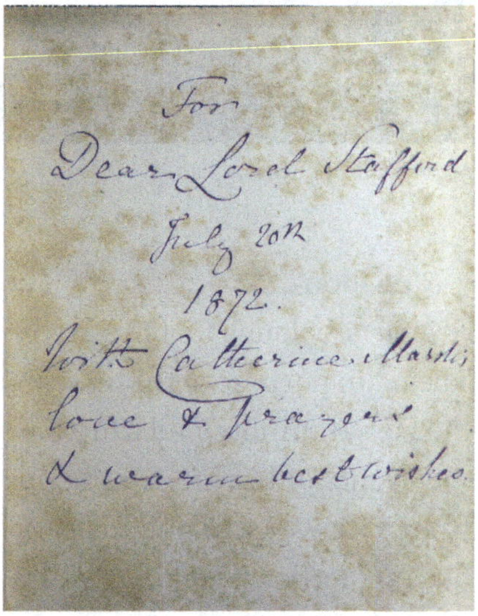

Handwritten inscription by the author

The NLM copy of *Memorials of Captain Hedley Vicars* is beautifully bound in blue morocco leather, embossed with gold tooling, decorated dentelles, and gilt edges reminiscent of the elaborate binding techniques often applied to rare and precious volumes for wealthy patrons a century earlier. The front flyleaf bears an inscription from the author to "Dear Lord Stafford" dated July 20, 1872, offering "love & prayers & warm best wishes." But what makes our copy of the book unique and special is a trait that you would not even know is there if you didn't know to look for it . . . a beautiful watercolor painting on the edge of the book, only visible if you fan the pages downward at just the right angle.

Known as a fore-edge painting, it depicts a hospital scene with Captain Vicars visiting a bed-ridden patient while nurses go about their business around the bed. This could represent any number of occasions described in the book where Vicars made the rounds through the hospitals, preaching, praying, and reading scripture with the sick and injured soldiers. There is also some speculation that Vicars is the patient in the scene, reflecting his brief hospitalization following the carbon monoxide incident. What is known is that hospital scenes are extremely rare in fore-edge paintings, making this one a treasured gem in our collections.

Fore-edge paintings were made by clamping the text block of the book with the pages slightly offset, so that a minute portion of the face of each page is exposed. The artist would carefully paint the scene, often illustrating a passage from the book but sometimes just a landscape, still life, or other image, on these exposed page edges. When the clamp is removed and the text block is shifted back to its solid rectangular form, the painting disappears into the pages. The edges would often be gilded

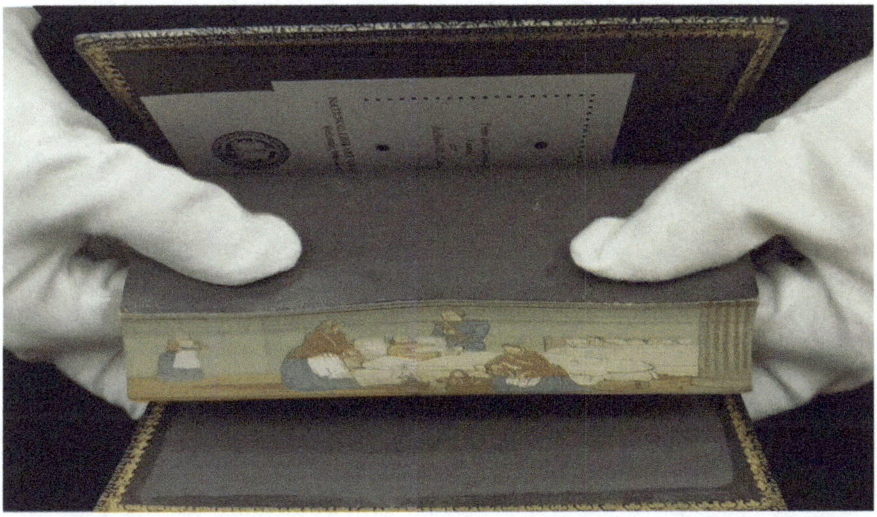

Edge painting reveal, *Memorials of Captain Hedley Vicars, Ninety-Seventh Regiment*, 1870

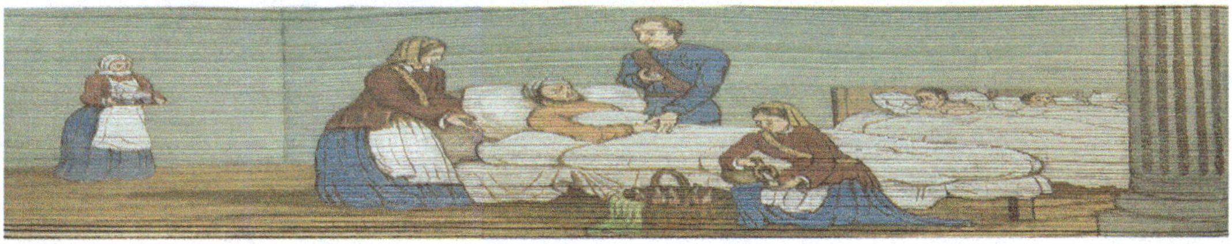

after the fore-edge was painted, ensuring that the image would not be visible when the book was in its normal, closed position.

Some varieties of fore-edge painting date back to the tenth century, but the "disappearing image" technique like the one seen here was not used until the mid seventeenth century. It was quite popular in England in the second half of the seventeenth century and throughout the eighteenth century, and as our book shows, it persisted through the nineteenth century. Sometimes the books would be decorated with double fore-edge paintings, meaning that different images would appear when you fanned the pages toward the front or the back of the book; the most elaborately painted books might also include images on the top or bottom edges. There are still a handful of artisans creating these unique works of art today, giving us a whole new reason to love our books.

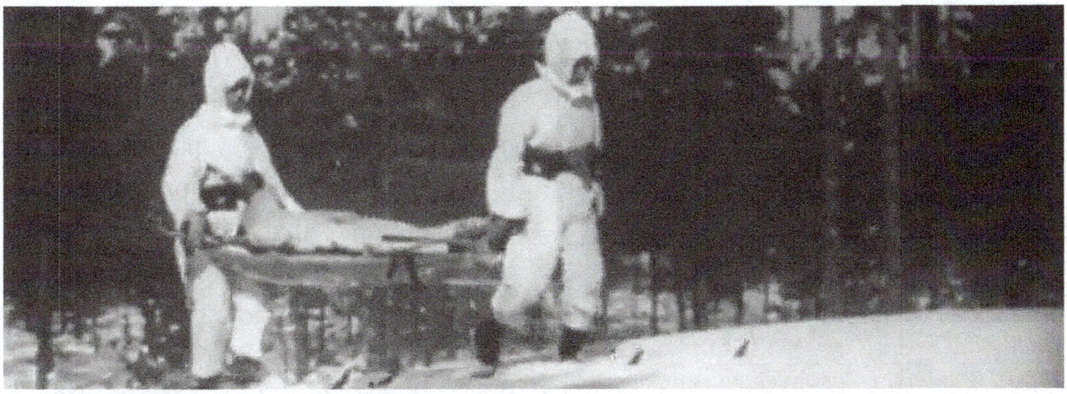

WINTER WOUNDS, PAPER DRESSING

https://circulatingnow.nlm.nih.gov/2015/02/24/winter-wounds-paper-dressing/

February 24, 2015 • Films & Videos

SARAH EILERS

It's a black and white film, but it's the white that overwhelms. A carpet of snow beneath Nordic pines, white uniforms head to toe, white planks used to construct a horse-drawn ambulance sleigh. Soon enough, an explosion, and the rising of white-clad figures from snow-covered foxholes, rifles at the ready. What is this?

With winter upon us, we searched the film vault for a title on cold-weather health concerns. What we found is an intriguing mystery: a VHS tape apparently duplicated from a 16mm film that itself is a copy of a copy. Given this lineage, the resolution is poor, but the military medicine depicted is clear enough.

The Medical Service of the Finnish Armed Forces in the Winter: The Utilization of Paper in the Care of Casualties appears to have been shot as a silent film in Finland in the late 1930s or early 1940s, probably by a Finnish military or medical agency. It shows Finnish troops in white winter

Watch the Video on YouTube

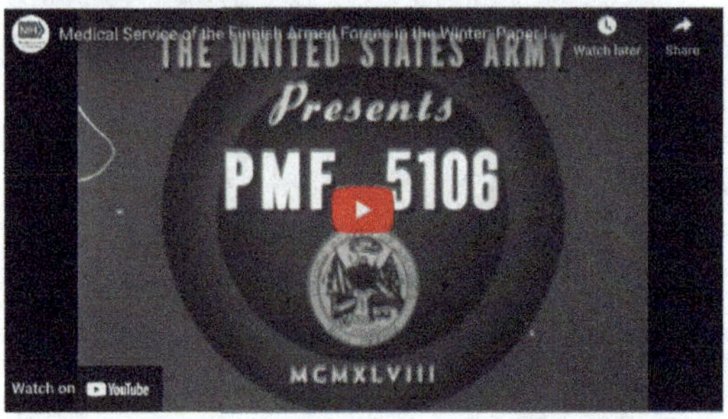

The Medical Service of the Finnish Armed Forces in the Winter: Paper in the Care of Casualties (1948)

uniforms on skis, demonstrating unusual techniques of emergency battlefield first aid. Soldiers use rolls of strong, reusable paper to make bandages, slings, even a stretcher. The film uses the terms crepe paper and kraft paper, and notes that, besides its durability as bandage material, the paper can withstand weights of up to 440 pounds when used to form the bed of a stretcher. Recall the time and place. In the Winter War of 1939–1940, Finland had shocked the world by repelling a Soviet military offensive, relying on skis, bicycles, complete familiarity with the landscape, and superb aim. This footage likely was shot around that time.

By March 1940, Finland had capitulated, signing the Treaty of Moscow and giving control of the Karelian Isthmus to the Soviet Union. The government soon allowed German troops on Finnish soil, forging a short-lived alliance with the Nazis as that army prepared to invade the Soviet Union. The lesser of two evils perhaps, with the Finns calculating that such an alliance might offer an opportunity to regain territory ceded to Moscow in 1940. In the end, that didn't happen.

An opening slide in the film reveals that a German version existed; perhaps the Nazi army somehow obtained the footage and re-made it as a German-language instructional film (no Germans appear on screen). After the war, with Germany under occupation, the American military confiscated the German version and re-made the remake, with narration in English. Somewhere along the way, an orchestral soundtrack was added, whether by the Finns, the Germans, or the Americans is not clear. Nor do we know the composer(s) of the pieces featured. The U.S. Army donated its English-language version to the National Library of Medicine in 1955.

As far as we have been able to determine, no Finnish collection has the film in its original version. One other repository in the United States, the University of California's Berkeley Art Museum and Pacific Film Archive (BAMPFA) has a copy of the German version. As in the English version, the film opens with a title slide and one additional scrolling slide describing what's to come, but contains no credits. The BAMPFA believes the film was donated by the Library of Congress, but has no other details.

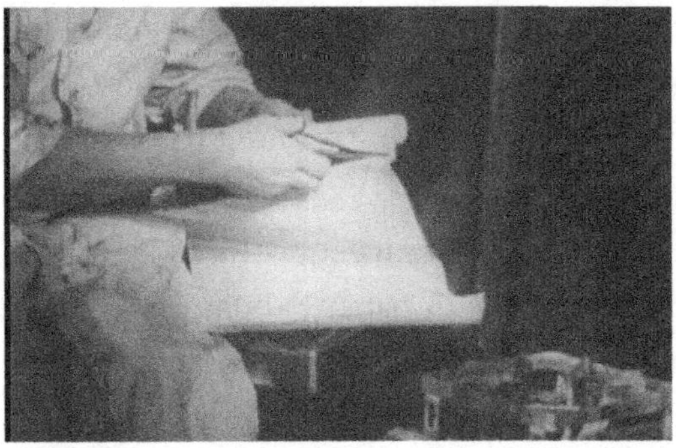

A doctor cutting paper

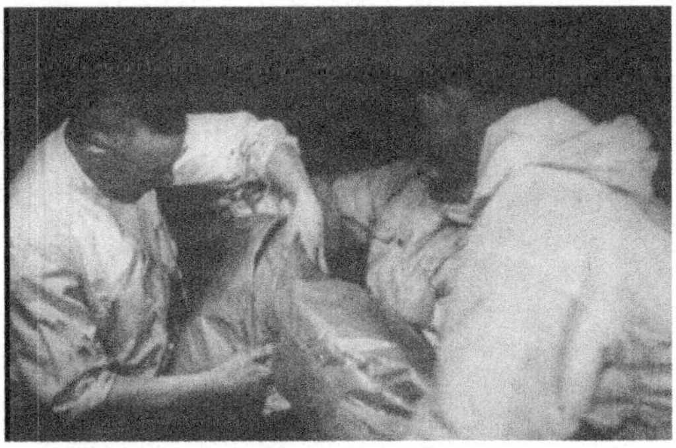

Paper bags

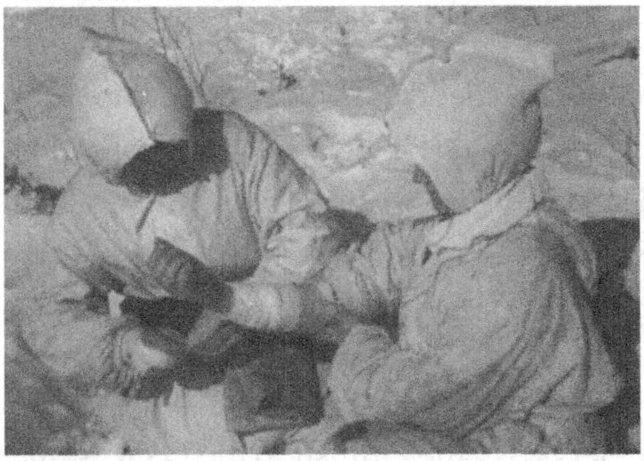

Bandaging with paper

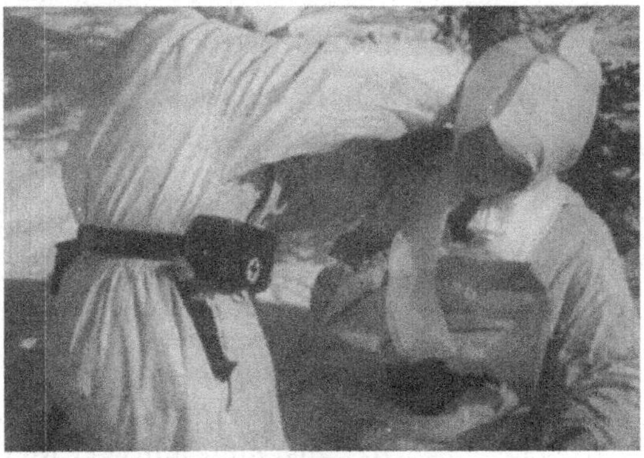

Bandaging with paper

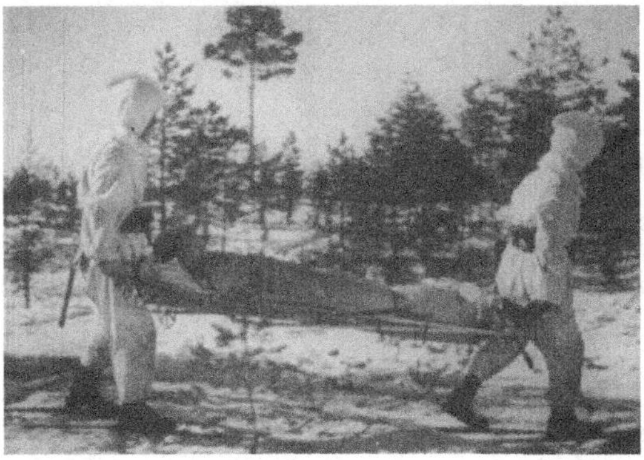

Transport

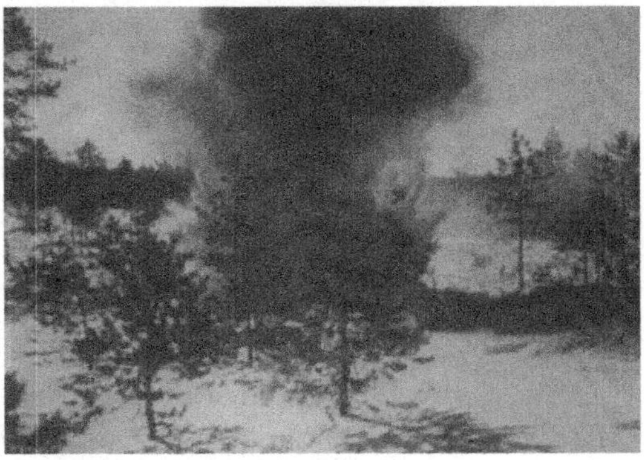

An explosion!

"Orphan" films such as *Medical Service of the Finnish Armed Forces* are not unusual in film archives. Titles may be passed from agency to agency with little attention paid to provenance, projected so often that pieces of the film break off, and revised with edits, soundtracks, and translations that may or may not be documented. For example, about fourteen minutes into our copy, the screen abruptly goes dark for about 10 seconds, then fires up mid-scene. We think a portion of film must have fallen away during handling and a clumsy splice inserted, but without comparing it to other versions, we don't know.

This film poses many questions; for instance, questions about the medical uses of paper: Was the technique of paper bandaging adopted by the U.S. and other militaries, and/or by civilian agencies? How did the Finns produce such durable paper? Wasn't paper scarce and expensive, even in a timber- and paper-producing country such as Finland? And questions about the film itself: Does a Finnish version still exist? Are there missing title slides, intertitles, or credits? Are the explosions staged? When was the orchestral soundtrack added, and who is the composer?

We hope an inquisitive reader may be able to help us learn more about the medical uses of paper and about the history of this rare and unusual film. If that reader is you, or someone you know, we invite you to share what you know about the film by commenting below.

•••

To watch more films like Medical Service of the Finnish Armed Forces *from the National Library of Medicine (NLM)'s historical audiovisuals collection, visit NLM Digital Collections.*

•••

Note: Since this post was published, five years ago, we have located the 16mm film reels during a reorganization of our offsite storage space. The reels were in a metal film can without identifying markings. The Library has had the film cleaned and digitized, and this crisp new copy, shown here, is now available for viewing. We shared a copy with KAVI, the National Audiovisual Institute of Finland, which holds all film materials of the Finnish Defence Forces. KAVI Film archivist Tommi Partanen told the NLM that they had never seen the footage, and while it "is Finnish Defence Force film material, there is no Finnish original version of this. Maybe Germans had some raw Finnish footage, which they used to make this film." Rare indeed. —Sarah Eilers, 2020

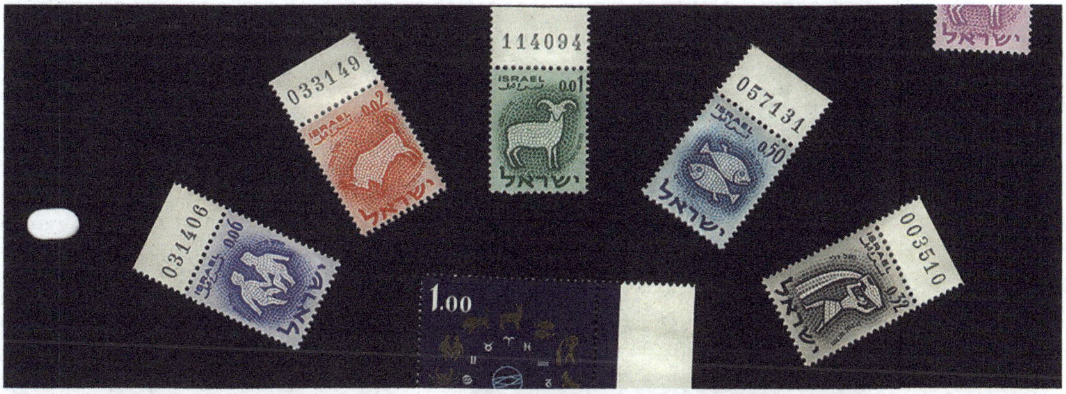

DR. SCHWARTZ'S STAMP COLLECTION

https://circulatingnow.nlm.nih.gov/2015/10/13/dr-schwartzs-stamp-collection/

October 13, 2015 • Prints & Photographs

GINNY A. ROTH

The Prints and Photographs collection in the History of Medicine Division at the National Library of Medicine holds many treasures that not only serve as research materials, but are also visually captivating. One does not need a trained eye in the arts in order to appreciate collection items that are as beautiful as they are informative. The following image is one page from a collection of medically themed stamps, which number in the area of 700,000 and fill 109 4-inch binders. The collection is a result of sixty years of collecting by Dr. Adolf W. Schwartz. Dr. Schwartz was born in Hamburg, Germany and received his MD at the University of Heidelberg. He later studied at the Mayo Clinic and practiced plastic surgery in Bakersfield California for over thirty years. Along with a lifelong interest in stamp collecting, Dr. Schwartz was also a world traveler, and many of the countries he visited are represented in the collection. Dr. Schwartz's daughter generously donated the collection to the Library in 2010.

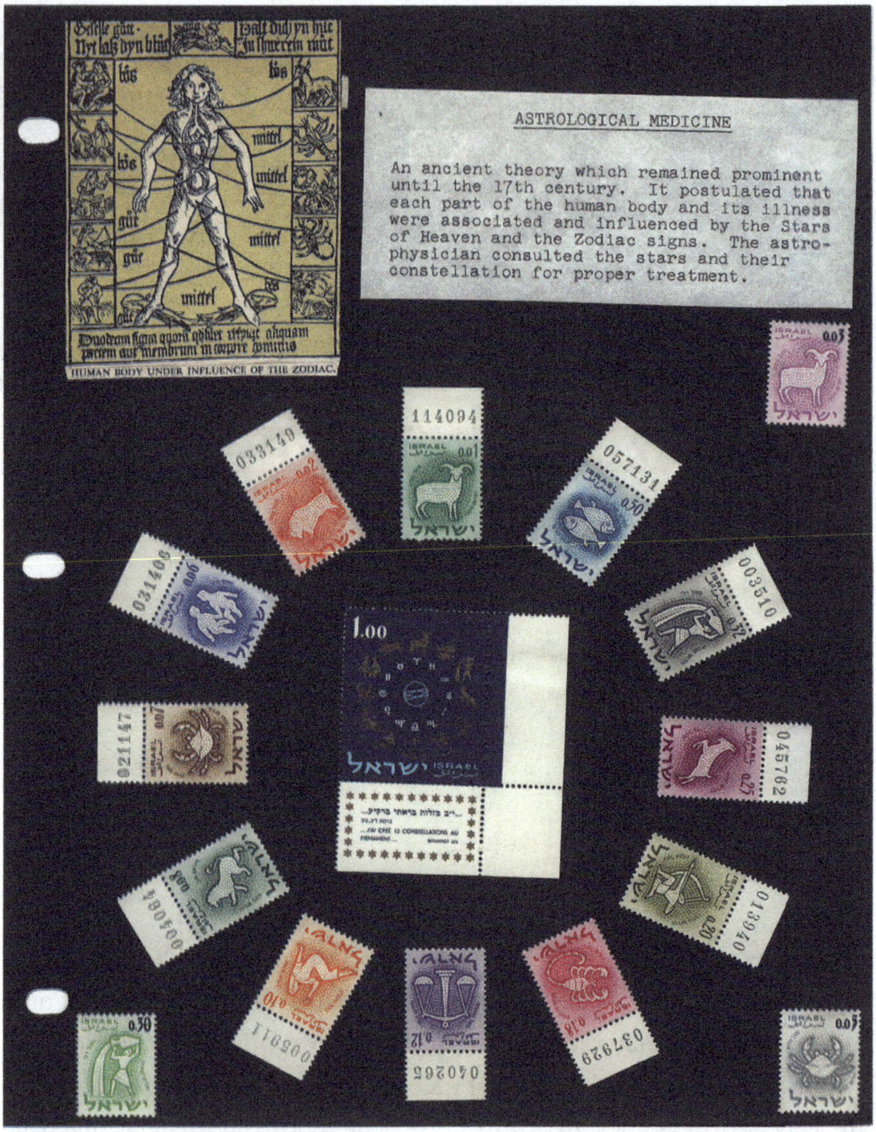

A page of stamps on astrological medicine from the medical stamp collection of Adolf W. Schwartz • *National Library of Medicine*

Subjects on the stamps include doctors, nurses, military medicine, dentistry, veterinary medicine, folk and mythical medicine, plants and herbs, inventors of surgical instruments, doctors serving in Congress, places named for physicians, and more. The stamps are canceled, non-canceled, commemorative, in postcard form, first-day issue, proofs, tax stamps, tobacco stamps, postal cancellations, and legal tender. Stamps feature, for example, Elizabeth Blackwell, Marie Curie, Wilhelm Roentgen, and Florence Nightingale, among thousands of others. The collection includes a series on the Nobel Prizes from the Federated States of Micronesia, as well as a series of special oversized cigar bands from the Canary Islands featuring Nobel Prize winners in Physiology or Medicine for the years 1901–1970, including Joshua Lederberg, James Watson, Francis Crick, and Marshall Nirenberg. The collection also includes sixteen books that Dr. Schwartz compiled containing biographical and historical information about the stamps and their subjects.

In 2014, the Library initiated an effort to preserve the collection and rehouse the stamps in archival pages and binders. As part of an ongoing project, Library interns with an interest in preservation have successfully rehoused half of the collection, carefully removing each stamp from its hinge and placing it on new acid-free mounting pages using clear photo corners.

The original order of the collection has been maintained throughout this process. Additionally, the entire collection, nearly 4,000 pages, has been digitized. Below is a gallery of images highlighting just a handful of the stamps that comprise this impressive collection.

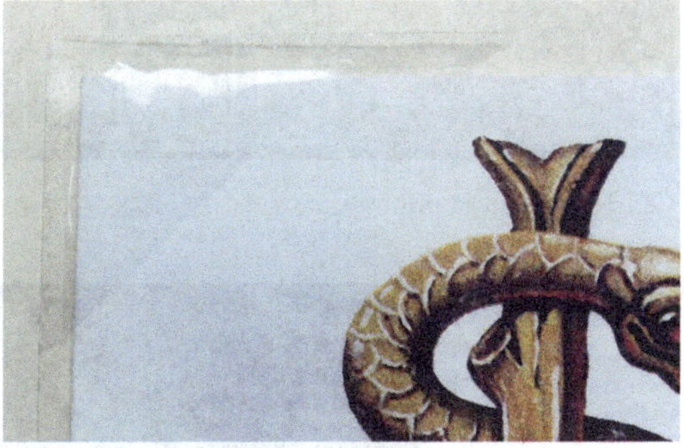

Close-up of a clear photo corner

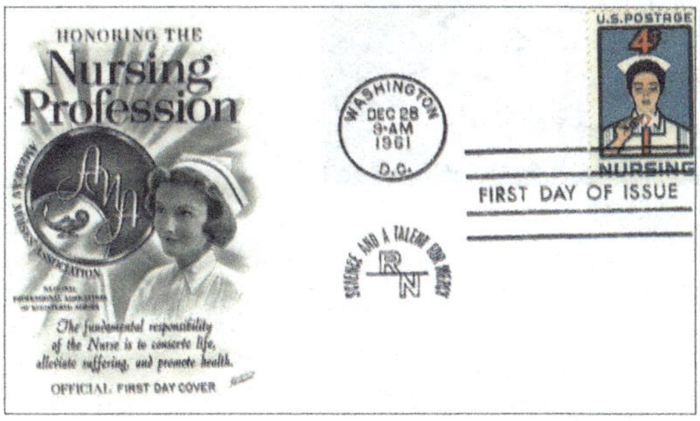

Nursing profession, United States, first day of issue, 1961

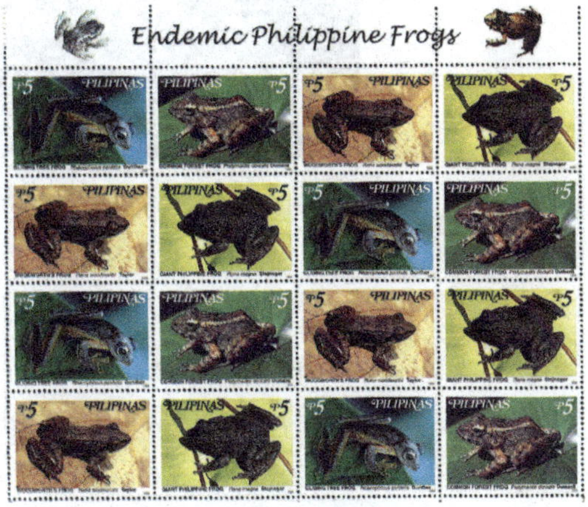

Endemic frogs, Philippines, 1999

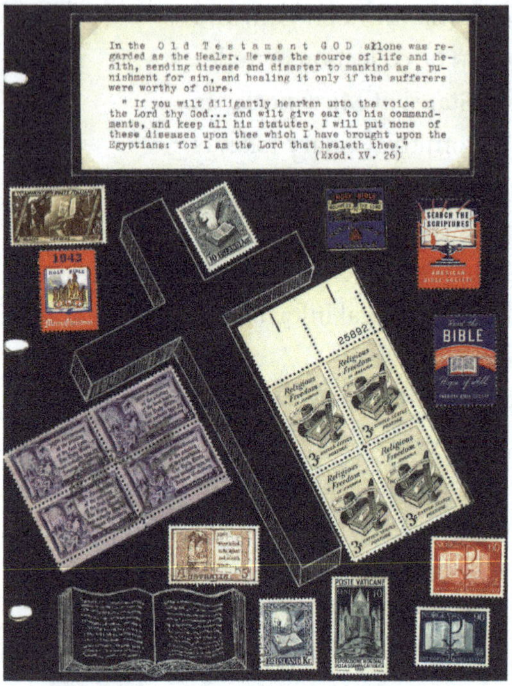

Old Testament stamps

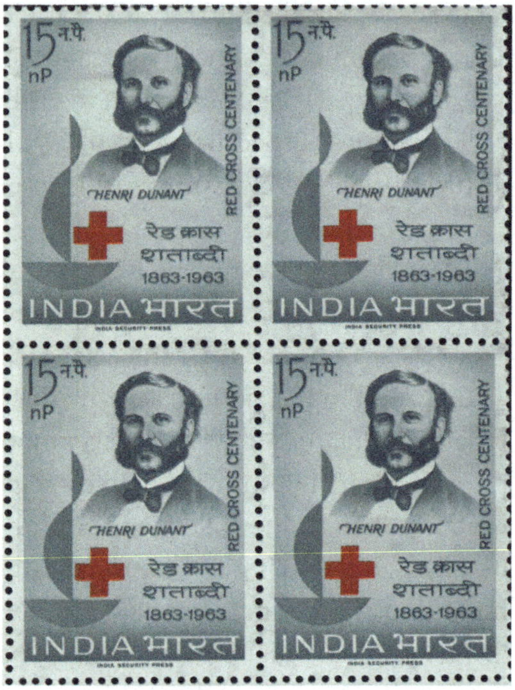

Henri Dunant, India, 1963

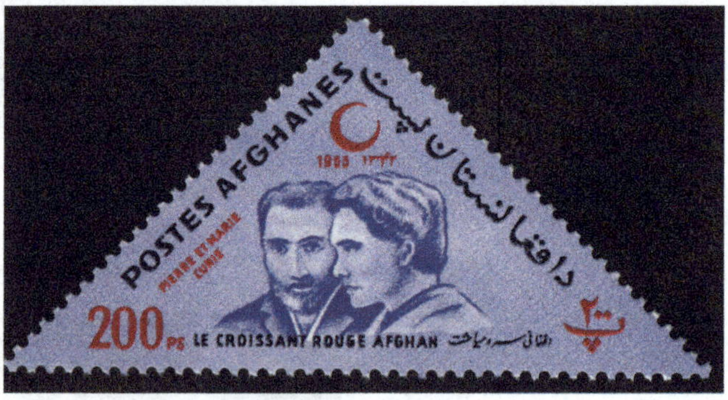

Pierre and Marie Curie, Afghanistan, 1953

• • •

Celebrate American Archives Month with Circulating Now. *Check out more posts from NLM's Prints and Photographs collection.*

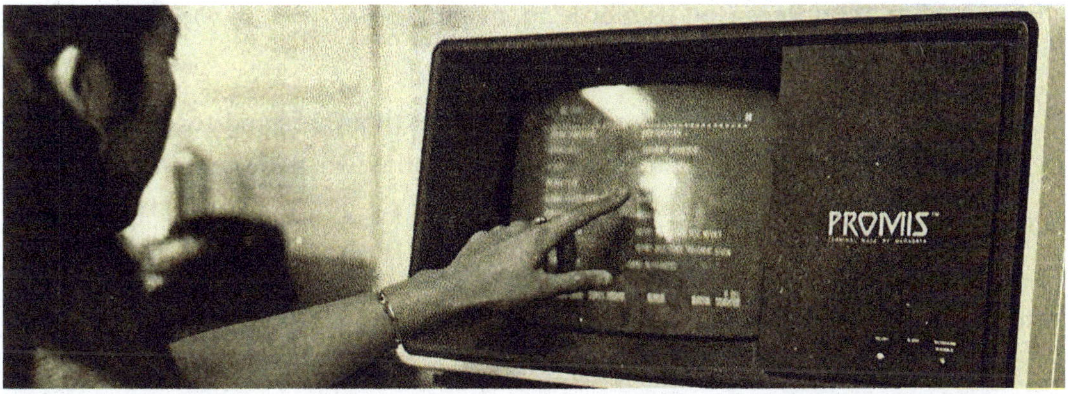

THE "PROMIS" OF COMPUTER-BASED MEDICAL RECORDS

https://circulatingnow.nlm.nih.gov/2019/06/27/the-promis-of-computer-based-medical-records/

June 27, 2019 • Archives & Manuscripts

JAN SCHULTZ

The National Library of Medicine (NLM) recently acquired the Patient/Problem Oriented Medical Record System Archives, a collection of materials related to the development of an early computer system for organizing patient data and diagnostic decision-making. Jan Schultz generously contributed archival materials from his work with Dr. Larry Weed at the PROMIS lab at the University of Vermont. NLM archivist John Rees asked Jan Schultz about his perspective on the early history of electronic medical records.

• • •

TOP Touch Sensitive Terminal used for storage and retrieval of patient records in the PROMIS system, ca. 1977, in "Automation of the Problem-Oriented Medical Record," 1977.

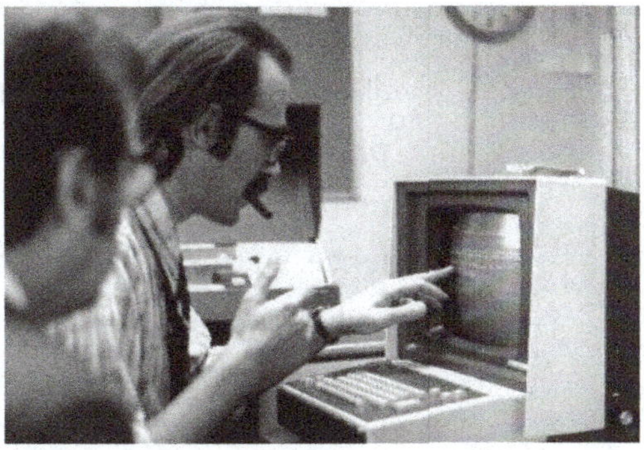

Jan Schultz using the PROMIS touchscreen terminal, ca. 1980, in *A History of Personal Workstations*, 1988. • *Courtesy Jan Schultz*

John Rees: Tell us a little about yourself. Where are you from? What's your background?

Jan Schultz: I grew up in Chicago in the 1940s and 1950s. I attended the University of Illinois, studying mathematics and very early computer science. I stayed at Illinois for a master's degree in math and also worked in an educational psychology computer lab developing SOCRATES, a very early computer-based teaching machine.

I moved to Cleveland and started working on a PhD in mathematics at Case Western Reserve University. I didn't last very long at Case. It turned out my main interest was computer science and not mathematics. Call it serendipity or maybe fate, but someone steered me to Dr. Lawrence Weed at the Cleveland Metropolitan General Hospital (CMGH). This was 1966 and I was twenty-four years old.

JR: You worked with Larry Weed for many years. What was he like? Who else worked with you? What was the lab trying to accomplish?

JS: Larry was brilliant, driven, and dedicated to providing good medical care while educating physicians. As the Director of Outpatient Clinics, Larry taught residents many things, including how to organize medical records. I worked in Larry's office with the head resident, Dr. Charles Burger, and saw first-hand how they managed the voluminous paper records of patients with numerous complex medical problems.

In the late 1960s, Larry and I worked together to envision a computer-based patient-oriented medical record (POMR). I developed a sample printed output for a "theoretical" electronic POMR, and Larry, Charlie and I reviewed it and discussed how to begin getting the data into the electronic record. We decided that the "information-originator," whether a physician, nurse, ancillary staff, or patient, could enter the record directly using a computer terminal. Glass teletypes were just coming into existence, so this decision was radical for the time.

Robert Masters of the Research Division of Control Data Corporation had developed an early system using a touchscreen CRT terminal, the Digiscribe, and a software menu editing and paging system. In 1967 we used a Digiscribe to prototype PROMIS and as a concrete example we showed that with properly structured branching-logic displays, a complete cardiovascular problem could be defined and then stored in what would become a patient's electronic POMR.

In 1968, Larry and I were Co-Principal Investigators on a grant from the National Center for Health Services Research entitled "Automation of the Problem-Oriented Medical Record" to develop a prototype system called PROMIS (Problem-Oriented Medical Information System)

Then, in 1969, Larry accepted a professorship in the medical school at University of Vermont (UVM) in Burlington, and our problem-oriented group moved with Larry to Burlington. We set up our computer room and offices at the Medical Center Hospital of Vermont (MCHV) and called the new computer lab PROMIS Laboratory. Larry and I worked together for twelve years at UVM. Over the years, the PROMIS lab had numerous visitors, so many that taxi drivers started calling us the "Promised Land."

JR: The PROMIS/POMR system was one of the first electronic health record systems. What was your role in its development? Can you describe how it worked? What problems was it trying to solve?

JS: It became clear that we needed to be able to manage a patient's complete problem list and for each problem be able to retrieve all of the associated data. All medical record data, once the initial workup was done, was problem-oriented. Larry wanted to be able to retrieve data from the electronic medical record (EMR) in many different ways: problem-oriented, source-oriented, time-oriented (chronological and reverse chronological) and be able to create dynamic flow-sheets for any data in the EMR. In 1970, we set up the initial operational POMR at MCHV on the OB-GYN floor.

Larry described the PROMIS system as removing dependence on user memory, capturing user logic using problem-orientation, coordinating care among all of the providers, and providing feedback for medical research. I described the PROMIS system as responsive: allowing 70 percent of all selections to be processed within 250 milliseconds. Because the system needed to be available 24/7, it had to be reliable, and, since a single system could not handle all of the terminals needed for a hospital, the system needed to be scalable. Here is a video demonstrating PROMIS in action. PROMIS was also fortunate to be identified as a landmark in the history of personal computing with a chapter in *A History of Personal Workstations*, 1988.

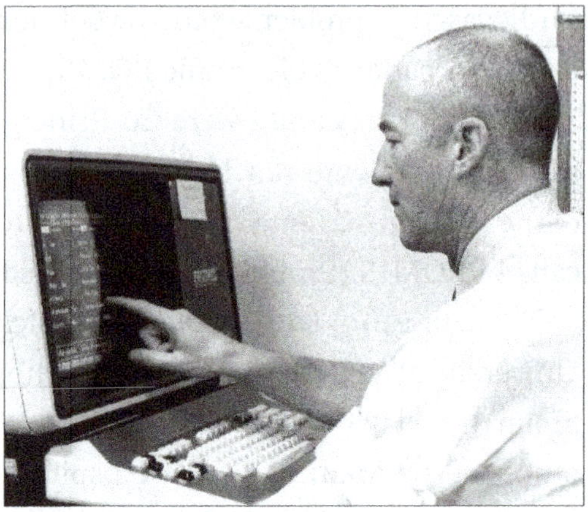

Larry Weed using the PROMIS touchscreen Megadata terminal, ca. 1980, in *A History of Personal Workstations*, 1988. • *Courtesy Jan Schultz*

In order to remove the dependence on user memory, PROMIS lab managed an ever-growing library of displays of medical knowledge. The final library had over 60,000 displays, and PROMIS lab had ten 'medical-content' domain experts managing and updating the library. Papers written by Mel Conway, a consultant hired by the National Bureau of Standards, and Larry describing the national library are included in the donated materials.

JR: How do today's EMR systems resemble the PROMIS system?

JS: The PROMIS system of touchscreen workstations connected to a scalable network of mini-computers using a hypertext interface for all clinical and administrative functions was in operation at the Medical Center Hospital of Vermont in 1977. At the time, touchscreens were very rare: most observers did not fully understand the complexity "behind the scenes" needed to make the system so easy to use. Many visitors went away after seeing PROMIS and tried to reproduce it. A group at Carnegie Mellon University experimented using PROMIS to enhance the human-usability of their ZOG hypertext architecture, but as far as I know, none were successful. Today, every mobile phone has a touch-screen with browsers using HTML hypertext-pages, and the major Silicon Valley hi-tech firms use services with multiple computers tied together in a high-speed network with very large distributed databases. Included in the PROMIS archive are notes related to two patent cases that I participated in, one relating to early hypertext systems and the other to distributed databases.

JR: Software preservation is a challenge for archivists and there is not a working PROMIS system anymore. Can you describe the materials in your donation and how they might contribute to the history of medicine and computing?

JS: While much is being written currently about physician EMR use, I am struck that contemporary EMRs are not looked at as clinical tools to manage a patient, but as an administrative and billing system that many clinicians feel that they are forced to use. PROMIS was a very early electronic medical record that was oriented around a patient, not around the hospital's billing office. The materials I contributed to the NLM can provide many of the technical and clinical details needed to create an electronic patient/problem oriented medical record that is focused on clinical care for a patient. The materials may be quite valuable if future software architects want to understand how Weed and the PROMIS group structured the electronic medical record and the computer system to support it. I still believe strongly in the soundness of the PROMIS approach and did not want to see the materials lost.

JR: We connected with each other almost accidentally before I came to Burlington to appraise the collection, learn about your work, and meet some of your former colleagues—everyone was so happy to see each other

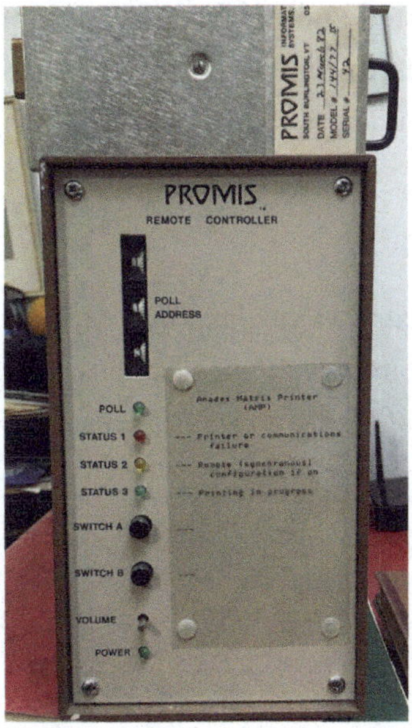

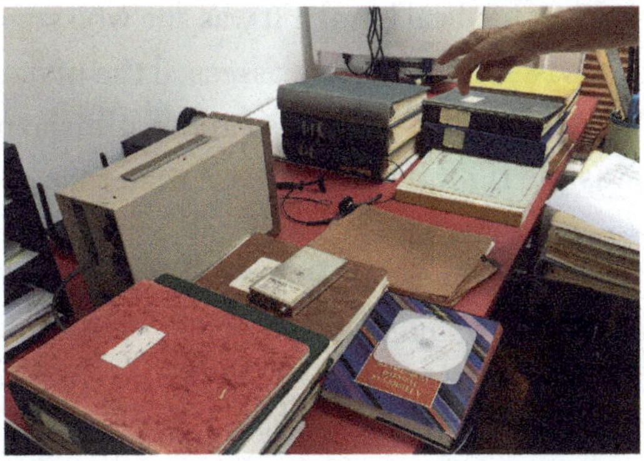

ABOVE Some of the archives in situ at Schultz's Burlington, Vermont, home office

LEFT The only surviving piece of PROMIS hardware is this printer controller that allowed users to print data from anywhere across the PROMIS network in a hospital.

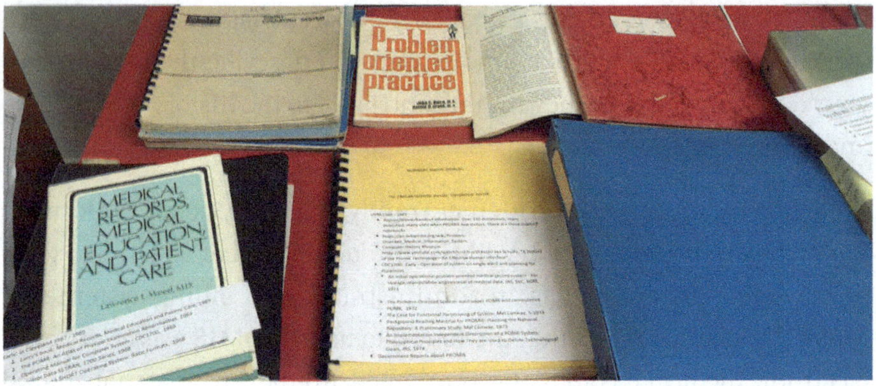

Some of the archives in situ at Schultz's Burlington, Vermont, home office

this mini-reunion seemed like old home week to me. Have you ever worked with archivists before? What was the donation experience like for you?

JS: This was my first time working with an archivist. It was an exhilarating experience. As I sorted through the PROMIS papers, I reconnected with several old PROMIS colleagues and the energy that got the project going. I remembered Larry at his visionary best. Larry was focused somewhat like a bulldog, and when I met him, I was a twenty-four-year-old bulldog, so we worked well together. Over the years, I've become mellower. I don't think the same can be said for Larry Weed!

Julie McGowan is a medical informatics expert who at one time headed UVM's medical library. It was she who suggested I talk to the NLM. When you visited Burlington, assessed the materials, and met several PROMIS folks, your thoroughness and enthusiasm made it clear that the NLM was the right home for these materials.

• • •

Explore the finding aid for this collection and learn more about our Archives and Modern Manuscripts collections. For questions about this collection please email archivist John Rees or contact the History of Medicine Division reference staff via NLM Customer Support.

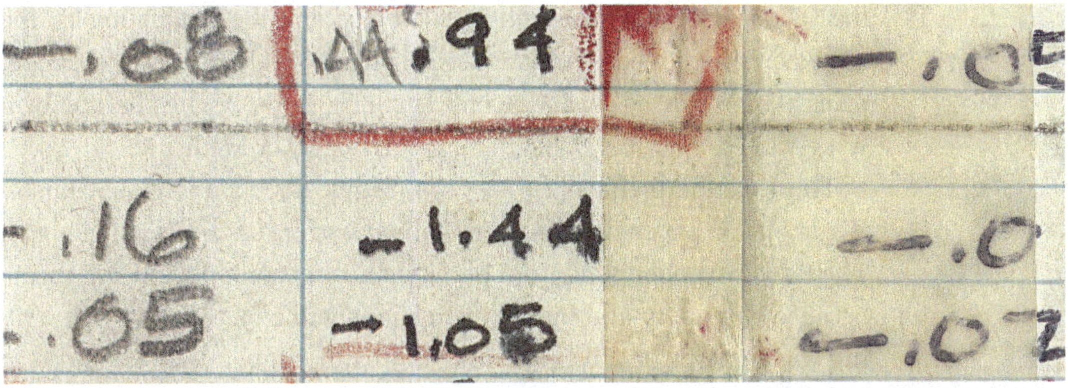

PRESERVING NIRENBERG'S GENETIC CODE CHART

https://circulatingnow.nlm.nih.gov/2014/09/16/preserving-nirenbergs-genetic-code-chart/

September 16, 2014 • Archives & Manuscripts

KRISTI WRIGHT AND HOLLY HERRO

The National Library of Medicine (NLM) is home to a series of very important documents in scientific history—Marshall Nirenberg's Genetic Code Charts. The charts contain original, handwritten data from experiments that determined how protein sequence was dictated by the sequence of precursor ribonucleic acids (RNAs). Conservators at the NLM have been studying the charts to determine the best methods of preserving them for the future.

The famous 1953 discovery of DNA's double-helix structure, which incorporated the work of James D. Watson, Francis Crick, Maurice Wilkins, and Rosalind Franklin, was a major breakthrough in genetic research, but it was just the start of our understanding of DNA. What was not known then was nature's genetic code: how a DNA sequence is translated into an RNA sequence that is in turn translated into a protein sequence. By 1965, Marshall Nirenberg, with help from his colleagues at the National Institutes of Health (NIH), had become the first to complete the sequencing of the code. The language of protein synthesis was understood, painstakingly worked out and recorded in these charts. As a result Nirenberg was awarded the 1968 Nobel Prize in Physiology or Medicine.

The Nirenberg charts consist of multiple sheets of 1950s Addison Wesley lined paper that has been joined with pressure sensitive tape. The tape is in poor condition, but it is an important part of the charts because Nirenberg and his lab technicians wrote on top of it. The writing was done in pencil, India ink, and ballpoint pen ink. The need to address the deteriorating state of the ballpoint pen ink on these unique documents became a driving force behind the most recent phase of our ongoing ballpoint pen ink research in the NLM conservation lab, in this case focusing on ideal rehousing methods.

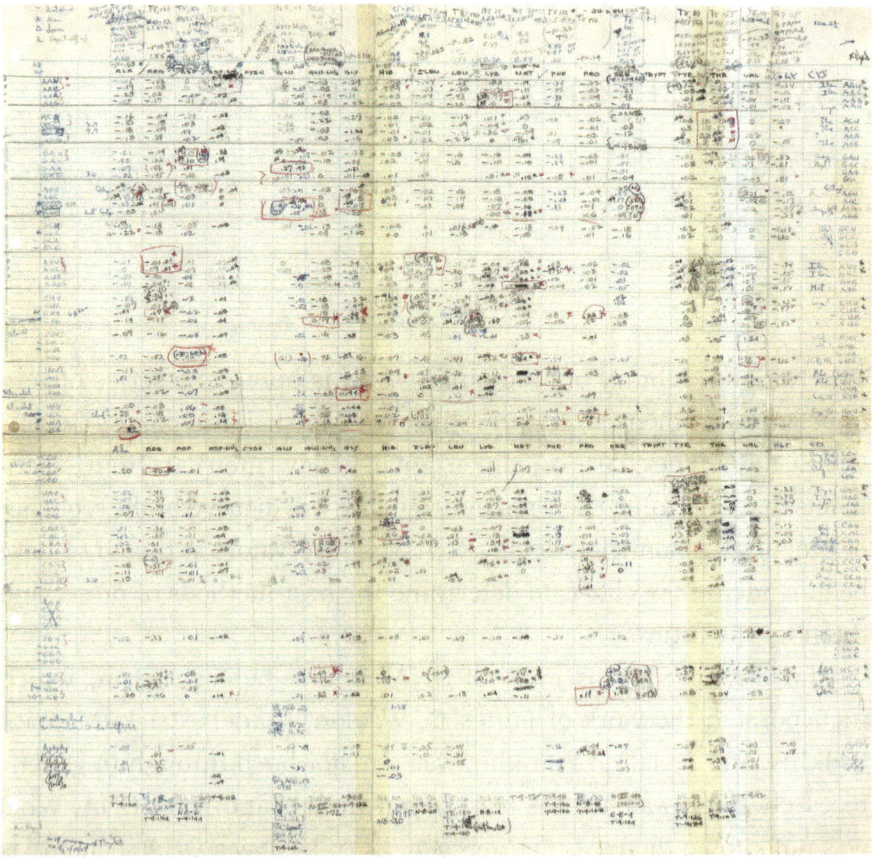

Marshall Nirenberg's Handwritten Genetic Code Chart, 1965 • Profiles in Science, *National Library of Medicine*

In order to determine the correct housing for the Nirenberg charts, we first determined what type of pens were used. Norma Heaton, one of Dr. Nirenberg's original lab technicians, told us that the genetic code charts were written with Skilcraft ballpoint pens. Next, we did some testing and researched the history of the Skilcraft pen ink and found the ink formula had not changed in forty some years. Then, we used a technique we've recently developed in-house called Photoshop Assisted Spectroscopy for the examination of different lighting and storage environments on this type of ballpoint pen ink. We set up a series of mock documents in a variety of enclosure types and exposed them to different lighting conditions for a period of three months. Before, during, and after the exposure period, we took scans of the documents and performed Photoshop Assisted Spectroscopy to see if and how the color of the ink had shifted.

Photoshop Assisted Spectroscopy is a technique to track color shift, which is a good indicator of deterioration in ink. Color shift is a change in the ratio of red, green, and blue (RGB) values in the color of a substance and occurs when the chemistry of a material, in this case of the ballpoint ink, changes over time and through reaction with its environment. To perform the technique, the document must first be digitized using equipment

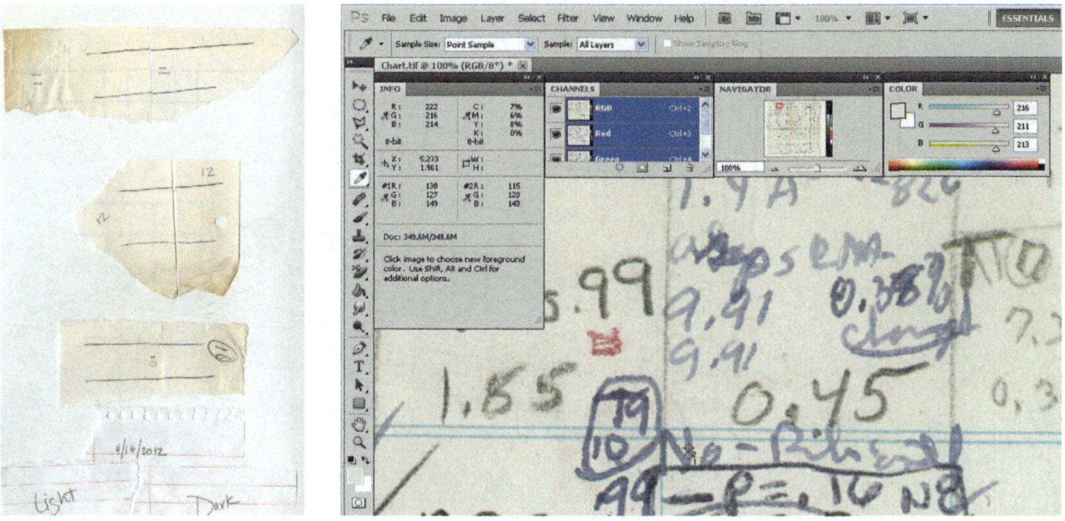

FROM LEFT TO RIGHT (1) A series of mock documents exposed to different lighting conditions **(2)** Reading the color values of a digitized document with Photoshop

calibrated for color accuracy. The technique uses the "info" window in Photoshop to retrieve the RGB values of individual pixels. By recording a series of these values, we are able to note the color of a document section at the start of the experiment. Later, a new scan is taken and the values for that section recorded again. The values from both scans are plotted on a three-dimensional graph with the X, Y, and Z axes corresponding to each RGB value. Graphing in this manner allows the direction of any color shift across the collected data points to easily be seen.

As a result of this study, we've determined that anoxic (oxygen-free) environments are ideal for documents written with blue and black Skilcraft brand ballpoint pens. We have therefore chosen to store the charts in an anoxic environment and, because we have the initial scans

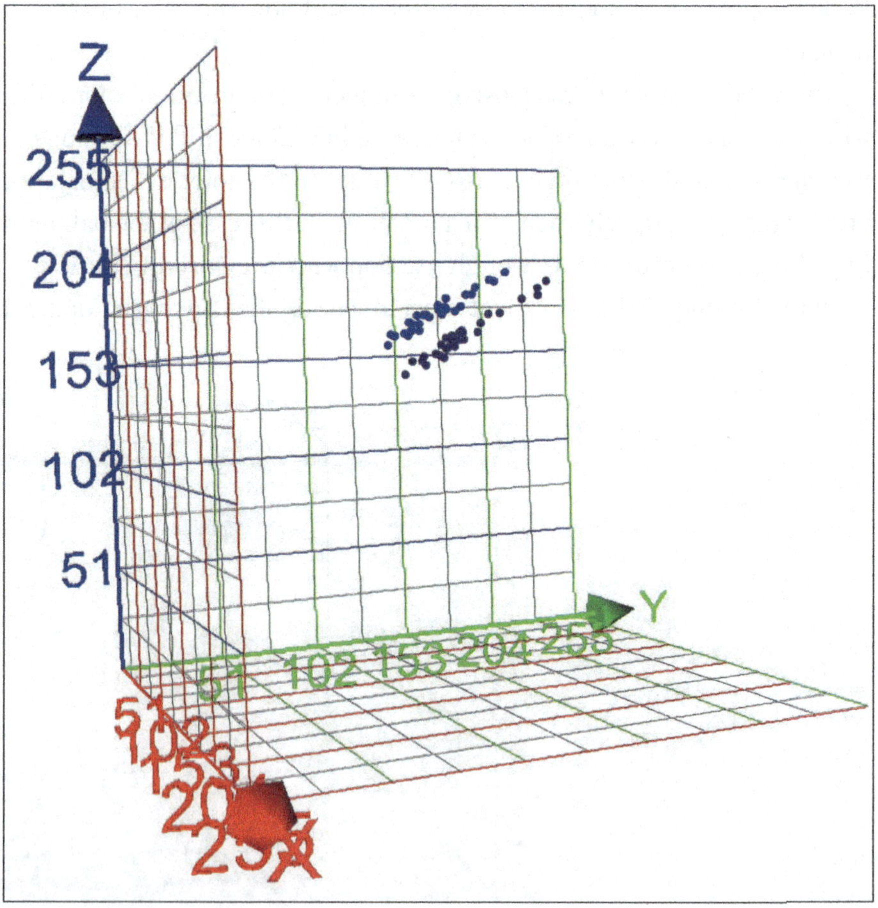

Values from before and after a test period are plotted on a three-dimensional graph with X, Y, and Z axes corresponding to each red, green, and blue (RGB) value respectively. This allows the direction of any color shift across the collected data points to easily be seen.

to create a starting point, we can monitor the charts long-term as a preventive method to detect any color shift while they are housed in their enclosures. We will also be working with the NIH Mechanical Design and Fabrication section to build an attachment that will allow us to monitor the environment inside the frames with existing equipment and ensure that the enclosures remain anoxic over time. Each frame will create a sealed microenvironment for the enclosed document, so while people will easily be able to view the charts, they will be protected against the damaging factors associated with a normal air environment and preserved for new generations of researchers.

• • •

This article is part of a series that commemorates the fiftieth anniversary of the Genetic Code Charts.

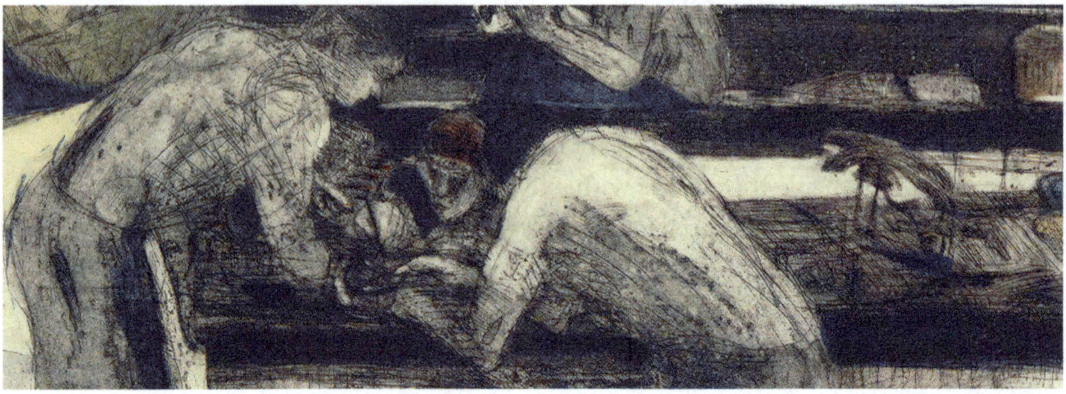

DOCTORING THE ART OF MEDICINE SERIES

https://circulatingnow.nlm.nih.gov/2013/11/08/doctoring-the-art-of-medicine-series/

November 8, 2013 • Prints & Photographs

LAURA MCNULTY

As an artist, May Lesser (1927–2001) seemed destined to produce works of art relating to the medical field—her father, brother, husband, and three of her four children were doctors. As a child, Lesser would secretly look at her father's anatomy books, admiring the drawings contained within. Lesser received her undergraduate degree in fine arts from the H. Sophie Newcomb College at Tulane University and went on to complete a graduate degree in painting at the University of Alabama. Lesser also studied anthropology at Columbia University and child psychiatry at Johns Hopkins University, after which Lesser moved to California and joined the art department at UCLA. While working in the art department, she turned to the anatomy department in order to learn more about bone and muscle anatomy.

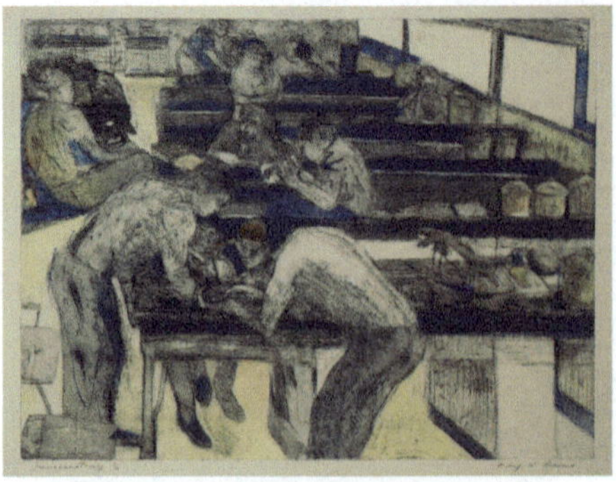

Working closely with the anatomy department in classrooms and laboratories, Lesser had the idea of observing and drawing students as they worked, rather than focusing just on anatomical specimens. Dr. Charles Sawyer, an anatomy professor, suggested that Lesser follow a class of students as they progressed through medical school. So, Lesser began observing and capturing the adventures of the UCLA medical school class of 1971. She would sit in lectures, laboratories, and operating rooms, sketching and engraving copperplates as she observed the students and their professors. She would then go back to her studio and print the plates in color. As a result, Lesser produced a different perspective of medical school; by focusing on the people rather than the tools and techniques, she made doctors and their work more human. As Lesser put it, "there is a loveliness in human beings helping another." The etchings produced in this period make up the bulk of the collection of May Lesser's work held at the National Library of Medicine (NLM).

In the summer of 2012, I was brought on as an eager, pre-program conservation student volunteer to clean and rehouse this collection of thirty-nine Lesser prints that were donated to the Library in 2011. Working closely with Ginny A. Roth, the Prints and Photograph Curator, and Holly Herro, the Conservation Librarian, I was responsible for removing the prints from the frames and then treating and rehousing them. The prints came to the Library in frames that did not create a stable environment for the works, so my first task was to get the prints out of the frames and assess the condition of each print. Most of the prints had been attached to support boards with starch- and acrylic-based adhesives.

After determining the best course of treatment, I went to work removing the tape carriers and adhesives from the etchings. Wielding a microspatula and a jar of methylcellulose, I became proficient at applying the methylcellulose to the starch-based adhesive residue, waiting for about ten minutes, and then carefully removing it.

Naturally, some of the starch-based adhesive left residue on the paper, and this is where I learned the importance of regular, old-fashioned spit in conservation practices. One of the natural enzymes in spit is known as amylase, which breaks down starches. With a little bit of spit on the end of a cotton swab, I gently removed the starch-based adhesive residue from the paper.

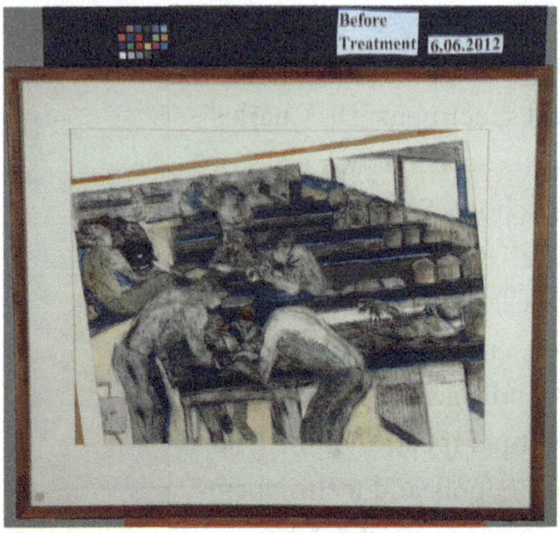

Neuroanatomy before treatment

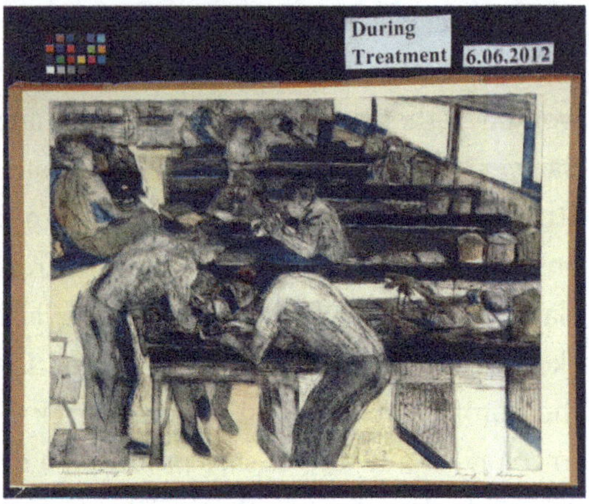

Neuroanatomy during treatment

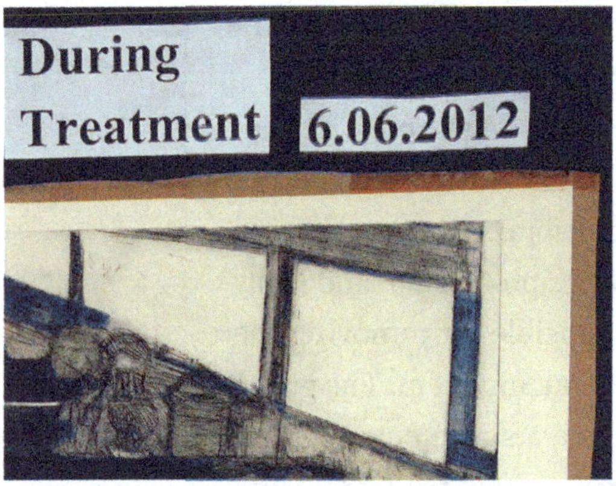

Detail of adhesive damage

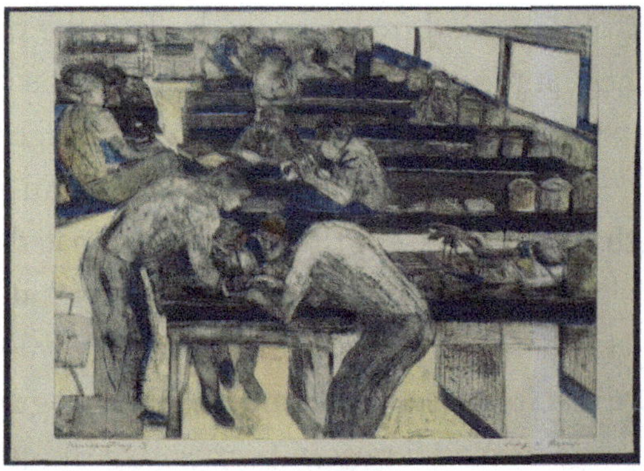

Neuroanatomy after treatment

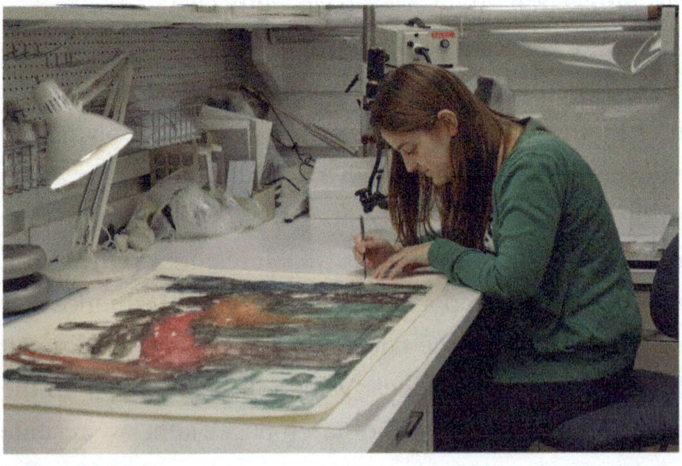

Laura at work

For the most part the starch-based adhesive was cooperative and cleanly came off the paper. But, the acrylic adhesive was more stubborn. With the most stubborn acrylic adhesive, I had to employ a heated spatula to remove the carrier, along with a slide-warming tray as a heat source, to swell the adhesive so that it would let go of the paper. Once the prints were cleaned, and after Holly and Ginny approved my work, I created a more stable housing environment for the prints. Using photo corners, I attached the prints to acid-free, lignin-free mat board, placed a piece of pH neutral tissue paper on top of the print, and then placed it into a Mylar sleeve.

These new enclosures create the stable environment for the works of art necessary to keep them in good condition for a long time.

Determined to see the collection processed from beginning to end, I returned to the NLM this summer as a student intern in the Pathways program. After adding call numbers to each print, I created catalog records for them, thereby making them available in the Library's online catalog. In addition, I am happy to report that the collection of thirty-nine prints can now be found in the NLM Digital Collections.

CHAPTER 3
COLLECTIONS AND COLLABORATIONS

INTRODUCTION • JILL L. NEWMARK

In *The Poet at the Breakfast Table,* Oliver Wendell Holmes, Sr., said that "many ideas grow better when transplanted into another mind than the one where they sprang up." When people work together, they can inspire and motivate each other, and their communities, to expand minds and spur invention, innovation, advancement, and beauty in literature, science, music, and art.

Throughout history, collaborations have created some of the most inspiring and innovative ideas and advancements. Alfred Blalock, Helen Taussig, and Vivien Thomas together developed a surgical technique that corrected blue baby syndrome in infants and saved countless lives; Wilbur and Orville Wright built an airplane that helped to make commercial air transportation possible; and Alice Paul and Lucy Burns, along with hundreds of other women, successfully worked to secure a woman's right to vote in America. These are just a few examples of people working together to create change and advance human society.

In the same vein, technology has expanded collaboration and accelerated the dissemination of information. Now individuals in different physical locations can work together to conceive and implement new ideas, no longer bound by the constraints of geography or physical constructs.

Over the past twenty years, collaboration has become a cornerstone of medical and scientific research as well as social and political change. Likewise, the National Library of Medicine (NLM) has partnered in a variety of ways to connect the diverse collections of the Library to communities of people: engaging minds; inspiring new ideas; and advancing research, advocacy, and public health. These collaborations form communities and collective resources that impact and influence how we live and how we learn. *Circulating Now* documents and celebrates these collaborations and their outcomes for the public.

The NLM has kept an eye on the future by collaborating with other institutions addressing the digitization and preservation of important and extensive analog materials and more contemporary born-digital materials. This critical approach to collecting, preserving, and making accessible important historical and scientific materials is a key point in several of the Library's posts in *Circulating Now*. One such collaboration was the NLM's participation with the National Digital Stewardship Residency Program featured in "Autism and Alzheimer's on the Web." Through this joint effort of the Library of Congress and the Institute of Museum and Library Services, Maureen Harlow, a resident of the program, created a thematic web archive collection for the NLM on "Disorders of the Developing and Aging Brain: Autism and Alzheimer's on the Web." Autism and Alzheimer's are two disorders that affect many people across the globe. Research is ongoing to gain an understanding of these disorders, as well as to improve treatments and patient care. This important resource provides a glimpse of the world's understanding of Autism and Alzheimer's at a particular moment in time, allowing current and future researchers a point of reference in the evolving understanding of these disorders through the eyes of scientists, physicians, caregivers, and people living with the disease. This project brought together a diverse group of born-digital materials to form a cohesive, documented, and accessible collection.

Access to and availability of medical history, research, and public health is key to the mission of the NLM and was at the forefront of its partnership with Columbia, Harvard, and Yale Universities, together with the Open Knowledge Commons, in the establishment of the Medical Heritage Library. This open access digital resource makes over hundreds of thousands of items relating to the history of health and medicine accessible to the public. The Medical Heritage Library gives readers an opportunity to "examine the interrelated nature of medicine and society, both to inform contemporary medicine and strengthen understanding of the world in which we live." "Making a Medical Heritage Milestone" celebrates the NLM's contribution of its 50,000th item to the digital library. The extensive collection of digitized materials is an invaluable resource that not only includes books and journals but also photographs and films providing free, global access to a diversity of collections and information for research, teaching, and learning to advance personal and collective health and well-being.

Collaboration can also illuminate the past to better understand the future. When HIV/AIDS came into the public eye in the 1980s, it overwhelmed the population of gay men who were among the first communities affected by the disease. In the beginning, little was known about HIV/AIDS and this uncertainty spread fear and confusion throughout the country. Homophobia fueled these fires leading to a failure of the government to acknowledge the disease or respond to it in a meaningful and effective way until it began to impact the general public. This inaction of the government devastated the gay community who were forced to take action on their own to provide care and information to those living with the disease. The opposing positions of the government and the gay community set off a social and political struggle that resulted in the politicization of HIV/AIDS. In "Remembering & Witnessing: AIDS35 and the NLM Exhibition 'Surviving and Thriving'," Thomas Lawrence Long explains how the University of Connecticut, using the educational foundation of the NLM exhibition *Surviving & Thriving: AIDS, Politics, and Culture* collaborated with several community-based institutions to create a network of informational outlets to educate the local community and student population on how "a health problem could be . . . insidiously ignored and politicized with disastrous effects on vulnerable populations." This effort helped a community learn from the past and use that knowledge as a bridge to inform the future.

Scholarship, understanding, and appreciation of beauty can also be advanced through collaboration. The cooperation between several curators and libraries, including the NLM, was central to the 2018 exhibition *Romance and Reason: Islamic Transformations of the Classical Past*, displayed at New York University. In "NLM Manuscripts on Loan to Romance and Reason," curator Roberta Casagrande-Kim explained how the exhibition displayed ancient manuscripts, including several on loan from the NLM, to illustrate the prominence of science in Islamic culture and society. These beautifully illustrated manuscripts helped visitors understand that "despite the divisions that existed between people and nations, the exchange of images and ideas was boundless." In this case, analog materials loaned by the Library offered illustrated texts that demonstrated the "Islamic interest in mathematics, astronomy, astrology, and medicine" and their use of Greek knowledge to advance the sciences. While these texts themselves highlighted the collaboration of people in the eighth to tenth centuries CE in the study and understanding of science and medicine, their loan by the NLM reflected one of the core missions of the Library: to make its diverse collections widely available to diverse audiences.

Through its varied collaborations, as reflected in the following selection of posts, the NLM not only embraces its mission of stewardship and interpretation of the Library's historical collections but also supports the Library's mission to be a platform for discovery that can reach more people in more ways through enhanced dissemination and engagement. As we move forward in the twenty-first century and embrace the global community through collaboration, the NLM will continue to be a leader in the advancement of research, advocacy, and public health.

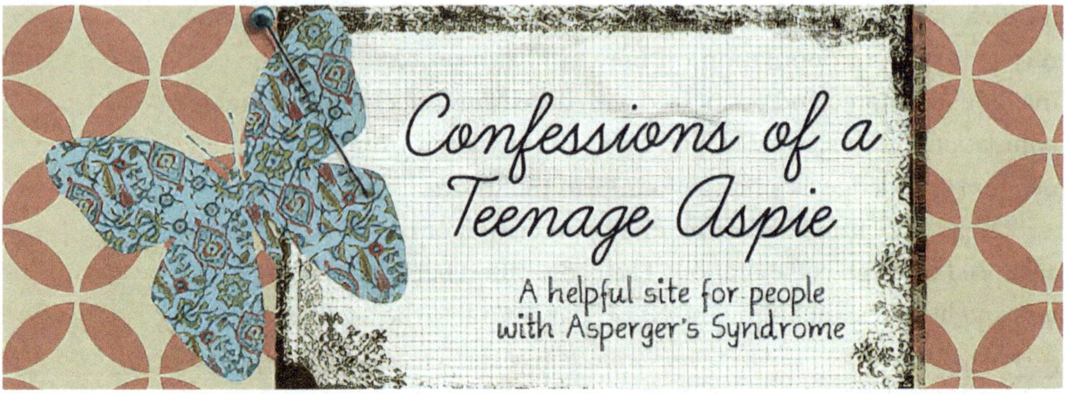

AUTISM AND ALZHEIMER'S ON THE WEB

https://circulatingnow.nlm.nih.gov/2014/05/30/autism-and-alzheimers-on-the-web/

May 30, 2014 • Archives & Manuscripts

MAUREEN HARLOW

Capturing websites and keeping copies of them for the future to represent how they looked and what they said at a certain moment in time ("web collecting") is an important activity for cultural heritage institutions because so much of our lives is now conducted online. Whereas in earlier decades, people regularly kept journals to document experiences and personal reflections, now blogs are a far more popular medium. Likewise, broadsides used to present information and give notice of important events to passers-by, but now those are all but obsolete and Twitter has filled that niche. Pamphlets used to be published frequently by all sorts of organizations, but now the same information is often published online as PDFs instead of printing and distributing several runs of print copies. While paper journals, broadsides, and pamphlets can be preserved fairly easily if handled well and stored in the proper conditions, digital content is at a far greater risk. Given the ephemeral nature of web content, National

Library of Medicine (NLM) staff are improving their capacity to capture this born-digital content, which will likely be as important to future researchers as their analog counterparts of the past.

Since September 2013, I have been embedded in the NLM as a National Digital Stewardship Resident (NDSR). The NDSR program is a joint effort of the Library of Congress and the Institute of Museum and Library Services. Ten projects hosted by institutions around the Washington, DC, area were chosen from a pool of applicants, and ten residents were similarly chosen to complete the projects. I was lucky enough to be chosen for a project here at the NLM to create a thematic web archive collection that would be added to the collections of the Library and serve as a model for future thematic web collecting at the NLM.

This project involved developing a theme, identifying content to capture, crawling the sites, and describing the collection. This work builds on the NLM's pilot Health and Medicine Blogs collection and a web collection documenting the response from the Department of Health and Human Services to the H7N9 avian Flu. After considering a number of themes, I eventually chose to create a collection documenting a representative sample of current perspectives on Autism and Alzheimer's called "Disorders of the Developing and Aging Brain: Autism and Alzheimer's on the Web." I felt that it was particularly important to collect on these diagnoses because they represent disorders whose understanding is currently undergoing a great deal of change. Both of these disorders are being researched heavily at the National Institutes of Health (NIH) and elsewhere, and our understanding of both is changing rapidly. In ten or fifteen years our collective understanding of Autism and Alzheimer's may have changed significantly, but it will be important for researchers to understand what we know at this moment in order to appreciate how it has changed over time.

"Disorders of the Developing and Aging Brain: Autism and Alzheimer's on the Web" consists of sixty-six unique websites that are split evenly between the two diagnoses and cover several different perspectives:

- current understanding
- patient perspective
- caregiver perspective
- research
- causes
- treatment
- prevention (for Alzheimer's only)

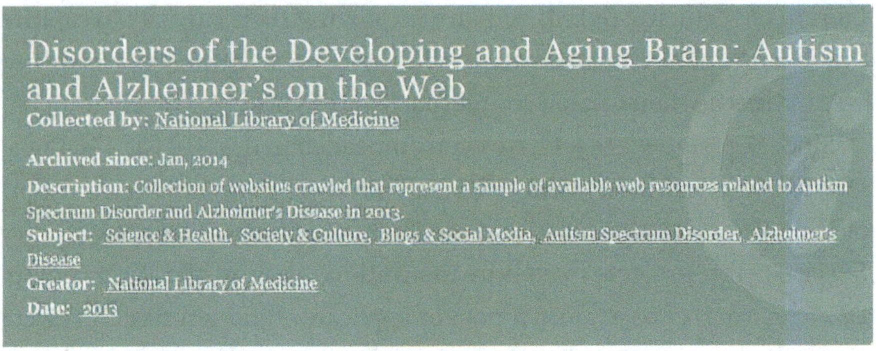

Disorders of the Developing and Aging Brain: Autism and Alzheimer's on the Web

The websites I identified for the patient and caregiver perspectives are first-person blogs, whereas many of the sites I selected for the other categories are resources created by non-profit research organizations, government agencies, and news sources. I did not directly collect prevention for Autism because there is no reliable consensus about how to prevent it, and capturing this debate was excluded from the scope of this particular collection. The controversy surrounding prevention and some of the theories about it may be reflected in other content in the collection.

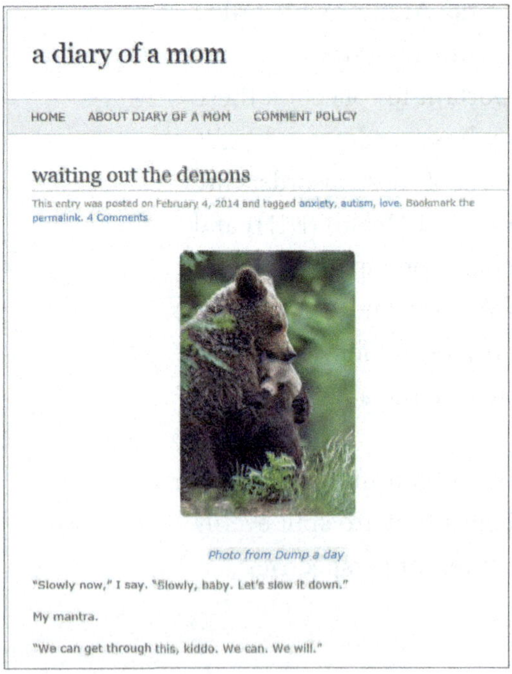

A Diary of a Mom blog

Here are two examples of the content about Autism that I identified for this collection:

A Diary of a Mom author Jess is a Boston-area parent with two daughters, one neurotypical and one autistic. The blog chronicles her experiences raising both children with her husband and the special challenges presented by her younger daughter's Autism.

Confessions of a Teenage Aspie is a blog created by a self-described "Aspie" (person with Asperger's) in her late teens, recently started at college. Her blog provides a front-row seat to the challenges of being a teenager with Asperger's who is just starting to live independently.

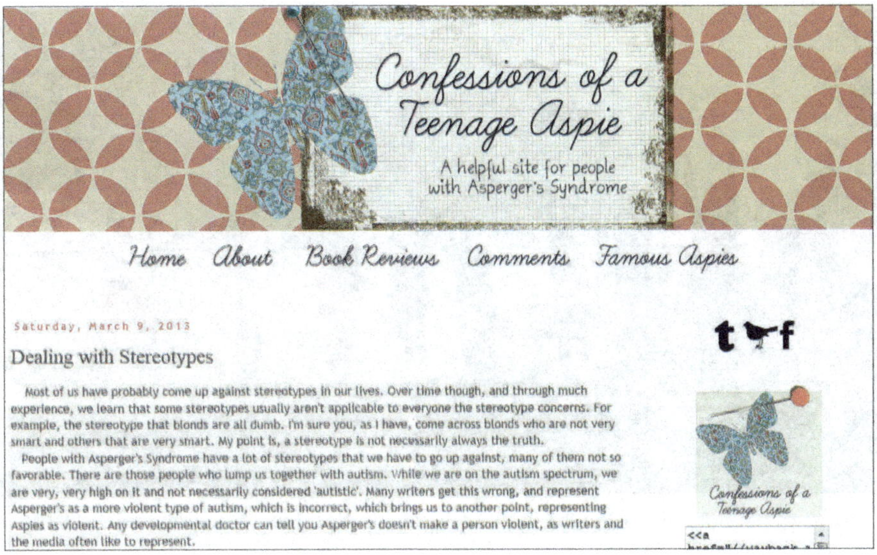

Confessions of a Teenage Aspie blog

After collecting the websites and performing quality assurance on them to ensure that the copies reflect as best as possible the desired content, I began the process of describing the collection. I wanted to describe each item selected as well as provide a means of describing the collection as a whole, grouping the various perspectives and types of content together. In many ways the model of a historical manuscript collection finding aid made sense. So, I talked to the archivist and digital resource manager in the NLM's History of Medicine Division, we settled on a plan of action, and I got to work!

In the end, I developed three levels of description to maximize the collection's findability: a robust Dublin Core metadata on the collection's Archive-It page, a catalog record so the collection can be searched in the general NLM catalog, and an Encoded Archival Description (EAD) finding aid so that the collection's full description can be found among the other NLM collections. This may seem like an extraordinary level of description, but it's actually only one more level than other archival collections get. The extra level is the item-level metadata on the collection's Archive-It page. The metadata I entered there simply makes it consistent with other NLM Archive-It collections, and allows users who access it directly from Archive-It to search it from the Archive-It interface.

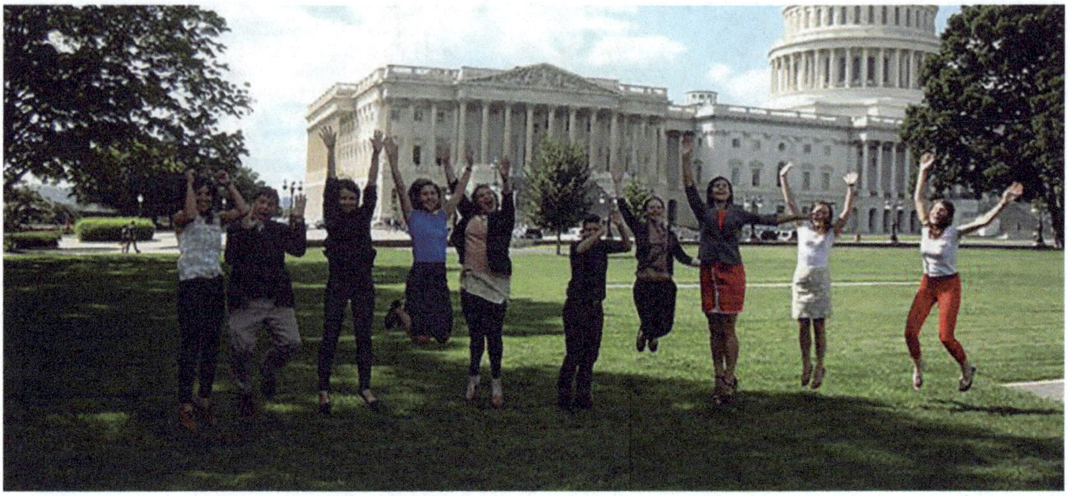

NDSR Graduation • The 2013 cohort of National Digital Stewardship Residency program celebrate their graduation. • *Photo by Ali Fazal, Library of Congress*

Working at the NLM has been an extraordinary experience, and one that I'll not soon forget. As a new archivist and an almost digital native, it is fantastic to see a library like the NLM on the cutting edge of web archiving. Sometimes, convincing people that websites are important historical artifacts is a hard sell, but the NLM has truly been in the vanguard of web archiving and thematic web collecting. I'm so glad to have had the opportunity to work on this collection and get it off the ground!

Reflection

As a National Digital Stewardship Fellow at the NLM in 2014, I was thrilled to have the opportunity to create one of the Library's first curated, fully described, thematic web collections. The collection focused on born-digital web resources about Autism and Alzheimer's. It was a fantastic learning opportunity about doing this type of collecting. In particular, I learned about web accessibility; features that were implemented irregularly have become much more common practice. Now, for example, social media platforms offer automated live captions as a matter of course.

After leaving the NLM, I moved to a position at PBS, the first major broadcaster to standardize and use closed captions consistently. I regularly draw on lessons learned during my time at the NLM and while curating the Autism and Alzheimer's web collection specifically, including the importance of accessibility through closed captions and descriptive video tracks.

Autism and Alzheimer's remain mysterious. Doctors and scientists still lack full understanding of these disorders and their best treatments. However, in the last eight years, remarkable progress has been made in identification, treatment, and diagnosis. Looking back at the *Circulating Now* posts I authored in 2014 reveals how much our knowledge has changed—and continues to change—regarding these disorders.

Reflecting on this experience, I appreciate the changes that have occurred yet remain cognizant about how much remains to achieve for Autism and Alzheimer's, accessibility, and web representation for all audiences. I'm eternally grateful for my time at the NLM and the opportunity to curate this collection. —Maureen Harlow, 2023

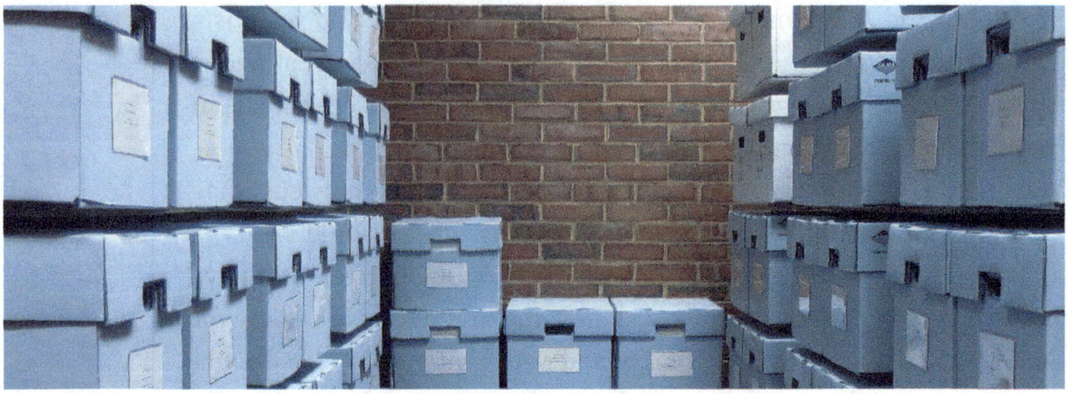

JOHN E. FOGARTY: FROM PROVIDENCE TO PROFILES

https://circulatingnow.nlm.nih.gov/2015/11/17/john-e-fogarty-from-providence-to-profiles/

November 17, 2015 • Archives & Manuscripts, Guests

RUSSELL M. FRANKS

Circulating Now *welcomes guest blogger Russell M. Franks, Librarian for Special and Archival Collections at the Phillips Memorial Library, Providence College, who relates some of the history of the John E. Fogarty Papers collection now featured on the National Library of Medicine (NLM)'s* Profiles in Science.

• • •

In July 2014, Rebecca Warlow, Head, Images and Archives Section, History of Medicine Division, NLM, made Providence College an offer that was too good to pass up.

For years, the College had sought ways to raise public awareness of its founding flagship collection, the papers of Congressman John E. Fogarty. So when Ms. Warlow, on behalf of the National Library of Medicine,

TOP Part of the Fogarty collection in the John E. Fogarty Room at the Phillips Memorial Library • *Courtesy Russell M. Franks*

invited the College's Phillips Memorial Library to participate in a collaborative project to digitize a portion of Congressman Fogarty's papers relating to his congressional work in promoting and advancing healthcare legislation, we immediately agreed. The culmination of this year-long collaboration can be seen on the National Library of Medicine's John E. Fogarty *Profiles in Science* website.

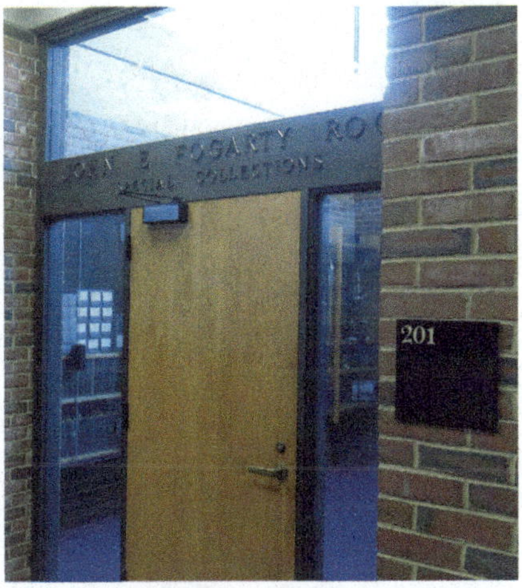

Entryway for the Special Collections John E. Fogarty Room at the Phillips Memorial Library • *Courtesy Russell M. Franks*

As a member of and later as Chairman of the House Appropriations Committee's Subcommittee for the Department of Labor and the Department of Health, Education, and Welfare (HEW), Congressman Fogarty increased the HEW budget exponentially and shepherded numerous health-related legislative bills through Congress during his tenure. His papers contain documentation on virtually every important piece of federal health legislation from 1949 to 1966.

When Congressman Fogarty passed away in January 1967, his wife, Luise, came to the conclusion a few months afterward that:

> Knowing how much he [*Fogarty*] thought of Providence College and being mindful of the fact that he was always so devoted to the people of Rhode Island, I decided that the best place for the record of his public life to be kept would be the library of Providence College. (In letter to William P. Hass, OP, President of Providence College) March 14, 1967

Thus, the first major manuscript collection was acquired by the then newly formed Providence College Archives, which was spearheaded by the College's archivist, Matthew J. Smith. Congressman Fogarty's collection, which is over 150 linear feet in length, contains not only his legislative papers, but also personal and constituent correspondence, photographs, public documents, and memorabilia from his time in Congress.

When the College received the collection, press releases were issued, on-campus public exhibitions using Congressman Fogarty's materials were mounted, and with an original grant from the National Library of Medicine, the collection was processed and a detailed 200-page finding aid

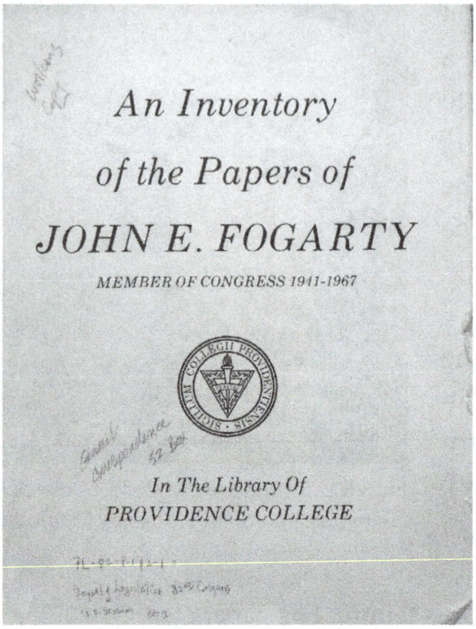

An Inventory of the Papers of John E. Fogarty • The original finding aid for the Fogarty Collection • *Courtesy Russell M. Franks*

was published and disseminated to interested parties and institutions. A special reading room on the second floor of the new Phillips Memorial Library was dedicated and named the John E. Fogarty Room to house the collection and to provide researchers a comfortable place in which to conduct their investigations. Over the years, the collection has been used extensively by various researchers for their particular projects, and the finding aid worked well for those researchers in the pre-digital era. For remote research, access was less than ideal.

The original finding aid for the Fogarty collection was one of the first legacy inventories we converted to the Encoded Archival Description (EAD) schema for online use. In addition, we also digitized more than 350 representative images from the collection for virtual use. Still, the use of the collection did not increase significantly through these efforts. Interestingly enough, when the nation was debating the Affordable Healthcare Act of 2010 a few years ago, there were very few requests for use of the health-related materials in the Fogarty collection. This was rather surprising since the framework for this landmark health legislation was first laid down decades ago by Congressman Fogarty and his colleagues in the Great Society programs of the 1960s.

The donation of Congressman Fogarty's papers, however, set the focus and collecting mission of the newly formed College archives. Since then, the College's archival collections development policy has generally been centered on acquiring and preserving the papers of mid twentieth-century Rhode Island politicians at the local and national level. These holdings by the College include the papers of Rhode Island Governor Dennis J. Roberts (1927–1970), Congressman Aime J. Forand (1918–1972), and Senator John O. Pastore (1907–2000) among others.

Rhode Island is proud of its native son, John E. Fogarty, and his legacy lives on through the work of The John E. Fogarty Foundation in advancing the quality of life for Rhode Islanders with intellectual and developmental

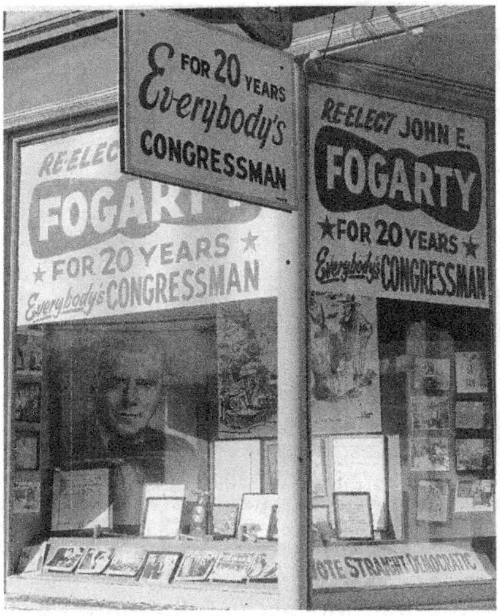

John E. Fogarty campaign headquarters in Providence, RI, 1960 • *Courtesy Phillips Memorial Library, Special and Archival Collections at Providence College,* Profiles in Science, *National Library of Medicine*

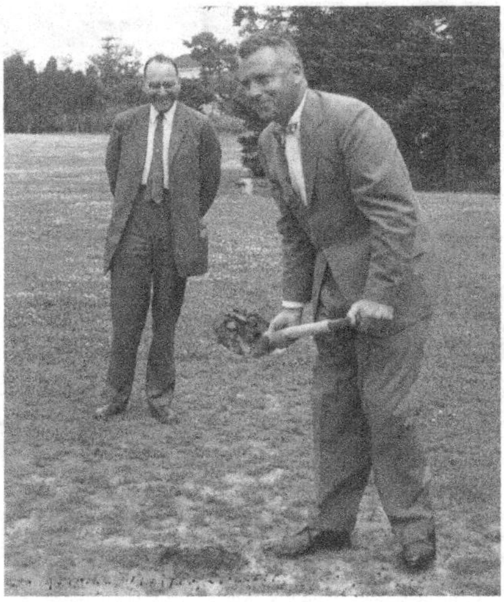

John E. Fogarty lifting a shovel at the Bradley Hospital groundbreaking in East Providence, Rhode Island, 1957 • *Courtesy Phillips Memorial Library, Special and Archival Collections at Providence College,* Profiles in Science, *National Library of Medicine*

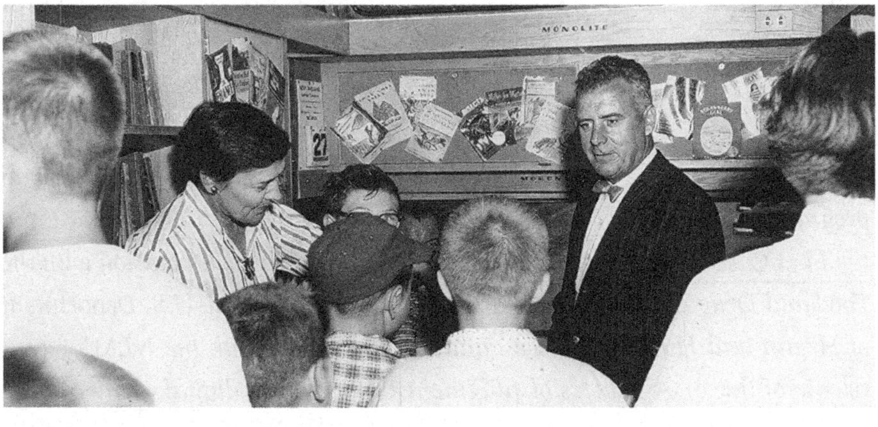

John E. Fogarty visiting a public library services bookmobile in Rhode Island, 1960 • *Courtesy Phillips Memorial Library, Special and Archival Collections at Providence College,* Profiles in Science, *National Library of Medicine*

disabilities. However, with the continued support of and collaboration with the National Library of Medicine through its John E. Fogarty *Profiles in Science* website, Congressman Fogarty's rightful place among the nation's pantheon of health pioneers has been finally acknowledged and is fully secured.

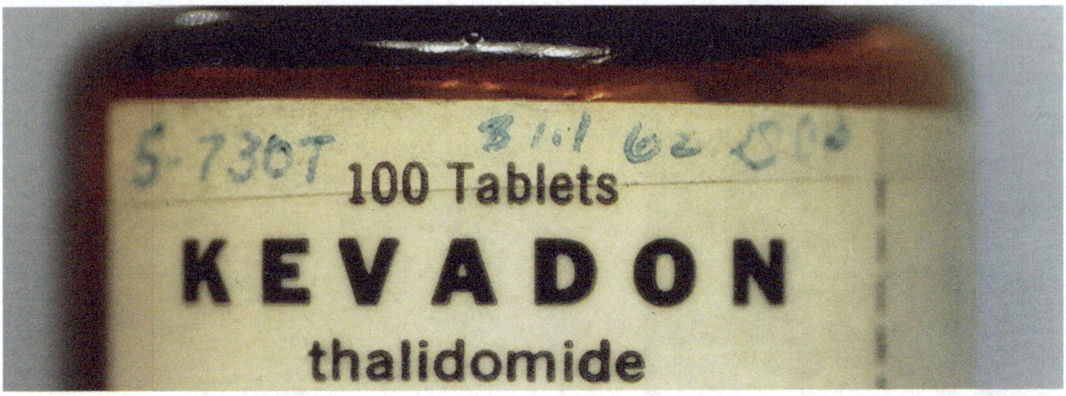

A HISTORY OF THE FDA NOTICES OF JUDGMENT

https://circulatingnow.nlm.nih.gov/2015/05/07/a-history-of-the-fda-notices-of-judgement-john-swann/

May 7, 2015 • Archives & Manuscripts

JOHN SWANN

On May 7, 2015, the National Library of Medicine (NLM) held a special program, "A History of the Food and Drugs Act Notices of Judgment—From the First Case of 1908 to the Digital Archive of 2014" in collaboration with the Food and Drug Administration (FDA) History Office of the U.S. Department of Health and Human Services, and in conjunction with the NLM's recent release of the FDA Notices of Judgment Collection, a digital archive of the published notices of judgment for products seized under authority of the 1906 Pure Food and Drug Act. The program included presentations from NLM Archivist John Rees and FDA Historians Suzanne Junod and John Swann. Circulating Now *interviewed the presenters and today we hear from John Swann.*

• • •

Circulating Now: Tell us a little about yourself. Where are you from? What is your typical workday like?

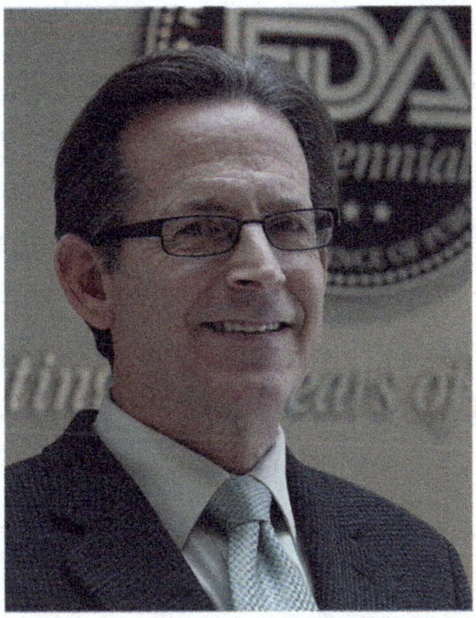

John Swann: I grew up in a small town in northeastern Kansas, Leavenworth, perhaps best known for a number of prisons located nearby. When I was a kid my baseball teams played some games at the honor farms at the federal and state penitentiaries, but that's about as close as I got! I did my undergraduate work at the University of Kansas (chemistry and history) and I received my PhD in pharmacy and in history of science at the University of Wisconsin. After a postdoctoral year at the Smithsonian I worked on an institutional history of the University of Texas Medical Branch in Galveston, then I came to Food and Drug Administration (FDA) in 1989.

As a historian at the FDA I have the opportunity to get involved in a wide range of activities: publishing historical work; speaking to new hires, visitors, and outside groups of all kinds; mounting exhibits (I'm currently working on an exhibit about the variety of ways and reasons why FDA has issued warnings to the public and professional audiences in the past); participating in agency decisions about the identification and preservation of historically significant records; documenting FDA's history through material culture; occasionally assisting in the development of legal briefs and other agency studies with historical background; interacting with outsiders such as scholars, the print and broadcast media, students at all levels of education, filmmakers, law firms, and others that have an interest in the history of FDA and its work. I don't get involved in all of these every day, but life can get interesting sometimes.

CN: This special event celebrates the completion of the digital archive of FDA Notices of Judgment Collection, 1908–1966, how did this collaboration come about?

JS: The FDA History Office has had a long collaboration with the History of Medicine Division (HMD) at the NLM since about the 1970s with our oral history program. The recordings of interviews we conduct, along with a copy of the transcript, are deposited in the archives in HMD.

This has worked out very well, and I think the prospect of having their interviews in the NLM for posterity has helped us when approaching retiring agency officials for oral histories. Of course, there have been many other occasions where we've worked with the NLM over the years. For example, Suzanne collaborated with the NLM on an exhibition about the history of tea and its regulation, I've served on the NLM history of medicine grants evaluation panels a few times, and we have a couple objects presently on loan to the NLM—treatments for leprosy from our artifact collection—for the current exhibition *Native Voices.*

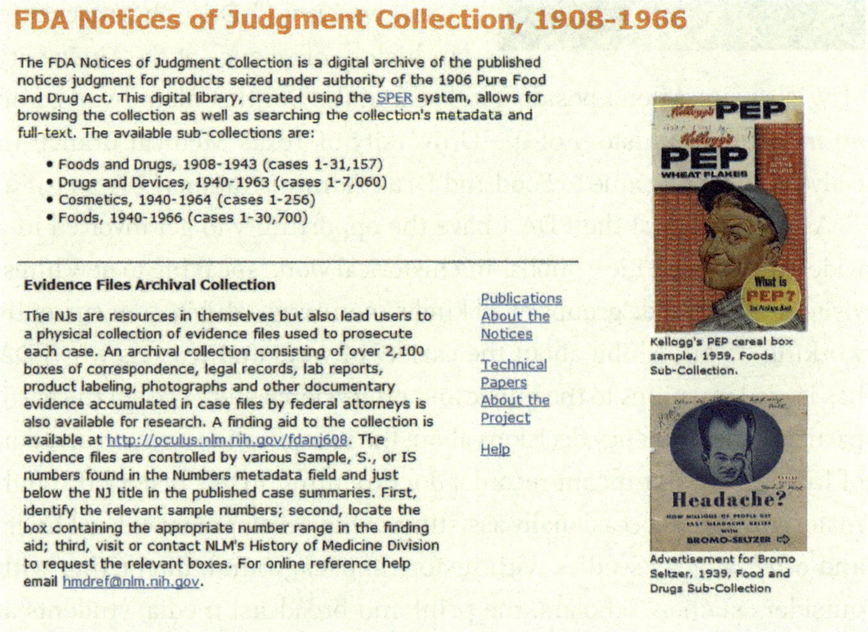

FDA Notices of Judgment Collection, 1908-1966

The FDA Notices of Judgment Collection is a digital archive of the published notices judgment for products seized under authority of the 1906 Pure Food and Drug Act. This digital library, created using the SPER system, allows for browsing the collection as well as searching the collection's metadata and full-text. The available sub-collections are:

- Foods and Drugs, 1908-1943 (cases 1-31,157)
- Drugs and Devices, 1940-1963 (cases 1-7,060)
- Cosmetics, 1940-1964 (cases 1-256)
- Foods, 1940-1966 (cases 1-30,700)

Evidence Files Archival Collection

The NJs are resources in themselves but also lead users to a physical collection of evidence files used to prosecute each case. An archival collection consisting of over 2,100 boxes of correspondence, legal records, lab reports, product labeling, photographs and other documentary evidence accumulated in case files by federal attorneys is also available for research. A finding aid to the collection is available at http://oculus.nlm.nih.gov/fdanj608. The evidence files are controlled by various Sample, S., or IS numbers found in the Numbers metadata field and just below the NJ title in the published case summaries. First, identify the relevant sample numbers; second, locate the box containing the appropriate number range in the finding aid; third, visit or contact NLM's History of Medicine Division to request the relevant boxes. For online reference help email hmdref@nlm.nih.gov.

Publications About the Notices

Technical Papers About the Project

Help

Kellogg's PEP cereal box sample, 1959, Foods Sub-Collection.

Advertisement for Bromo Seltzer, 1939, Food and Drugs Sub-Collection

Our collaboration on the unpublished seizure case files and the Notices of Judgment developed out of a concern for the preservation of the case files. Typically, regulatory records such as these have not been identified as permanent records, perhaps in part because of their volume. However, they shed light on so many elements of the development of American business, culture, health, and of course regulation, that we felt it necessary to find a home for this collection. Not an easy task, since the records date from about 1908 to the 1960s, and beyond. The HMD Chief at the time, Dr. Elizabeth Fee, and Dr. Paul Theerman, who oversaw the archives then, appreciated the historical research value of this collection, received the support of the Library leadership, and made the commitment to take these on—and in the process substantially expand the size of the HMD archives! So, the FDA and the NLM developed a Memorandum of Understanding for the transfer of current and future seizure files.

CN: Would you tell us about the research you presented in your lecture today?

JS: I explained why these records came about in the first place, under both the 1906 Food and Drugs Act and the 1938 Food, Drug, and Cosmetic Act, as a statutory obligation to inform the public about the work the Bureau of Chemistry and the Food and Drug Administration was doing to oversee these important consumer protection laws. Since John Rees and Suzanne delved into examples of the nature of the inquiries that the Notices of Judgment and case files can address, I tried to focus a bit more on the challenge in finding a safe haven for this enormous collection and the challenges inherent in that enterprise.

CN: What sparked your interest in working with this collection? Are there any items that stand out for you as particularly useful in your research, or for which you have special interest?

JS: I knew the collection was a gold mine from about the moment I arrived at the agency. James Harvey Young, the historian of food and drug control whose personal papers are now a part of the archives at the NLM, told me about their usefulness. Certainly, these were an important resource in Harvey's research and publications that I had followed long before I came to FDA. When I learned that these records—records dating back to 1908—could be destroyed, it was obvious something had to be done to prevent that. But not just to avoid their destruction; these had to be made available in a venue where researchers could make use of them, and where the records would receive proper care.

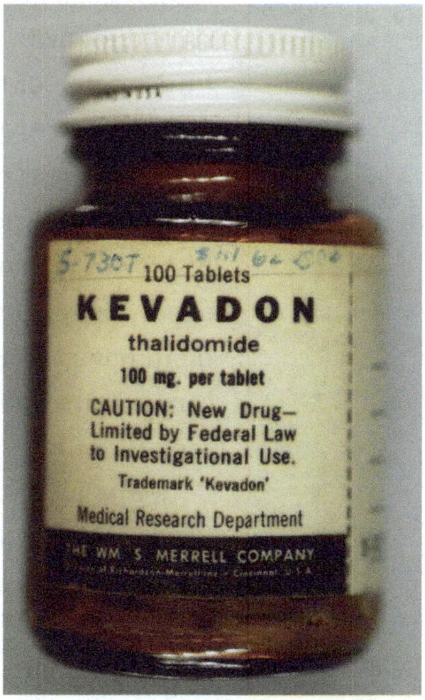

A seized bottle of Kevadon (thalidomide) • *Courtesy FDA*

I have used them in my own research, of course. For example, in work I did on the history of a very dangerous diet pill from the 1930s called dinitrophenol (DNP)—a byproduct of the munitions industry—the case files, and the Notices of Judgment that introduced me to the most relevant of these files, really helped me understand the challenge for FDA of dealing with a product that was killing people yet slipped through the loopholes of the 1906 Act. Indeed, DNP served as one of the more high-profile components of the *Chamber of Horrors*, a traveling exhibit assembled by FDA to illustrate the need for a new law. The seizure case files helped me gain an understanding of the regulatory history of this hazardous drug.

CN: How did you originally become interested in the history of pharmaceutical and drug regulation? What inspires you in your work?

JS: I had an early interest in the history of pharmaceuticals per se since the time of my graduate work, though my introduction to the evolution of drug regulation really did not start in earnest until I arrived at FDA. As I started to investigate the subject it fascinated me more and more. While I miss some of the research I was engaged in prior to coming to FDA, looking at networks of research and how they interact with one another, FDA is a great place to work and its history is an unending source of amazement. And now that there are so many scholars interested in the history of pharmaceuticals and regulation, being at FDA gives me an opportunity to learn about their work, discuss my own, and possibly help them navigate the confusing records terrain of the agency. But when it comes to the seizure files and Notices of Judgments, I know where I can send them.

Being at FDA has given me the chance to learn things I otherwise would never have had the chance to if I were working outside the agency, and some of these things do give me pause. For example, I never would have been called by the person in Oregon, wondering if I knew anything about some diet pills back in the 1960s that she heard had killed her mother. Upon investigating I discovered a story that, in itself was a horrible episode in medical history, but delving deeper I learned that it was part of an ongoing history that has drawn me in ever since.

• • •

Stay tuned this week as Circulating Now *brings you interviews with the presenters of the special program, "A History of the Food and Drugs Act Notices of Judgment—From the First Case of 1908 to the Digital Archive of 2014."*

Reflection

Collaborating with the collegial staff of the NLM has always been a great pleasure for me. Perhaps that is because of our shared interest in medical history, or our common purpose as public historians, archivists, and librarians, or our organizational ties in the Department of Health and Human Services and our close physical proximity in Montgomery County, Maryland. Or perhaps it is knowing that my colleagues at the NLM are among the best in their fields. Elizabeth Fee and Paul Theerman quickly recognized the great value of the enormous collection of seizure case files generated under two of the most important consumer protection laws of the twentieth century. So did the NLM leadership. Their transfer to the NLM represented an extraordinary increase in the Library's archival holdings, but the alternative was the strong possibility that these records would not survive. Unfortunately, this collection has not yet attracted the attention of the broad community of American historians that it deserves: it is a treasure trove of primary source material on the consumer's everyday problematical experience with the medical and nutritional marketplaces. To say that research into this extensive collection is facilitated by the online database of Notices of Judgment does not come close to doing justice to them or the efforts of John Rees to create this resource containing summaries of each of the tens of thousands of cases pursued against violative consumer commodities. I hope scholars, the press, National History Day students, and others will discover the Notices of Judgment for themselves and appreciate that the NLM has preserved and made this collection available to all of us. —John Swann, 2023

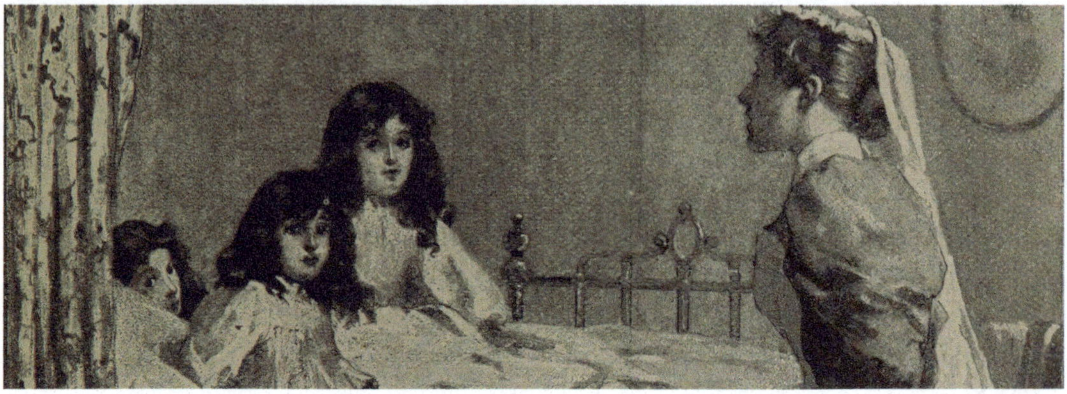

MAKING A MEDICAL HERITAGE MILESTONE

https://circulatingnow.nlm.nih.gov/2014/02/04/making-a-medical-heritage-milestone/

February 4, 2014 • Rare Books & Journals

MICHAEL J. NORTH

The Medical Heritage Library (MHL) has achieved an important milestone by adding the 50,000th item to its online collection housed in Internet Archive. The MHL was formed in the summer of 2009 when curators of historical collections at the medical libraries of Harvard, Yale, Columbia, and the National Library of Medicine (NLM) together with the Open Knowledge Commons collectively received a start-up grant of $1.5 million from the Alfred P. Sloan Foundation to digitize over 30,000 books relating to the history of health and medicine from their collections over the following three years.

As it turned out, it was the National Library of Medicine that scanned and uploaded that 50,000th item: Alvarado

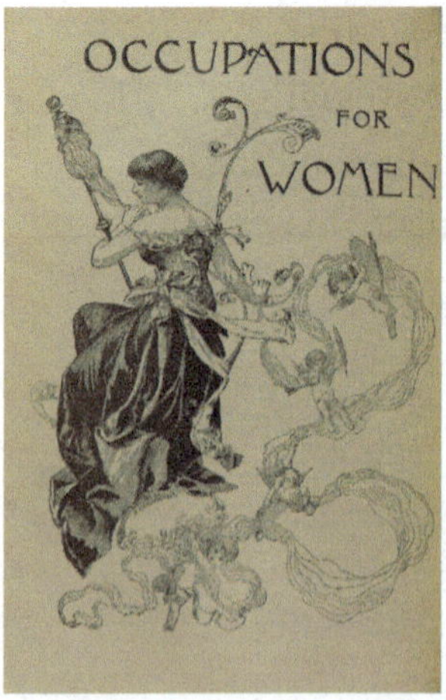

The Doctor's Advice, 1898 • *National Library of Medicine #63610540R*

Middleditch's *The Doctor's Advice*, published in Philadelphia in 1898. This popular advice guide for families, most likely designed as a gift book, contains a treasure trove for cultural historians of the American Victorian household, with chapters on topics such as: "how, when and what to eat and drink, how to secure good health and long life, . . . what mothers and nurses ought to know, how to care for baby, and give our boys and girls the best moral, mental, and physical culture, when and whom to marry, and how to choose a wife or husband, and how to be happy."

Included are over twenty illustrations showing ideal middle class Victorian family scenes and elaborate chapter headings, such as this one for "Occupations for Women," whose text begins, "Our girls—Shall we educate our girls to be genteel, and shall gentility mean to us only idleness, helplessness and a lolling men?" The author, Alvarado Middleditch (1829–1909), was a physician based in Waterloo, Iowa, where he was a general practitioner and known for his skill in electrotherapeutics.

The Medical Heritage Library was formed with the goal of creating a vast digital library of historical materials relating to health and medicine. Since then, many libraries have joined the MHL or contributed important digital collections. And they aren't all printed books: the University of California San Francisco contributed over 3,000 videos relating to the tobacco industry in the United States, ranging from commercials produced during the 1950s to newscasts about the progress of anti-smoking campaigns from the 1990s.

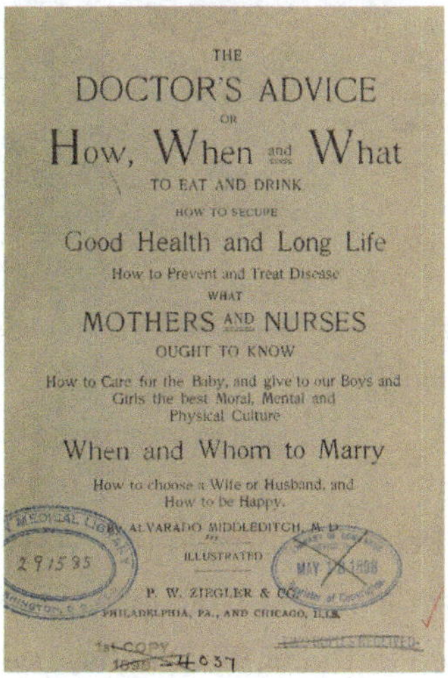
THE
DOCTOR'S ADVICE
OR
How, When and What
TO EAT AND DRINK
HOW TO SECURE
Good Health and Long Life
How to Prevent and Treat Disease
WHAT
MOTHERS AND NURSES
OUGHT TO KNOW
How to Care for the Baby, and give to our Boys and Girls the best Moral, Mental and Physical Culture
When and Whom to Marry
How to choose a Wife or Husband, and How to be Happy.
ALVARADO MIDDLEDITCH, M.D.
ILLUSTRATED
P. W. ZIEGLER & CO.
PHILADELPHIA, PA., AND CHICAGO, ILL.

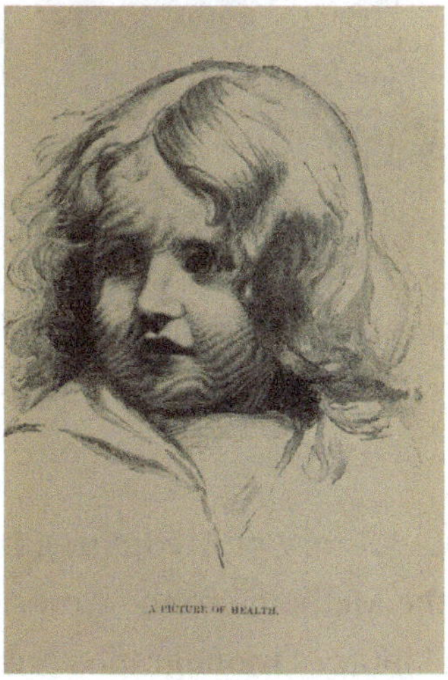

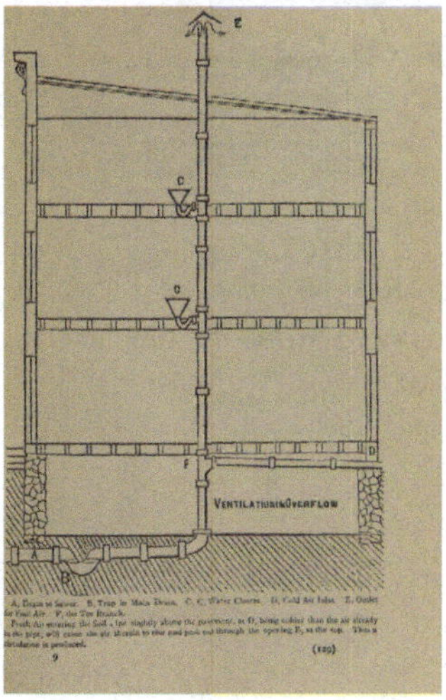

LEFT TO RIGHT (1) The Doctor's Advice • *National Library of Medicine #63610540R* **(2)** A Picture of Health • *National Library of Medicine #63610540R* **(3)** Ventilation & Overflow • *National Library of Medicine #63610540R*

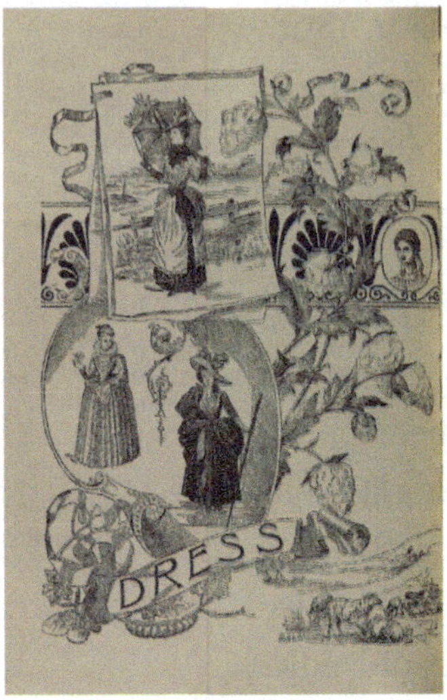

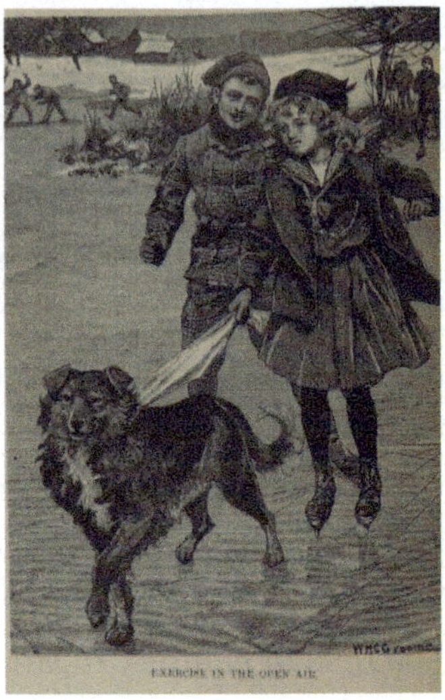

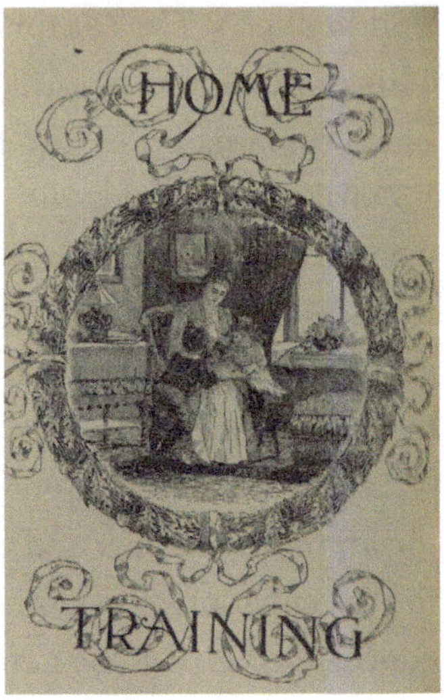

LEFT TO RIGHT **(1)** Dress • *National Library of Medicine #63610540R* **(2)** Exercise in the Open Air • *National Library of Medicine #63610540R* **(3)** Home Training • *National Library of Medicine #63610540R*

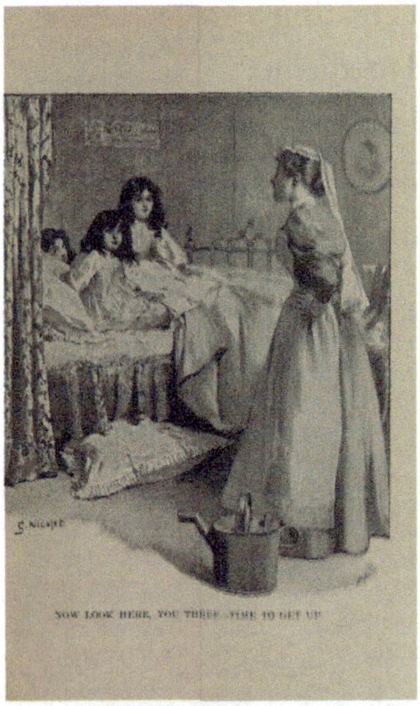

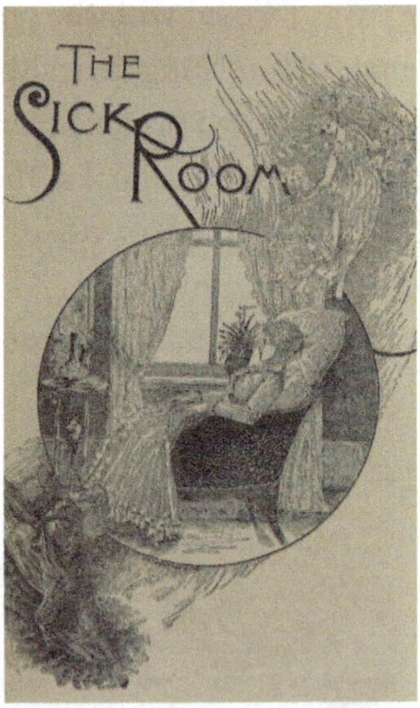

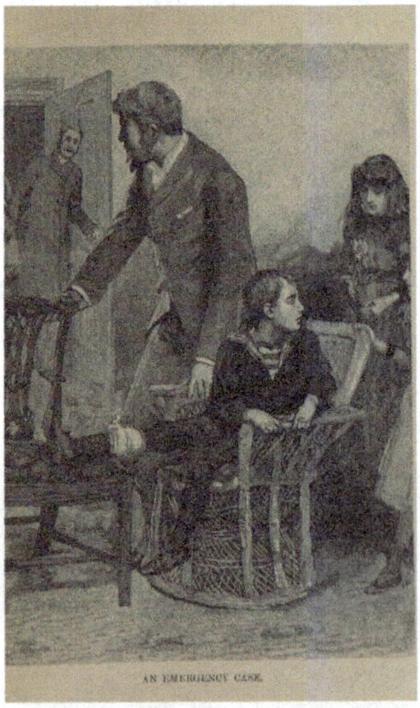

LEFT TO RIGHT **(1)** Time to Get Up • *National Library of Medicine #63610540R* **(2)** The Sick Room • *National Library of Medicine #63610540R* **(3)** An Emergency Case • *National Library of Medicine #63610540R*

The National Library of Medicine's initial contribution to the MHL endeavor was the Medicine in the Americas project, whose scope was to digitize all the Library's monographs published in the U.S., Canada, and Latin America up to the year 1865: a total of over 8,000 items and over 1.5

million pages, most of which can be seen on the NLM's Internet Archive Collections page. Since the completion of that project, the NLM has begun the second phase of Medicine in the Americas: scanning American books dating from 1866 to 1900. Additionally, the Library has just completed a project to digitize all NLM Publications going back to the 1860s.

The NLM is proud to have contributed this interesting title to the Medical Heritage Library and to continue scanning and uploading many more in the coming years. This book and over 9,000 more digitized by the NLM are also available in our Digital Collections, and new items are added regularly as we continue our digitization efforts.

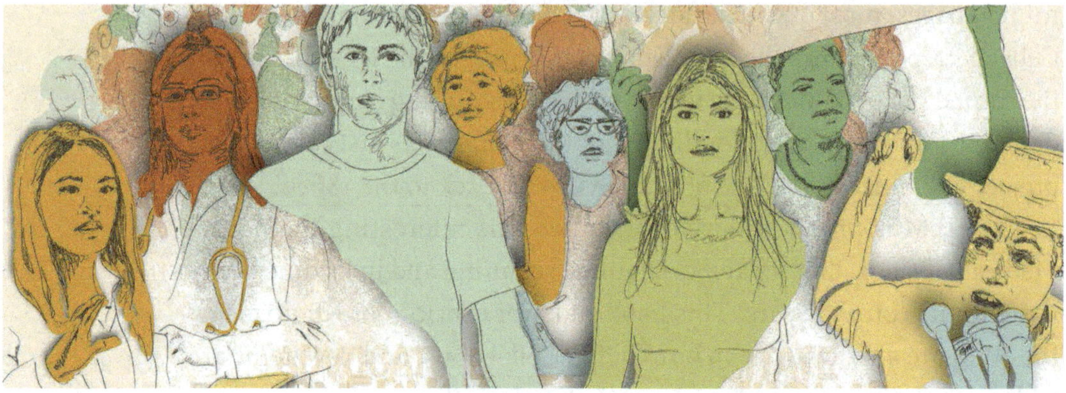

POWER TO THE PEOPLE: WASHINGTON GIVES BACK

https://circulatingnow.nlm.nih.gov/2016/08/09/power-to-the-people-washington-gives-back/

August 9, 2016 • Exhibitions, Guests, News

JENNIFER BRIER, ANNE ARMSTRONG, JULIE KUTRUFF, ERIN CARLSON MAST, AND PATRICIA TUOHY

Exhibitions

Creative individuals and institutions in Washington, DC, have moved beyond what often comes to mind when people think of "Washington museums." *Power to the People: Washington Gives Back* was a panel featured during this year's annual conference of the American Alliance of Museums, which met in Washington, DC, May 26–29. Leaders from four cultural organizations—two historic sites, a national library, and a museum—shared how their core storylines and programs respond to humanitarian challenges and strive to improve the health, well-being, and opportunities of the different communities they serve.

Jennifer Brier, professor at University of Illinois Chicago, moderated the panel. Dr Brier runs a project called History Moves that encourages community members to think of themselves as and act as history makers. She framed the session's conversation as one about *health* as more than the absence of disease and how exhibitions and programming can make that understanding visible to visitors and community members. This is especially needed in a place like Washington, DC, where institutions have national obligations and audiences and, also, very real local obligations to address the profound and historical inequalities and segregations that exist in the nation's capital.

Starting the Conversation: The Panelists

Anne Armstrong serves as deputy director of the National Guard Educational Foundation and director of the National Guard Memorial Museum, Archive, and Library. The National Guard Memorial Museum is situated in the shadow of the nation's Capitol Building—a location notorious for stress and a fast pace. Reflecting the evolution of American soldiers and their unprecedented service since 9/11/2001, Ms. Armstrong's museum hosts a Memorial Wall, dedicated to the Fallen. The Wall room provides

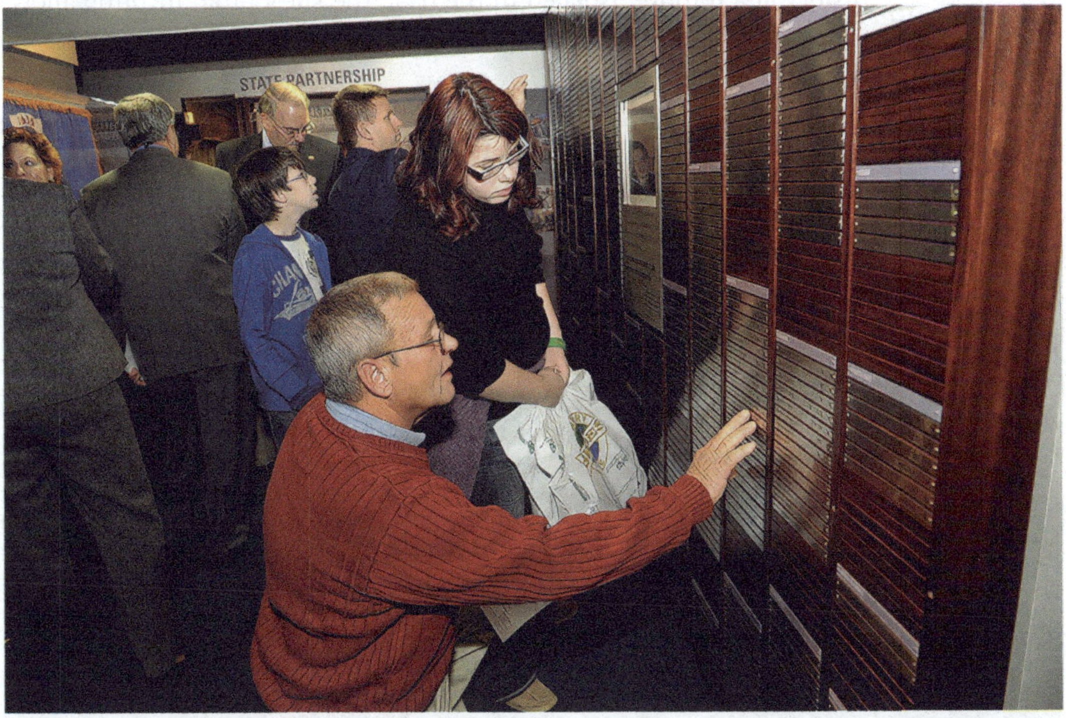

Visitors to the National Guard Memorial Museum respond to the Memorial Wall of the Fallen. • *Courtesy National Guard Educational Foundation*

the local community with a safe haven to come in out of the elements and to contemplate the sacrifices made on behalf of the nation. In so doing, the National Guard Memorial Museum contributes to the well-being and health of the Capitol Hill community.

Julie Kutruff is the Community Outreach and Partnership Coordinator for National Capital Parks-East, which manages the Frederick Douglass House, in the Anacostia neighborhood of Washington, DC. Programs and practices at the house share the legacy of Frederick Douglass to a broad audience from all over the country however the site has been making targeted efforts to reach out to the surrounding community. Ms. Kutruff spoke about the dynamic changes that shaped National Park Service programming to recover and rebuild community engagement with the site.

Erin Carlson Mast is CEO and Executive Director at President Lincoln's Cottage at the Soldiers' Home, a historic site where Lincoln made nation-changing decisions about freedom and democracy. Mast illuminated how honest conversations about the past and present empower us to heal ourselves and the communities we serve. Rather than presenting history at a remove, isolated in the past, the site's programming allows

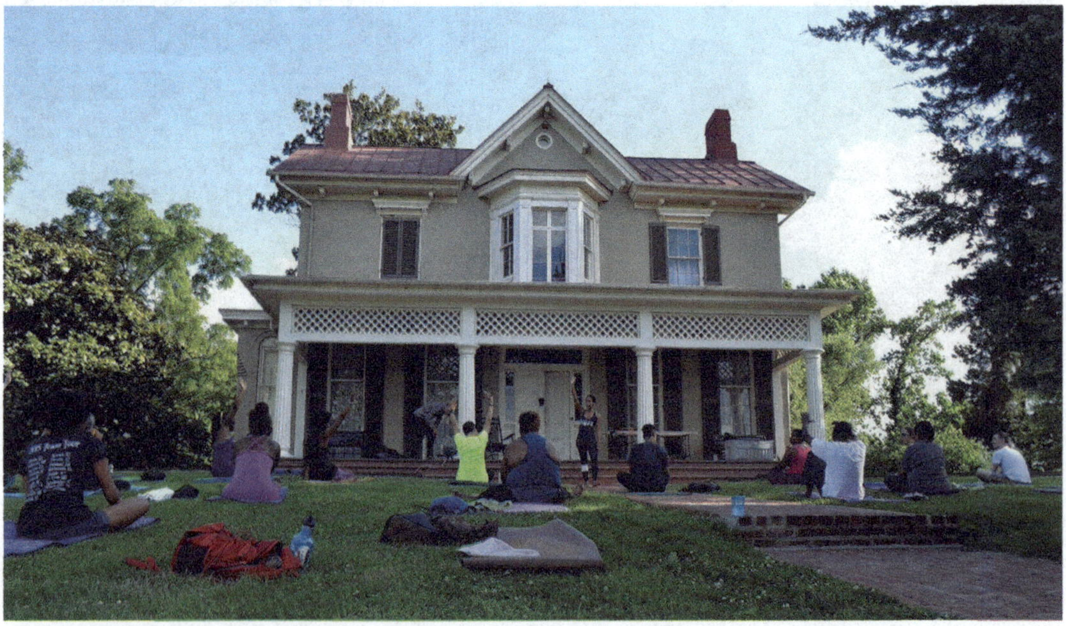

A community yoga program at the Frederick Douglass House • *Courtesy Frederick Douglass House*

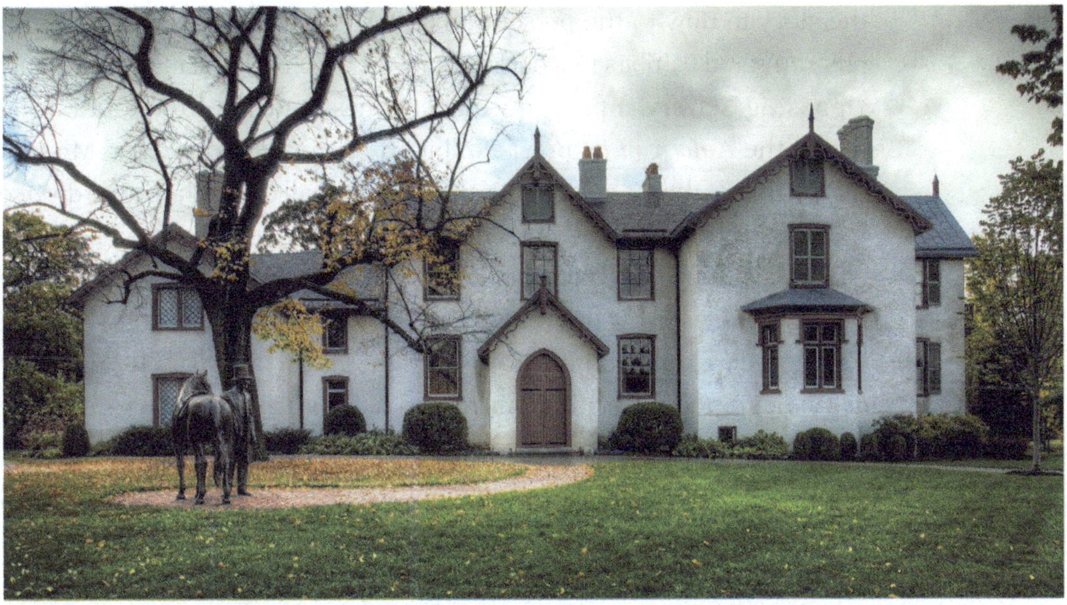

President Lincoln's Cottage at the Soldiers' Home • *Courtesy President Lincoln's Cottage*

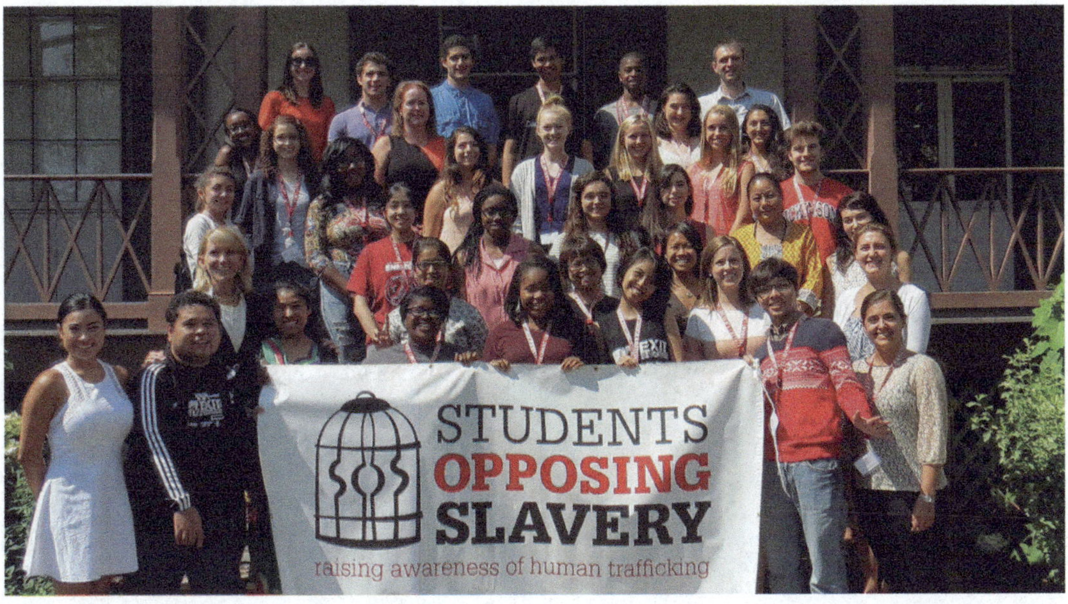

Young people who are part of President Lincoln's Cottage Students Opposing Slavery program • *Courtesy President Lincoln's Cottage*

the story to flow to the present. Ms. Mast shared stories about several programs and exhibits that demonstrate this approach, including Students Opposing Slavery, a program that engages students from around the world; the *American by Belief* exhibit on immigration; and the Mission Advancement through Special Events program, all of which require diverse collaborations to succeed and support cultural health and well-being.

Patricia Tuohy is head of the Exhibition Program in the History of Medicine Division at the National Library of Medicine. The Exhibition Program develops exhibitions that explore the social and cultural history of medicine and raise questions related to health as a human right. With a portfolio of more than a dozen traveling exhibitions, Ms. Tuohy called attention to a recent project about how a cohort of nurse activists, working together during the 1980s and 1990s, confronted the larger medical profession's inability to recognize domestic violence as a medical issue.

Confronting Violence: Improving Women's Lives highlights a manuscript collection, recently acquired by the National Library of Medicine, that contains research studies, reports, published articles, letters, early publications, and presentation slides from two of the nurse activists, Jacquelyn Campbell and Daniel Sheridan, and some of their cohort.

This traveling banner exhibition is currently scheduled to go to fifty libraries across the country over the next several years. When libraries host the exhibition, they will develop programming responsive to and

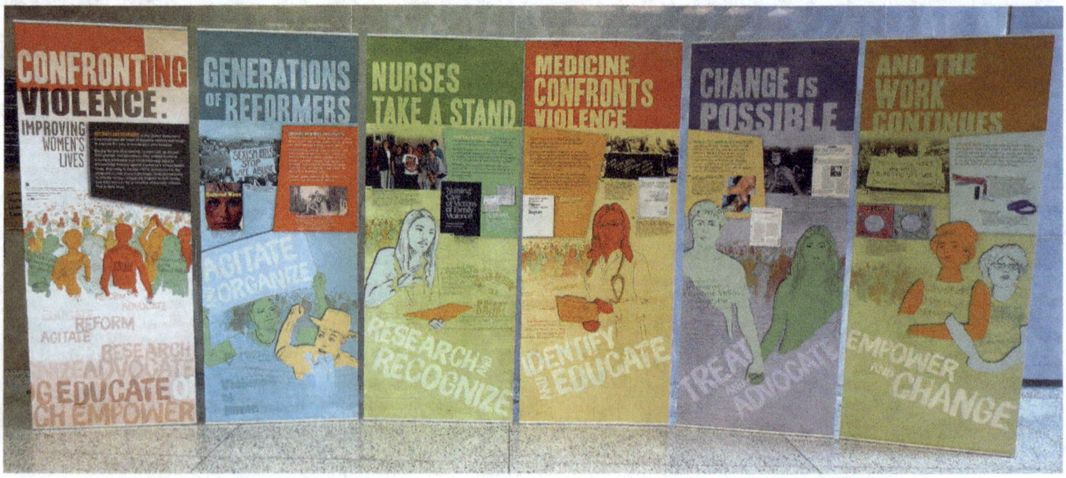

The Traveling Exhibition *Confronting Violence: Improving Women's Lives* • *National Library of Medicine*

in support of their communities' needs. In this way, National Library of Medicine exhibitions can become catalysts for change.

Read more about the history of these activists nurses and the anti-domestic violence movement of the 1980s, in this series of posts by exhibition curator Catherine Jacquet, PhD, assistant professor of history and women's and gender studies.

Continuing the Conversation

The larger conversation with the audience following the presentations explored the different forms of historical and contemporary violence, how it is unequally felt and experienced in our present and past. There were no easy answers. Violence followed by silence, though, only exacerbates the wounds and prevents healing. The presentations gave concrete strategies from four institutions for addressing the health and well-being of communities.

AIDS35

REMEMBERING & WITNESSING: AIDS35 AND THE NLM EXHIBITION "SURVIVING AND THRIVING"

https://circulatingnow.nlm.nih.gov/2017/10/19/remembering-witnessing-aids35-and-the-nlm-exhibition-surviving-and-thriving/

October 19, 2017 • Exhibitions, Guests

THOMAS LAWRENCE LONG

Circulating Now *welcomes guest blogger Thomas Lawrence Long from University of Connecticut School of Nursing. Drawn from a presentation given as part of a bimonthly webcast series hosted by the Network of the National Library of Medicine called "NNLM Resource Picks," this post is third in a series of four exploring how libraries around the country build programming around National Library of Medicine (NLM) traveling exhibitions.*

• • •

In 2016, the thirty-fifth anniversary of the first published reports of what would come to be called "HIV" and "AIDS" (or "SIDA" in much of the world) provided the University of Connecticut's School of Nursing with an opportunity to educate its students about the history of the epidemic and to reach out to the local community (on campus and off). Our program AIDS35 featured the NLM's traveling exhibition *Surviving & Thriving: AIDS, Politics, and Culture*—a visually engaging and informative exploration of the early days of HIV/AIDS, which we supplemented with archival and artifact material from the school's Josephine Dolan Collection of Nursing History.

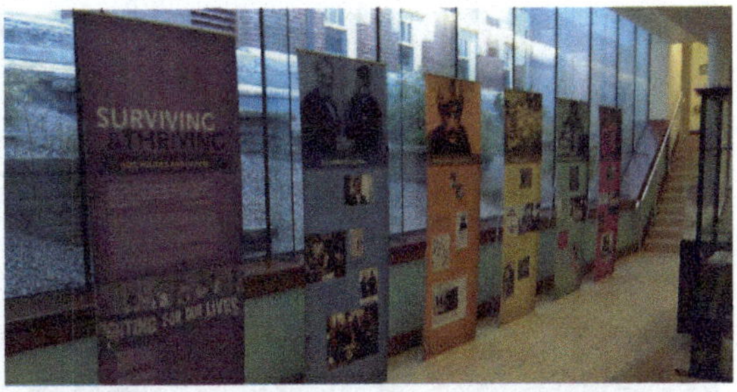

Surviving and Thriving on display as a part of Uconn's School of Nursing's AIDS35 program

For most of today's undergraduates, including nursing students, HIV is just a pharmaceutically manageable infection and an AIDS diagnosis a rare occurrence. The introduction of multi-drug antiretroviral therapy in 1996—before some students were born—curtailed the disease's progression to AIDS, characterized by certain opportunistic infections and low T cell counts. Many students are oblivious to the social and political struggles surrounding HIV/AIDS in the 1980s. They need to be made aware that a health problem could be so insidiously ignored and politicized with disastrous effects on vulnerable populations.

Several years ago, the approach of the thirty-fifth anniversary gave us an occasion to prepare. First, we reserved the NLM exhibit for a month in the fall of 2016. Then, we began to recruit campus-wide and local stakeholders to develop broader programming. The NLM traveling exhibition and supporting materials, including an informational brochure and a large poster, provided a solid educational foundation for our AIDS35 exhibits.

The UConn School of Nursing's Dolan Collection

Our nursing school's new Widmer Wing features a large, well-lighted, and high-ceilinged atrium where the banners could be displayed easily. In addition, free-standing vitrines for nursing history artifacts and archival materials gave us an opportunity to focus on nursing's role in the HIV/AIDS epidemic.

These Dolan Collection exhibits included early journals and indexes featuring nursing research on HIV and AIDS care. Ephemera, like safer sex pamphlets and condom and personal lubricant packs, were loaned by a doctoral student who has been an HIV clinician for most of the epidemic.

Recruiting Partners on Campus and in the Community

Finding other partners was more challenging. The term "broadcasting network" comes to mind because we had to invite over a dozen prospective

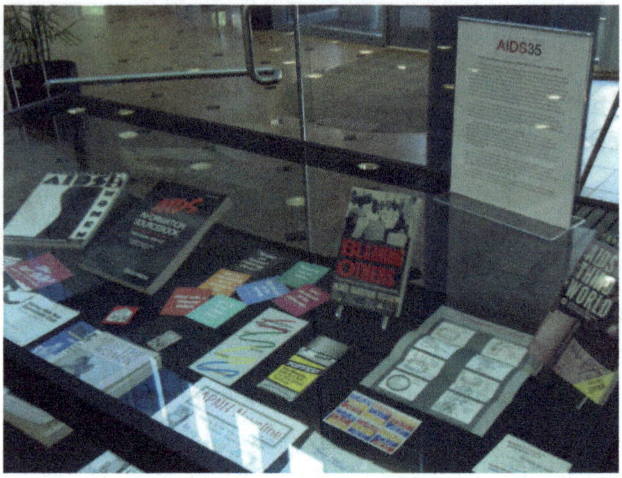

Books and ephemera display for AIDS35 at UConn

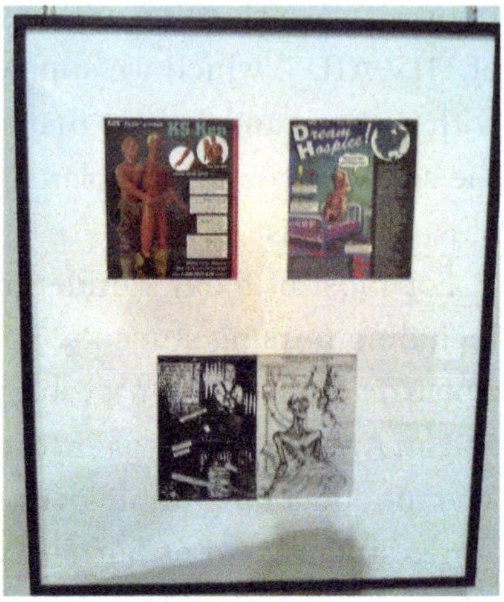

Zines on display for AIDS35 at UConn

partners in order to secure three: the UConn William Benton Museum of Art on the Storrs campus; the University Libraries' Archives and Special Collections; and Connecticut's public broadcasting, WNPR and CPTV.

The Benton Museum associate curator Jean Nihoul, working with the Dolan Collection curator Thomas Lawrence Long, identified graphics, photographs, and other visual arts from the 1980s and 1990s. Dr. Long supplemented these with material from his own collection of AIDS zines and demonstration graphics from the same period. Entitled *Visual AIDS*, the exhibit was open throughout the fall 2016 semester.

UConn's Archives and Special Collections includes substantial holdings in alternative publications, many of which were produced during and in response to the worst years of the AIDS epidemic, between 1981 and 1996. Archivist Graham Stinnett assembled ephemera (brochures and flyers) and more traditional publications (novels and non-fiction books) that were displayed in the Thomas J. Dodd Research Center. (Read more about the display here.)

Finally, University Communications was instrumental in securing broader publicity for these exhibits. In addition to writing an article for *UConn Today,* Kenneth Best secured an interview on WNPR's morning interview program, *Where We Live*. This interview was aired live, subsequently re-aired in "archive editions," and afterward, excerpts were featured as cultural spots promoting the Benton exhibit.

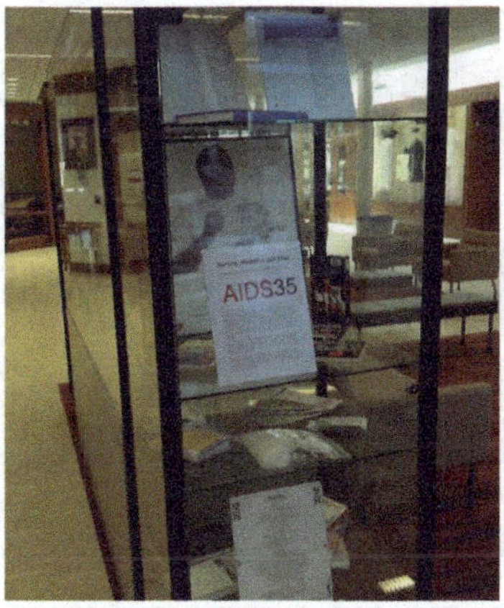

A display case for AIDS35

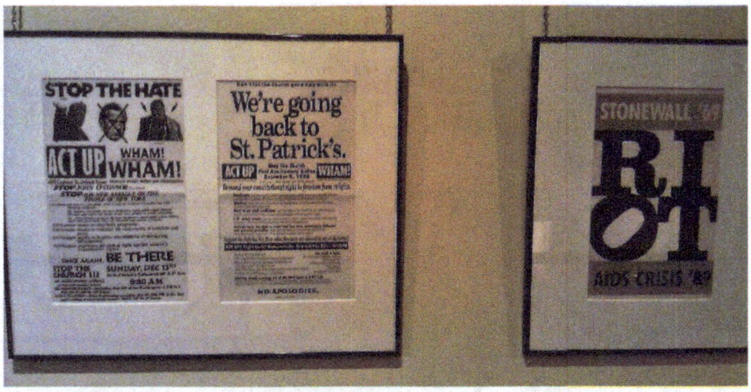

HIV/AIDS ephemera on display

Reflections on AIDS35 and NLM Traveling Exhibitions

Our collaboration in AIDS35 engaged a variety of resources, but the educational foundation was provided by the NLM's traveling exhibition. Culture and education organizations small and large can benefit from NLM traveling exhibitions regardless of their locations and budgets. Advanced planning is essential, however. Identifying a significant anniversary as we did or connecting the exhibition with other local events or interests and building partnerships that will leverage publicity take time and thoughtful effort. But the benefits to the organization and its constituents can be great.

• • •

In late 2016, the University of Washington, based in Seattle, Washington, which serves as the Pacific Northwest Region National Network library, hosted a brief questionnaire, using SurveyMonkey, asking librarians what they would want to learn about hosting a National Library of Medicine traveling banner exhibition. Over 250 representatives from libraries across the country responded with questions, ideas, and preferences. Their replies shaped this webinar.

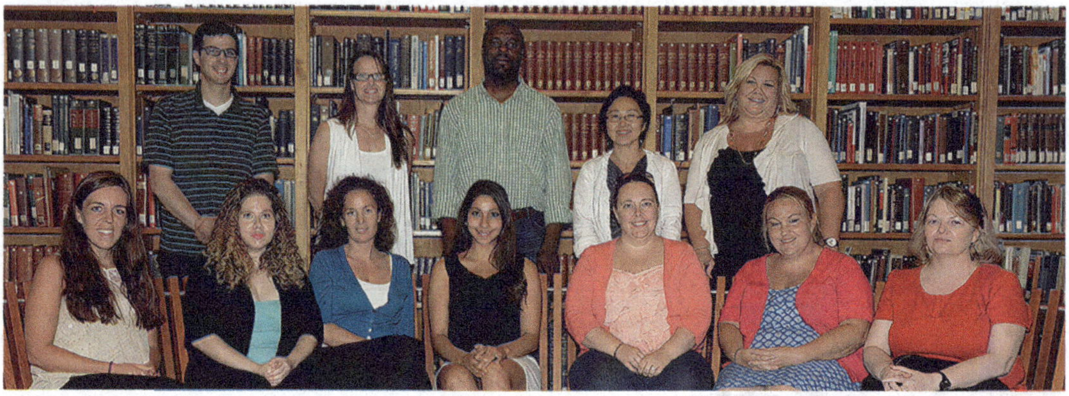

BY THE TEACHERS, FOR THE TEACHERS

https://circulatingnow.nlm.nih.gov/2013/07/30/by-the-teachers-for-the-teachers/

July 30, 2013 • Exhibitions

ERIKA MILLS

In June, the Exhibition Program welcomed nine educators from the Washington, DC, area for a Teacher Institute: a four-day workshop during which participants left their K-12 classrooms and school libraries behind to immerse themselves in National Library of Medicine collections, resources, and professional collaboration. A major part of the Exhibition Program's work is developing multidisciplinary lesson plans, higher education modules, online activities, and onsite education programs that draw on the historical and contemporary collection of the Library. This summer, we invited local teachers and media specialists to come learn about our educational offerings and help us create new ones.

ABOVE Teacher Institute participants with Exhibition Program and NIH staff. • Standing (l to r): Peter SanGeorge (Exhibition Program Pathways student), Robin Biser, Carson Wise, Jiwon Kim (exhibition educator), Kim Sidorick. Seated (l to r): Shannon Burden (NIH employee), Sarah Elwell, Emily Sigman, Samantha Candia, Lory Gardner, Amber Leber, Lisa Kellert

Jiwon Kim, the Exhibition Program's educator and lead exhibit specialist, developed the Teacher Institute, which provided presentations and tutorials that familiarize participants with our collections and online resources and facilitated collaborative work sessions for creating new lesson plans and activities related to our exhibitions.

During group discussions, teachers considered how to incorporate National Library of Medicine resources like MedlinePlus, our consumer health information site, into their work during the school year and facilitate their colleagues doing the same. Lory Gardner, a humanities and language arts teacher at Montgomery Village Middle School, appreciated availability of many visual materials through IHM, which provides online access to over 70,000 images in the Library's historical collections: "I'm glad to have some place to send my kids other than Wikipedia."

The educators brought expertise in different grade levels and subject areas—middle and high school, science, social studies, and humanities. The lesson plans and activities they created reflect the diversity of the group, and apparently not a moment too soon, as teachers are under increasing pressure to use a multidisciplinary approach in the classroom. For Sara Elwell, a library media specialist, and Carson Wise, a science teacher at McKinley Technology High School, the Institute was an opportunity to work with a colleague in another department. Carson

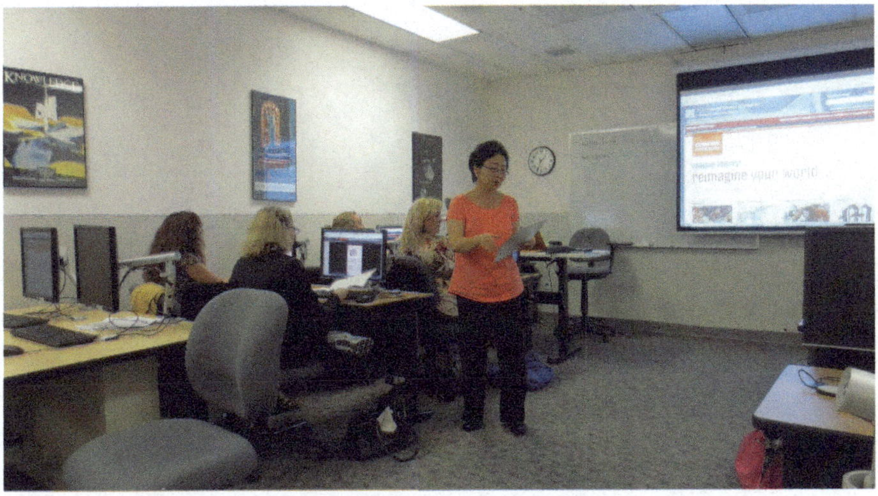

Jiwon Kim, the organizer of the Teacher Institute, leads a workshop activity.

Wise appreciated this. "I got to collaborate with a coworker I never got to collaborate with before. Now, I have someone that I can present ideas with." Sara Elwell plans to introduce more teachers to our resources. "I'm excited to share because I conducted a survey of teacher needs at my school and your materials seem to answer those needs."

We thank the Teacher Institute participants for their contributions! The Exhibition Program is always working on new education resources and we'll be sure to keep you abreast of new developments.

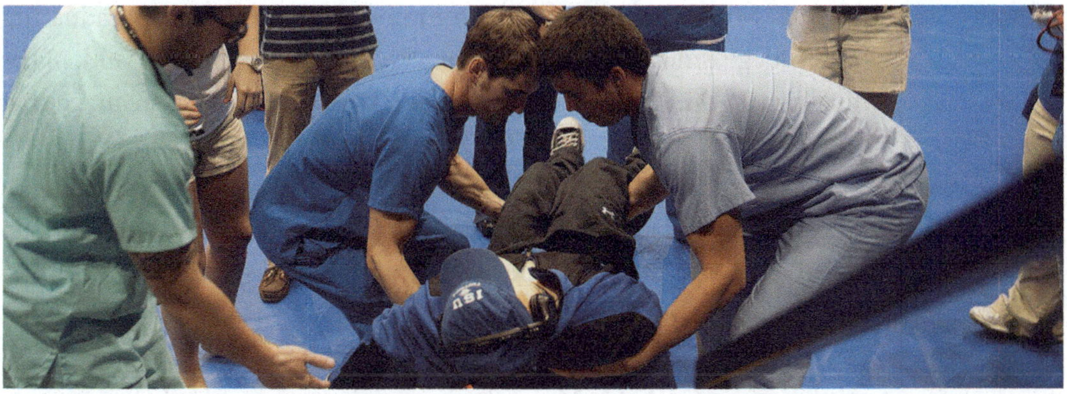

COLLABORATION AND CURATION

https://circulatingnow.nlm.nih.gov/2017/02/07/collaboration-and-curation/

February 7, 2017 • Exhibitions, Guests

LOREN E. MILLER

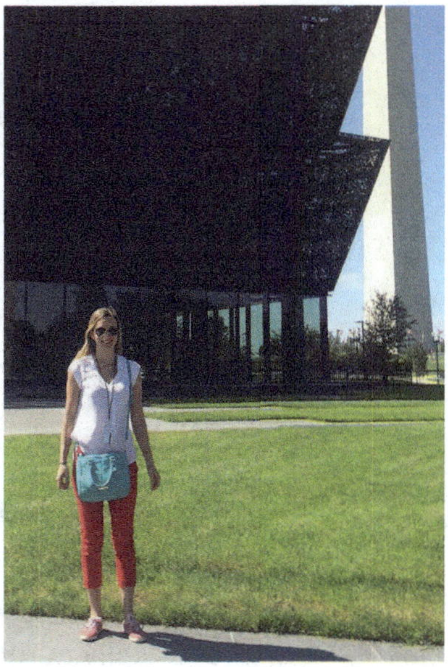

Loren E. Miller, PhD, will speak at 2 p.m. on February 14 at the NIH Natcher Conference Center on "Collaboration and Curation: Creating the Exhibition Collaboration and Care." Dr. Miller is guest curator of the National Library of Medicine (NLM)'s exhibition Physician Assistants: Collaboration and Care *and a curatorial assistant at the Smithsonian National Museum of African American History and Culture.* Circulating Now *interviewed her about her work.*

• • •

Circulating Now: Please tell us a little about yourself. Where are you from? What do you do? What is your typical workday like?

Loren E. Miller: I am originally from northern NJ, but after graduating from college I moved to Washington, DC, because I wanted to work in the museum world. Ten years later, I am lucky enough to have realized that dream. In 2015 I earned my PhD in history from American University and went on to serve as the Mellon Curatorial Fellow at the Smithsonian Museum of African American History and Culture. When the fellowship ended, the Museum hired me as the Curatorial Assistant for the Center for African American Media Arts (CAAMA). In this current position, I help the Curator of Photography and Film develop, plan, and mount exhibitions in CAAMA. My work varies each day; however, I often execute tasks such as performing research, selecting photographs for exhibitions, writing exhibit labels and content, and acquiring new collections. I feel lucky every day to be part of such an important museum.

CN: On February 14, 2017 you'll be at the NLM to talk about "Collaboration and Curation: Creating the Exhibition Collaboration and Care." Could you give us a little preview of your lecture?

LM: As you can probably tell from the title of the exhibit, collaboration is a key theme of *Physician Assistants: Collaboration and Care*. What might be less obvious is that it was also essential to my work as the curator of the show. My lecture will explore how the different parties involved in the project—the Physician Assistant History Society, the National Library of Medicine, and I—worked together to create a successful show that everyone was proud of. When I began considering lecture topics, I thought it would be interesting to explore the collaboration that occurred while developing the exhibition, because people don't generally think about the process of creating a show. As a curator, I see collaboration as an essential element of success. Curators must be good listeners and expert moderators to ensure that all the stakeholders in a project feel understood, as well as that everyone is proud of the final product.

CN: What did you find most interesting about this subject?

LM: One of the most interesting things about physician assistants (PAs) is how the profession developed rapidly in such a short period of time and continues to expand today. The first three PAs graduated from Duke University in 1967, and within fifty years the number of certified PAs has

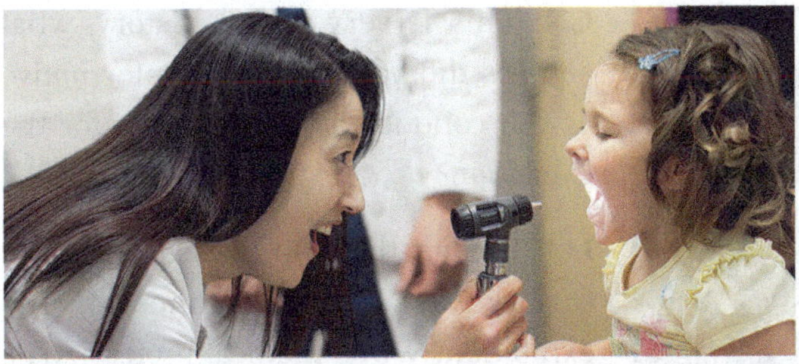

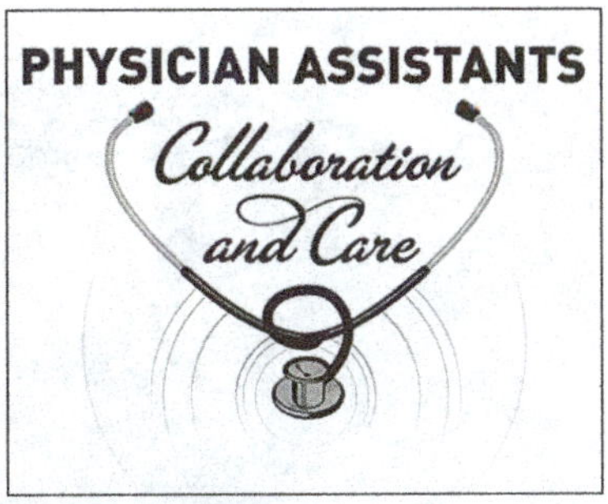

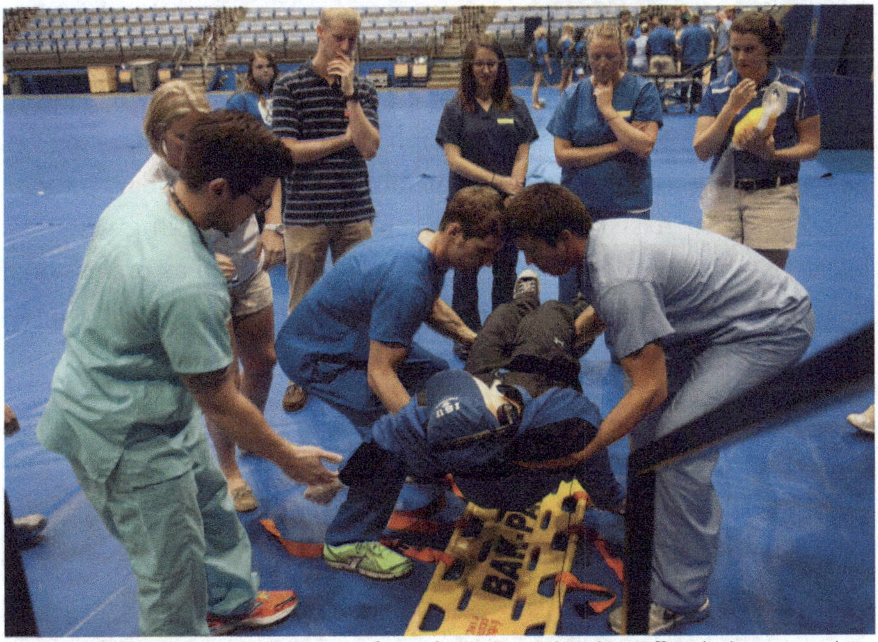

Collaborative training exercise to care for a "football coach" who suffered a heart attack on the sidelines of a game, Terre Haute, IN, 2013 • *Courtesy Indiana State University*

grown to over 100,000 in the United States alone. There has also been a significant amount of international expansion, with PA studies programs opening around the world. Over this fifty-year period, the leaders of the profession faced challenges such as identifying the new occupation's place within the larger field of medicine, standardizing and regulating the field, and responding to the country's changing medical needs. However, I believe the profession's success is largely based on PAs' abilities to listen, respond, and adapt to changing patient needs. For example, as science and medical technology have progressed over the years, PAs have expanded beyond general internal medicine by specializing in a variety of areas such as surgery, dermatology, and obstetrics and gynecology.

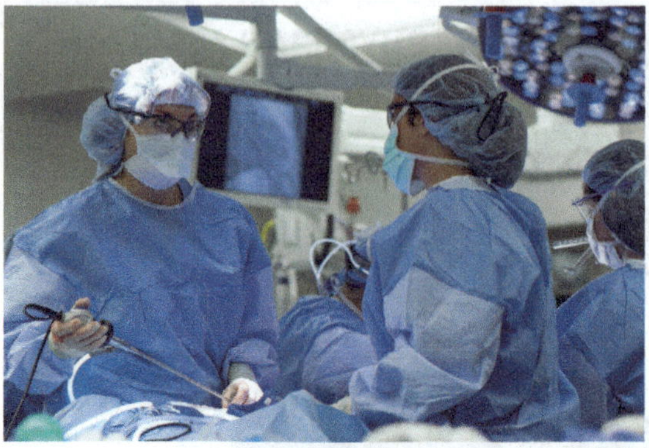

Collaboration with New Partners • At the Cleveland Clinic, Raisa Polacek, PA-C (left) assists during an open-heart surgery, Cleveland, OH, 2015. • *Courtesy Cleveland Clinic*

CN: This is very recent history, what sources did you find most informative as you conducted your research for the exhibition?

LM: The fact that PAs have such a recent history was a unique element of this exhibition. While medical professionals have written books and articles about PAs from a health perspective, there are few historical analyses. This challenge meant that I relied heavily upon primary sources during my research to supplement medically oriented secondary sources. The Physician Assistant History Society was an amazing resource, because it has a wide range of primary sources, such as professional documents, photographs, videos, and oral histories. The Society's book, *The Physician Assistant: An Illustrated History*, was also very helpful,

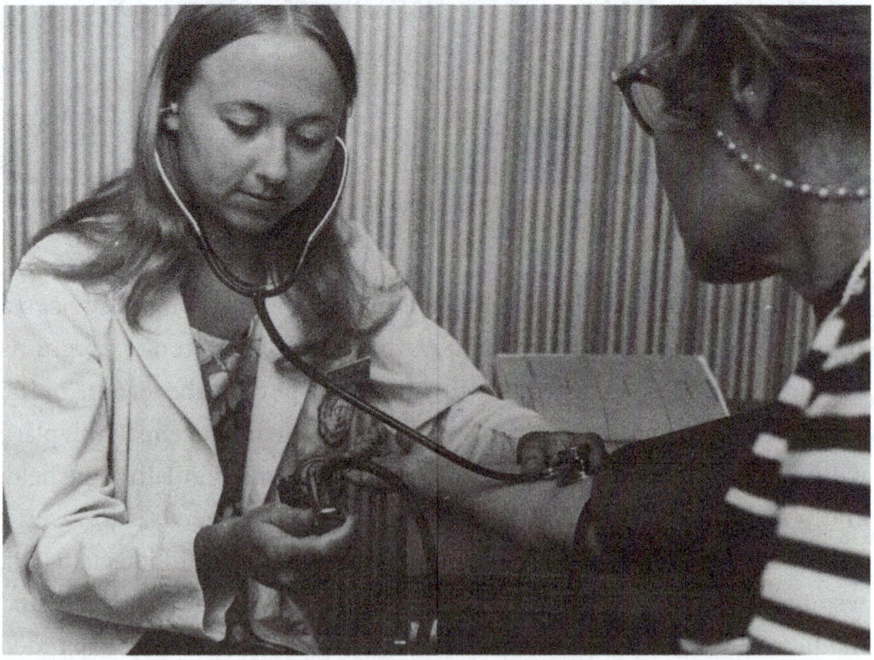

Diversity Makes a Difference • At the School of Allied Health Sciences, University of Texas Medical Branch, Kathy Lester (left) practices taking a patient's blood pressure during her clinical training, Galveston, TX, 1972. • *Courtesy National Library of Medicine*

because it provided a basic overarching history of the profession and biographies of notable PAs. One of my favorite sources at the National Library of Medicine was a collection of early photographs of PAs in the Prints and Photos Collection. Finally, I also used newspaper articles and stories in professional publications, such as the *PA Professional,* to learn about recent events, people, and stories in the field.

CN: In your research for this project, were you drawn to any particular individual's story?

LM: During my research, I was particularly drawn to Joyce Nichols, PA-C, due to her tenacity, perseverance, and generosity. Nichols was the first woman to become a PA, and she overcame many hardships to earn her degree. She grew up on a rural tobacco farm in North Carolina without enough money to pay for her education. At a time when most PA students were White, male, veteran corpsmen, Nichols was a married African American woman with young children. Additionally, during her first

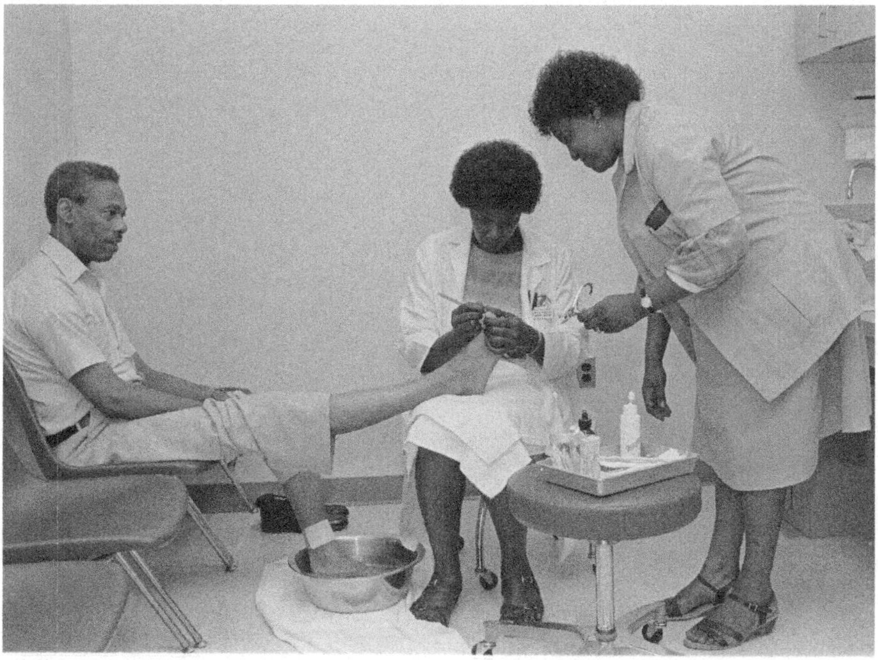

Joyce Nichols, 1983 • Joyce Nichols, PA-C (center) and aide Shirley Thompson (right) treat Raymond Hayes at the Lincoln Community Health Center's foot clinic, Durham, NC, 1983. • *Courtesy University of North Carolina Archives*

year in Duke University's PA studies program, her house burned down and her family lost everything. Despite this setback, Nichols graduated from the program and devoted her career to serving her community and those in need. She created one of the first rural, satellite health clinics in North Carolina dedicated to aiding underserved poor, rural, and African American people. I believe that Nichols' commitment to serving her community and bettering the lives of others truly embodies the values of the profession.

• • •

Dr. Loren E. Miller's presentation is part of our ongoing history of medicine lecture series, which promotes awareness and use of the National Library of Medicine and other historical collections for research, education, and public service in biomedicine, the social sciences, and the humanities. All lectures are live-streamed globally, and subsequently archived, by NIH VideoCast. Stay informed about the lecture series on Twitter at #NLMHistTalk.

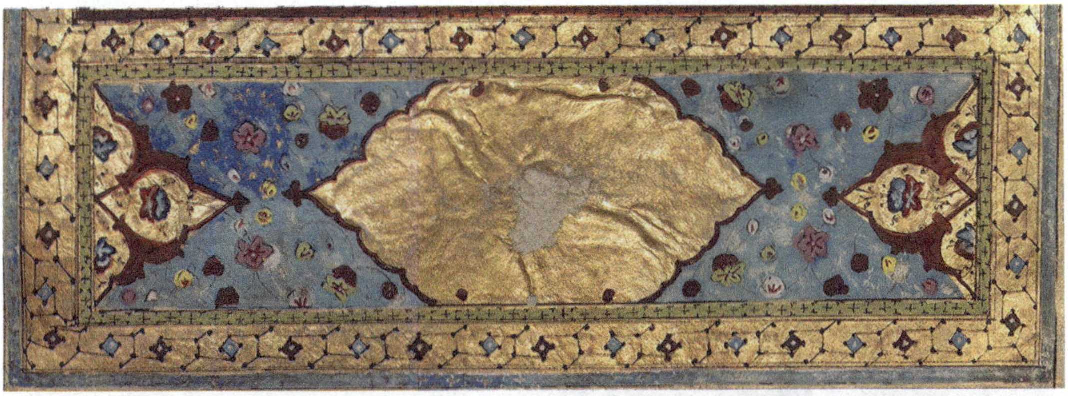

NLM MANUSCRIPTS ON LOAN TO ROMANCE AND REASON

https://circulatingnow.nlm.nih.gov/2018/03/22/nlm-manuscripts-on-loan-to-romance-and-reason/

March 22, 2018 • Rare Books & Journals

ROBERTA CASAGRANDE-KIM

Dr. Roberta Casagrande-Kim is research associate at the Institute for the Study of the Ancient World and assistant manager of exhibitions and publications at the Onassis Foundation USA. She is the co-curator of a new exhibition Romance and Reason: Islamic Transformations of the Classical Past *that opened recently at the Institute for the Study of the Ancient World (ISAW) at New York University. Several early manuscripts from the National Library of Medicine (NLM) historical collections are on display. This is the* *largest and most significant loan* *of collection material by the NLM to a cultural institution for exhibition.* Circulating Now *interviewed Dr. Casagrande-Kim about the exhibition.*

• • •

Circulating Now: Please tell us a little about yourself. Where are you from? What do you do? What is your typical workday like?

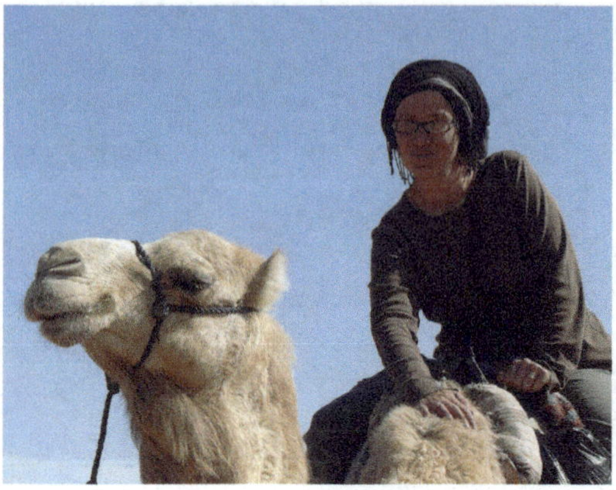

Roberta Casagrande-Kim: I was born in Turin, Italy, and I moved to New York in 2001 to pursue a PhD in Roman art and archeology at the Department of Art History and Archaeology at Columbia University.

I currently work for the Onassis Foundation USA where I manage the planning and implementation of exhibitions of ancient art as well as the production of their accompanying catalogues. In my free time I enjoy curating exhibitions (when I get a chance to). *Romance and Reason* is a perfect example of a stimulating collaboration with two co-curators, as well as among many museums, libraries, and cultural institutions.

I am also actively involved in archeological excavations: since 2006 I have been part of the team excavating the late antique site of Amheida, the ancient capital of the Oasis of Dakhla, in the Egyptian Western Desert. Since 2016, I have also been working at the site of Kinik Höyük in Southern Cappadocia (Turkey), where I investigate the Hellenistic phases of a site that originated in the Hittite period.

In the little time left, I study and publish on a variety of topics that draw my interest: my last two publications are an article on gem collecting during the Roman period, and a monograph, together with other scholars, on the graffiti at the basilica of Smirna (modern Izmir, Turkey) dated to the Imperial and Late Antique period.

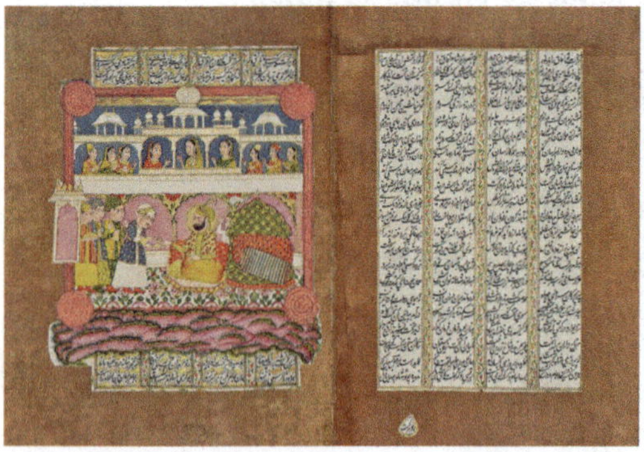

Khamsa by Nizami Ganjavi; Iskandar Served Kay Khusraw's Magical Goblet (jam-i jahan bin), seventeenth century, illustrations possibly later • *From the collections of The National Library of Israel*

CN: You've just finished work on the exhibition, *Romance and Reason*, that opened recently, what sparked your interest in curating this exhibition?

RCK: I was immediately intrigued by the transformation of Alexander the Great into Iskandar in the Persian epic poems. I wanted to explore to what degree Islamic culture assimilated true and fantastic aspects of Alexander's life and adventures as narrated in ancient Greek and Roman historical treatises and, more importantly, in the so-called *Alexander Romance*. I also was captivated by the degree of "persianization" of the character of Iskandar: the manipulation of the stories about Alexander created a new character that reflected the interests and aspirations of the Persian ruling dynasties.

The subject of Islamic assimilation of the ancient past pushed me to also look beyond Alexander, thus opening the exhibition to the investigation of the role of ancient exact sciences in medieval Islam.

CN: Tell us something we probably don't know about Alexander.

RCK: One interesting aspect of the adoption and incorporation of the character of Alexander in medieval Persian epics is the association, both in ancient Greek and Roman times and in later Islamic secular and religious literature, of Alexander/Iskandar as the "two horned one."

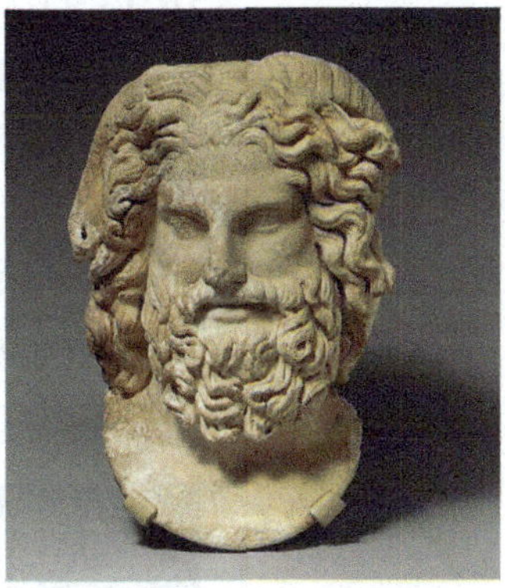

Marble head of Zeus Ammon, ca. 120 to 160 CE • *Courtesy The Metropolitan Museum of Art*

The historian Arrian of Nicomedia (ca. 86–160 CE) describes in his *Anabasis* a trip that Alexander took in February 332 BCE to the oasis of Siwa, in the Lybian desert, to consult the oracle of Ammon, a Lybian divinity. Ammon was usually shown with the horns of a ram and entered the Egyptian pantheon as a manifestation of the Egyptian god Amun. While Alexander's question to the oracle remains unknown, Arrian reports that he received "the answer that his heart desired." As a result of the trip, Alexander presented himself as the son of Ammon: coins and statuettes were produced portraying him with ram's horns. The episode of the oracle of Ammon was included in the *Alexander Romance*.

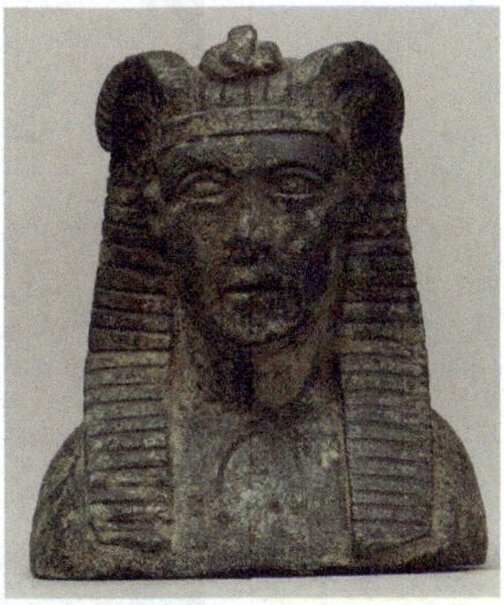

Bust of Alexander, with ram's horns, 150 BC to 200 CE • *Courtesy The Metropolitan Museum of Art*

This tradition of the horned Alexander also appears, in a different guise, in the Quran. In the exhibition we display a copy of Chapter eighteen (*Surat al-Kahf* [the Cave]), which refers to a cryptic figure known as "the Two-Horned One" (in Arabic, *dhu al-qarnayn*). The text relates that "the Two-Horned One" traveled east and west, meeting different peoples, and built a metal wall to protect against Gog and Magog—all motifs that were taken up in the later Persian

Alexander epics. Most medieval Islamic commentators have identified *dhu al-qarnayn* as Alexander the Great. Though the Quran only devotes sixteen verses to the story of "the Two-Horned One," the reference is amplified and expanded in Muslim literature where Alexander is transformed from conqueror to faithful prophet and mystical seeker.

In the late Persian prose work *The Story of Iskandar, The Two-Horned One*, which draws on the Quranic story and its commentaries, the Persian epics, and popular folktales, Iskandar is even depicted as having actual horns.

CN: More broadly, the exhibition explores the exchange of images and ideas between people and nations between the eighth and tenth century CE, what do these texts tell us about medieval Islamic culture?

RCK: The exhibition is an eye-opener, for people like me who do not have a background in Islamic studies, on the fundamental and defining role of medieval Islamic scholars in the assimilation and reformulation of Classical scientific knowledge as well as of Classical culture. More broadly, the manuscripts on view in the exhibition show how Islamic thinkers and artists conveyed, conceived, and reimagined—in words and in pictures—the ancient Greek classical heritage.

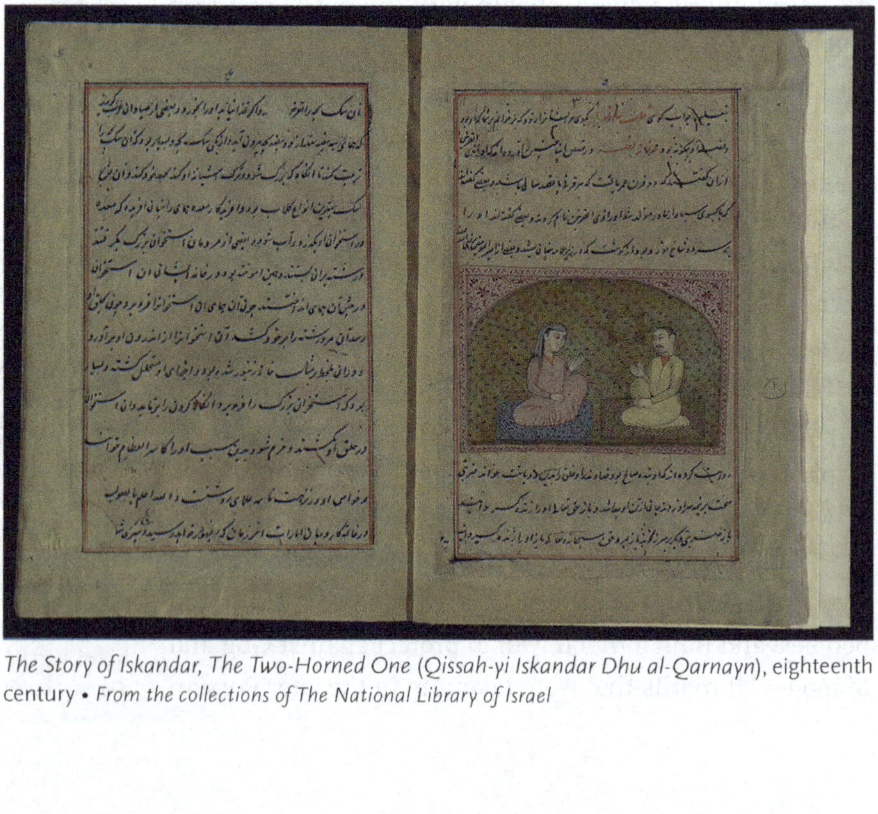

The Story of Iskandar, The Two-Horned One (*Qissah-yi Iskandar Dhu al-Qarnayn*), eighteenth century • *From the collections of The National Library of Israel*

Romance and Reason aims to show how the Islamic engagement with the classical intellectual heritage—in translation, commentary, integration, and full-throated debate—was in no way passive or derivative. Islamic thinkers actively expanded, and even argued with, the body of Greek knowledge. Moreover, that active engagement was not unified, but multiple, changeable, and diverse—truly "transformations" rather than a singular "transformation."

CN: The National Library of Medicine is pleased to have loaned eleven early manuscripts for the exhibition, what part of the narrative of *Romance and Reason* do these works inform?

RCK: The manuscripts generously loaned by the NLM constitute the core of the exhibition's investigation on the exact sciences, presenting to the public a series of images and texts that cover the Islamic interest in mathematics, astronomy, astrology, and medicine.

On display is one of the only four complete Arabic copies of *Canon of Medicine* by Avicenna, an encyclopedia that systematized, critiqued, and developed the traditional Greek Galenic medical theory. Widely read among Islamic physicians, it was commonly used in its Latin editions as a textbook for medical training in European universities, and inspired a new medical literature of abridgments, epitomes, and commentaries. This copy is decorated with illuminated openings made at one of the many flourishing Iranian workshops where manuscripts were copied, compiled, and illuminated, often for the libraries of the Timurid rulers (1370–1507 CE), who were great patrons of the art of books.

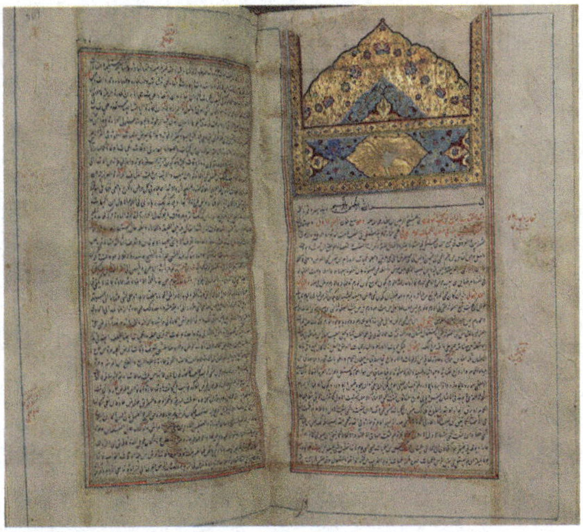

Arabic copy of *Canon of Medicine* by Avicenna, early fifteenth century • *Bruce M. White, photographer, 2017, National Library of Medicine #940377*

In the exhibition is also the third-oldest known Arabic manuscript, dated to November 30, 1094, comprising the third section of the *Comprehensive Book on Medicine* by Abu Bakr Razi, a prolific writer of texts on medicine, alchemy, astronomy, and philosophy. This treatise was posthumously assembled as a notebook collecting extracts of Razi's

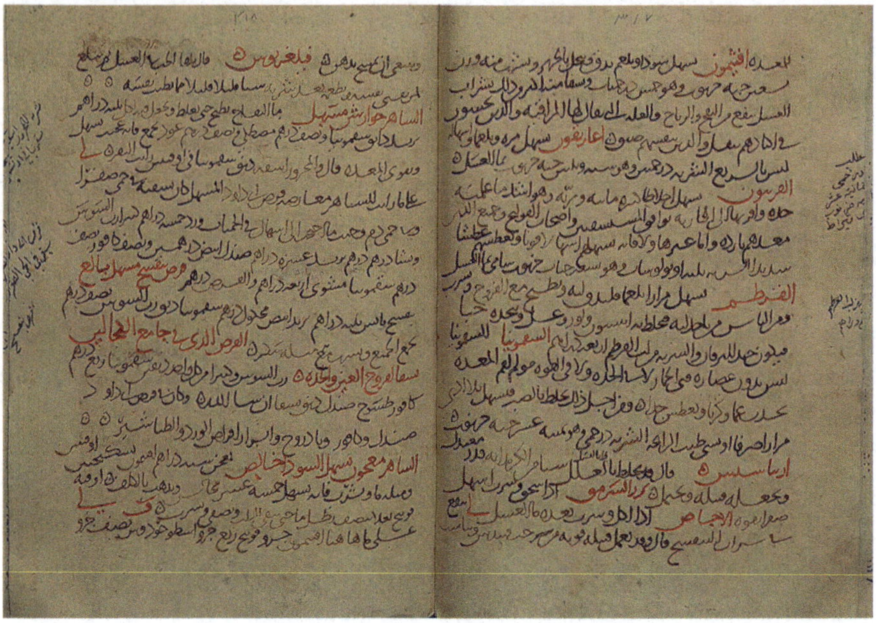

The third-oldest known Arabic manuscript, dated to November 30, 1094, comprising the third section of the *Comprehensive Book on Medicine* by Abu Bakr Razi • *Bruce M. White, photographer, 2017, National Library of Medicine #9404682*

works on diseases and therapies, as well as his personal observations and interpretations of clinical cases.

Among the most intriguing images in the "scientific" part of the exhibition, are two representations of the human body (illustrations of the venous and skeletal systems) from two NLM copies of the *Mansur's Anatomy*. Full depictions of various body systems first appeared in Islamic medical literature as illustrations to Mansur ibn Ilyas of Shiraz's Persian treatise on surgery. His *Anatomy* was influenced primarily by Galen's anatomical studies and Aristotle's embryological theory. Comprising five books, ibn Ilyas's work focused on the bones, nerves, muscles, veins and arteries, and compound organs. All five books were accompanied by diagrams of the body that were possibly inspired by medieval Latin Western works rather than earlier Greek sources.

CN: You're an archeologist, what's it like to work on a project entirely based on books?

RCK: I believe that "digging" in a library or museum looking for books or artifacts to populate an exhibition's checklist is not that different from

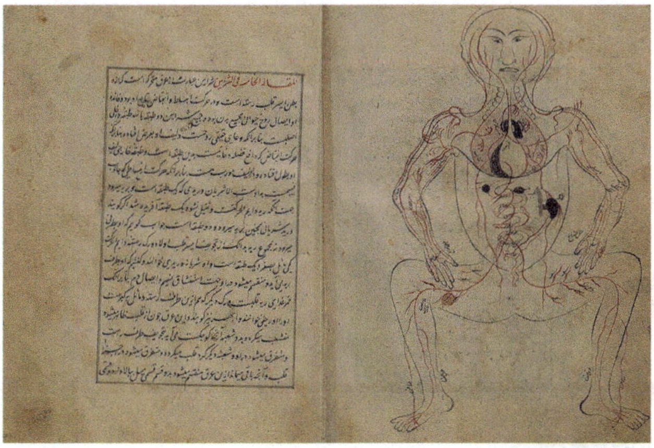

Representation of the human venous system in *Mansur's Anatomy*, December 8, 1488 • *Bruce M. White, photographer, 2017, National Library of Medicine #9403778*

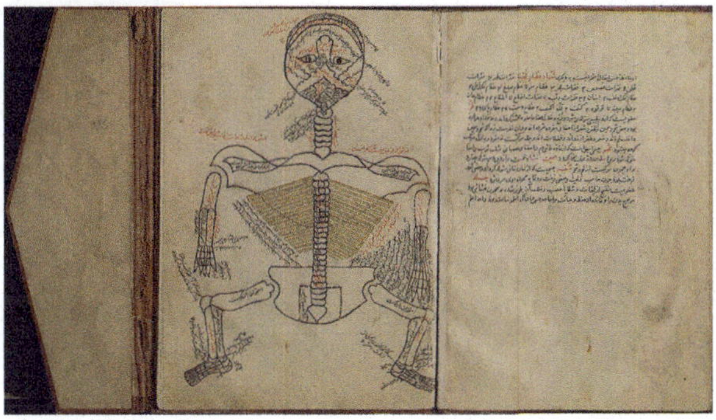

Representation of the human skeletal system in *Mansur's Anatomy*, ca. 1400s • *Bruce M. White, photographer, 2017, National Library of Medicine #9403778*

digging in the field. In both instances, we are looking for answers to specific questions we have about the past. In both instances, the results of our quest are objects (or architectures, in the field) that speak to us of cultures, civilizations, and societies that continue to play a major role in shaping what are today's traditions and cultural and moral values.

Also, exhibitions and excavations (especially if they result in sites open to the public) are two ways in which scholars of antiquity share their knowledge of the past, or of aspects of it, with the general public.

• • •

Visit Romance and Reason: Islamic Transformations of the Classical Past *at the Institute for the Study of the Ancient World at New York University now through May 13, 2018.*

CHAPTER 4

DATA IN THE DETAILS

INTRODUCTION • JOHN REES

"I believe . . ."

In 1969, two physicians presented their beliefs as they debated divergent conclusions about the use of smallpox vaccines drawn from the same data. The debate occurred as part of a film series produced by the National Medical Audiovisual Center at the National Library of Medicine (NLM), as a forum to explore health and medical concerns of the day, and was highlighted in the *Circulating Now* post "Revealing Data: Concepts and Controversies in Modern Medicine, 1969–70." The post recalls George Canning's adage, "I can prove anything by statistics except the truth."

Exploring beliefs, understanding truths (both comfortable and uncomfortable), recreating the past, asking questions about ourselves and the world around us—these are all the province of the historical enterprise writ large. Work is conducted by seeking and evaluating data, both qualitative and quantitative, to argue a case for generalizable knowledge about a person, a place, a controversy, a cause, or an event. *Circulating Now* has commissioned and published a series of posts designed to "reveal data" in the historical collections of the NLM in the context of the historian's craft and the work of librarians and archivists who build collections in large part to support history. In the posts that constitute this chapter, we see both old and new themes in the context of data. These themes include understanding our work through the lens of data science, showcasing the historian's labor, and finding new stories from "old data."

"Revealing Data: Explorations of Data in Collections" launched the series for *Circulating Now* in May 2017, to support one of the NLM's key 2017–2027 strategic plan initiatives as "the new home of data science at the National Institutes of Health (NIH)." Here, Christie Moffatt synthesizes the conversations and debates of archivists around what data means to the archival enterprise and in the context of a strategic plan. She also communicates what it means to be a collecting organization in the service of the historical enterprise employed to the labor of history and our mission to collect, preserve, and provide access to the unique collections that allow inquiring minds to discover newness about the human condition. Yes, we are surrounded by the "data" of our collections just as we have been throughout our life as an organization. Moffatt's post helpfully reveals a tension in traditional archival collecting relative to the overarching, rapidly expanding digital world. How are we thinking more critically about our role in collecting observational scientific data and therefore changing the direction of our labor? Equally, how are we thinking critically about the implications of that change in direction? Given the sheer scope of the historical collections of the NLM, to what extent should we substitute "collections" with "data" as a semantic exercise without addressing these key questions and pursuing new opportunities? Or is there a happy middle ground that archivists can reasonably occupy and from which we can advance our traditional enterprise while embracing and advancing the new trajectory of the Library?

I believe the answer is "yes, and"—that yes we can re-contextualize the "data" that has always been in our collections, and we can collect new kinds of archives and provide them in new formats to aid discovery, re-use, and computational inquiry. The expertise archivists and librarians bring to describing and contextualizing our collections as data sources for new and interesting uses is at the core of our labor. "Revealing Data: Why We Need Humans to Curate Web Collections" is an example of the traditional value informational professionals bring to the table in a new arena. Some NLM staff may not become data scientists, but they can nonetheless embrace the work of the data science enterprise in the context of the historical enterprise. Computer scientist Alexander Nwala uses machine learning algorithms to explore a classification question. He created a new dataset, using the NLM's selection process approach to website collecting, to test a computational model that provided statistically valid answers to the question, "Can automated unsupervised computer processes select more relevant websites than human curators?" In another example of Canning's adage, the answer was a qualitative "yes" in that it depended on the context of the question, whether it matters to your desired outcome to have a web archive collection with a deep, long tail that requires many resources to develop, or you are interested in a quick snapshot of a current event that took fewer resources to collect, but also contains some irrelevant content. Also, Nwala's selection approaches are biased and not equivalent—his computers only generated search results from search engines associated with Google, Twitter, etc., which themselves are algorithmically biased, whereas NLM curators use a much broader set of selection sources. *Circulating Now* surfaces these cost-benefit questions that archivists and librarians ask every day across all our collecting activities. These questions point to examples of how we might use data-driven results as elements in the complex business management processes chain that drives our collection development work.

For generations, historians and legions of graduate assistants have mined historical content including census records, election polling data, ship passenger logs, and estate inventories to produce numerical datasets for statistical analysis as evidence to prove qualitative historical theories. Compiling these data are the science and labor behind the art of crafting an engaging historical narrative. Posts by professors E. Thomas Ewing and Sarah Runcie are two clear examples. Ewing's "Revealing Data: Measuring Mortality during an Epidemic" is a classic example of the traditional hard labor tasks required to generate numerical data from the free text. Using these numerical data enables Ewing to create new charts and graphical visualizations that reinforce his narrative, create a more convincing argument, and make it all the easier to understand the factual data deeply embedded in narrative texts published across a long timeframe, in this case the Russian influenza epidemic of 1889–1890. It is a wonder that contemporary public health officials were able to make decisions having to wade through such complex narratives. Hopefully Ewing's task was made easier by leveraging the digitized full-text contents of the *British Medical Journal* through PubMed Central, but no amount of artificial intelligence or machine learning could magically solve the problem of converting numbers-as-narrative to data.

Sarah Runcie's interview, "Naming, Networks, and Power in Histories of Medicine in Africa," is an important contribution along with the work of her many colleagues who participated in the 2018 *Viral Networks* research workshop hosted by the NLM, funded by the Office of Digital Humanities of the National Endowment for the Humanities, and organized by Virginia Tech. Not only does Runcie's work illustrate the historian's labor needed to derive statistical data from archival records, she embraces new data science tools and techniques to tell a story, but most importantly to use data science to uncover the lost and silent voices of colonized Africans. It is common to see data visualizations that illustrate or validate known assumptions about a topic, but it is rare to see them used in the historian's craft as null-hypothesis experiments—to surface and ask questions about what and who are missing from a narrative. Runcie and other twenty-first century digital humanists/historians are thinking like computer scientists, flipping hypotheses and asking, "What is missing from my data, what gaps in the historical record are my data revealing?" This is important, if uncomfortable, work that scholars and memory-preserving institutions need to prioritize to surface and recognize aspects of cultural and social hegemony biases that exist in the collections of our largely White memory institutions.

Finally, Ashley Bowen's "Revealing Data: Rain, Epidemics, and Life on the Docks in 1918" is the type of classic historical craftwork that led me to pursue a career in the humanities. Bowen explores one of the Library's Marine Hospital Station Journals whose day-to-day entries serve as a diary that allows us to partially re-create and re-live the everyday life of individuals whose voices are likely to not be documented otherwise. In my past life as a cultural historian, I wondered what life was like for the yeoman farmer of colonial Virginia. When I read Rhys Isaac's *The Transformation of Virginia, 1740–1790* (1982) and David Hackett Fischer's *Albion's Seed* (1989) in graduate school, the wonder of exploring data hidden in the material culture recorded in estate tax inventories, traced in the foot-trail maps between farm and church, and echoed in the voice of architecture opened a world not captured in the biographies of politicians and statesmen. Bowen's storytelling about the daily comings and goings of the day's weather, of ships, cargo, base repairs, and immigrants and how these seemingly ordinary people were affected (or in this case, not affected) by the 1918 flu pandemic is the kind of scholarship I want to read. Similar to Sarah Runcie's work, Bowen's post exposes the story missing from the available data as much as it explains what is recorded. It is why I show off these station journals in every collections tour I give. The blog posts in this chapter demonstrate the value our existing collections have always contributed to the scholarly enterprise as well as asking what more can or should we be doing to satisfy the information needs of future historians. I continue to think that the archival program should leave data warehousing and computational data science to our expert colleagues in the National Center for Biotechnology Information and the many other domain-based data repositories that exist across academia and industry, but we can and should collect the papers of figures like Jack Wennberg, the pioneer healthcare researcher, and others who use data to explore, critique, and solve the big issues of their times and provide the context for why data is important to the history of medicine and the health sciences. We can find new ways such as web archiving to document and preserve the quieter voices left behind by "traditional" archival collecting. We can digitize more of our analog collections and better advertise their availability to make collections computationally-ready to some small degree, if messy. We can preserve the born-digital contents of our collections, the floppy disks and hard drives, in their original state to be re-used as data. We can add value by transforming messy data into more data science ready formats when the business needs and resources allow. "I believe . . ." we will see *Circulating Now* continue to publish the work of many more researchers who use our collections to expand the boundaries of the archival and historical enterprises.

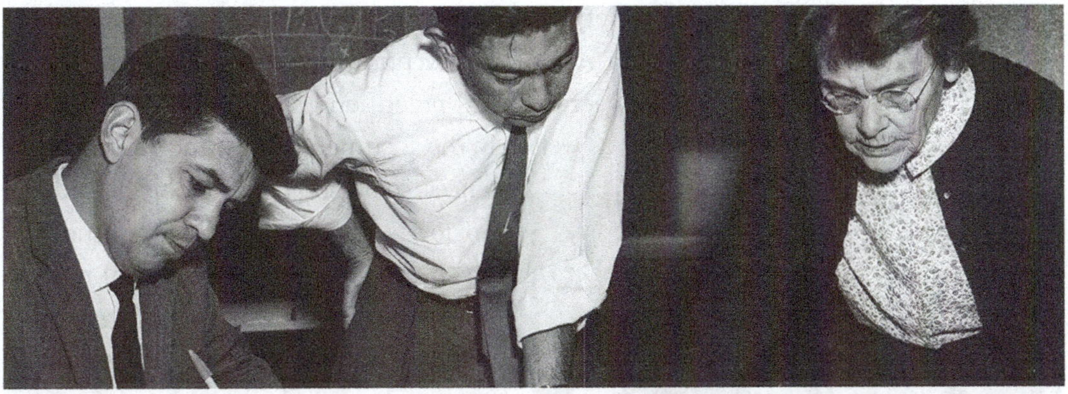

REVEALING DATA: EXPLORATIONS OF DATA IN COLLECTIONS

https://circulatingnow.nlm.nih.gov/2017/05/17/revealing-data-explorations-of-data-in-collections/

May 17, 2017 • Revealing Data

CHRISTIE MOFFATT

We hear about data every day. In historical medical collections, data abounds, both quantitative and qualitative. In its format, scope, and biases, data inherently contains more information than its face value. This series, Revealing Data, explores how, by preserving the research data of the past and making it publicly available, the National Library of Medicine (NLM) helps to ensure that generations of researchers can reexamine it, reveal new stories, and make new discoveries. As the NLM becomes the new home of data science at the National Institutes of Health (NIH), Circulating Now *explores what researchers from a variety of disciplines are learning from centuries of preserved data, and how their work can help us think about the future preservation and uses of the data we collect today.*

• • •

Within the NLM's historical collections there are formal recordings of data in scientific laboratory notebooks, charts, logs, drawings, photographic images, and in a variety of other formats. The collections also include a wide range of data recorded informally, in jotted-down notes and correspondence between medical practitioners and scientists of many disciplines and fields, as well as in the documentation of individual experiences, in personal diaries, blogs, and oral histories. In addition to presenting data itself, this diversity of material reflects the many ways in which data is gathered, visualized, analyzed, and shared among personal networks, members of a team or lab, the broader scientific and medical community, and with the public, in lectures, reports, speeches, posters, moving images, and social media.

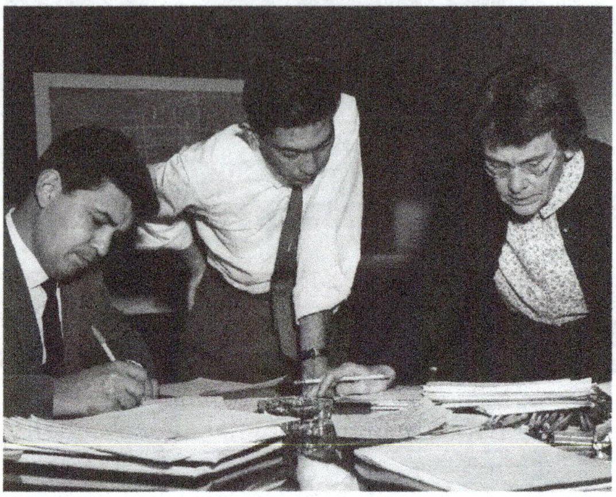

Discussing Data • Almiro Blumenschein, Angel Kato, and Barbara McClintock with research notes, 1966 • *Courtesy American Philosophical Society,* Profiles in Science, *National Library of Medicine*

Often these recordings of data include important details and observations that reflect the larger world around the data and its collector, including biases; ethical norms; and technological, physical, or other challenges that reflect the state of research and research practices of the time. Examining these observations carefully, one can begin to discern the bigger stories behind the data: the what, when, where, why, and how the research was done. And when we collect and preserve materials related to data-specific sources—like correspondence between Barbara McClintock and collaborators while researching the origins of maize in South America, and Joshua Lederberg's laboratory notebooks documenting his experiments on the genetics of bacteria, research that led both to later earn a Nobel Prize—we can achieve deeper understanding of these big stories. Together, these different but complementary kinds of historical materials help to document research processes, as well as the myriad medical, social, and cultural contexts in which data is recorded, analyzed, discussed, and reported.

Marshall Nirenberg and his research team, for example, collectively and painstakingly prepared a chart as they discovered how sequences of DNA, known as "triplets," direct the assembly of amino acids into the structural and functional proteins essential to life, a first summary of

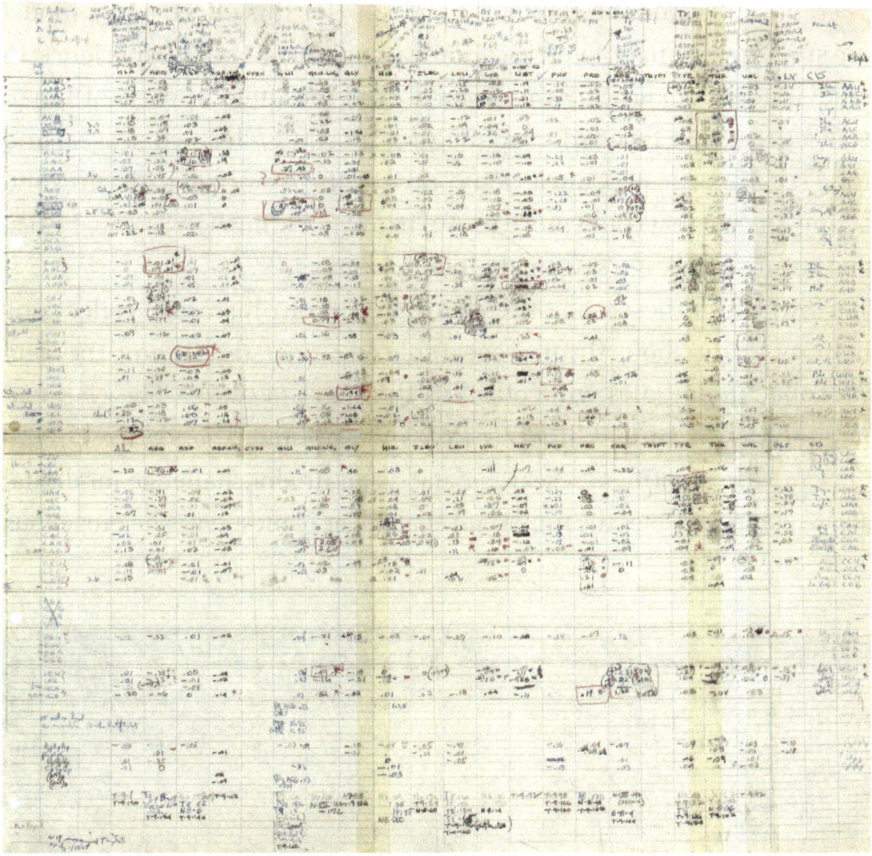

Recorded Data • Nirenberg's Handwritten Genetic Code Chart, 1965 • Profiles in Science, *National Library of Medicine*

the genetic code. But the chart is in a code all its own. Specific notations refer to laboratory notebooks: "N7-88," for example, refers to the laboratory notebook labeled "Norma, book 7, page 88." Experiments referring to "T" are in the laboratory notebooks of Theresa Caryk. The Library's collection of Marshall Nirenberg Papers contains the context, in oral histories, notebooks, letters, photographs, and other documentation, to translate not only the data in the chart, but the process and impact of the discovery.

In another example, detailed instructions for inspectors in Fred Soper's Yellow Fever Service operation in Brazil show how data was collected, describes the tools used, and includes sample forms, including definitions of terminology, used to track inspections and advise action. Soper literally "wrote the book" on effective eradication procedures and personnel management; the Yellow Fever Service manual of operations became the standard handbook for this effort, and a model for subsequent malaria eradication campaigns. Soper's experience in studying and eradicating the *Aedes aegypti* mosquito in parts of Brazil was a great step forward in managing mosquito-borne diseases, and the Fred Soper Papers are a rich source of the history of gathering and acting on data that could prove useful in today's campaigns against Zika, and future campaign's against other epidemics.

How might these and other examples in our historical collections help us think about future research and understanding of the data we collect today, and will collect in the years to come? The National Digital Stewardship Alliance's (NDSA) National Agenda for Digital Stewardship identifies "research data" as an urgent challenge for digital stewardship, and cites the important challenges of preserving heterogenous

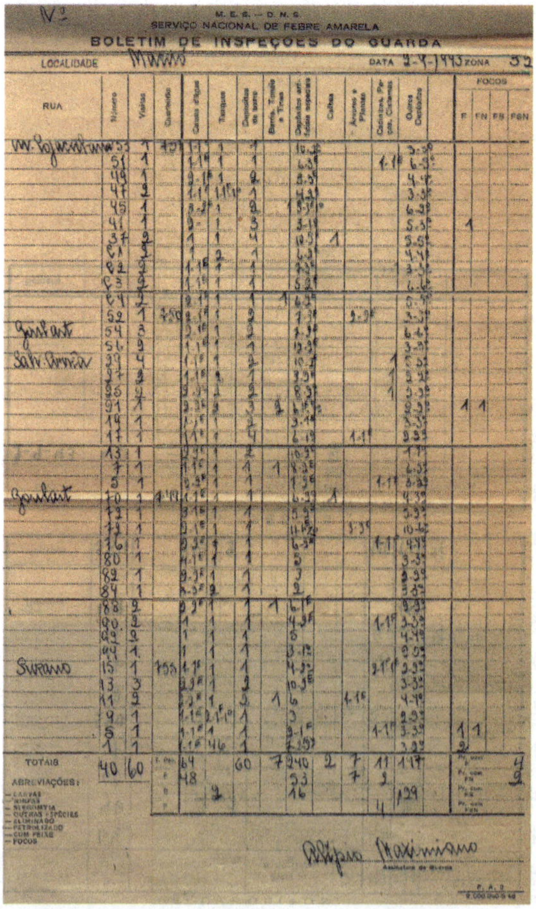
M. E. S. — D. N. S.
SERVIÇO NACIONAL DE FEBRE AMARELA
BOLETIM DE INSPEÇÕES DO GUARDA
LOCALIDADE
DATA
ZONA
RUA
FOCOS
TOTAIS
ABREVIAÇÕES:

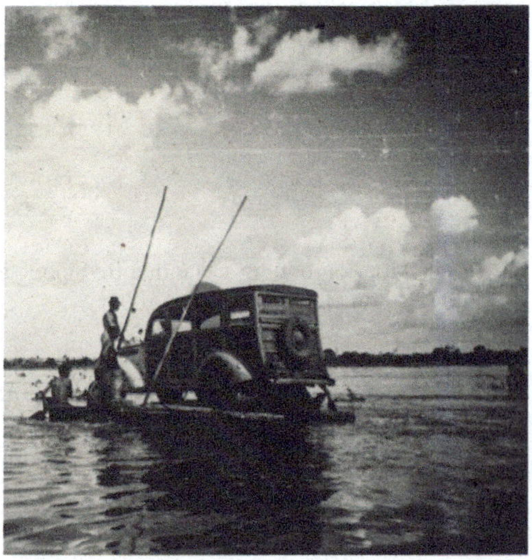

RIGHT Collecting Data • Jaguaribe river in Ceara, Brazil, ca. 1930s • Profiles in Science, *National Library of Medicine*

LEFT Data Tables in *Boletim De Inspecoes Do Guarda*, 1943 • Soper's field manual contains this, the Yellow Fever Service report form used by Brazilian inspectors, whose title translates to "Officer's Record of Inspection." • Profiles in Science, *National Library of Medicine*

data, different information standards and management practices across scientific disciplines, and the sheer volume of material being generated. In addition to preserving research data itself, scientific and cultural heritage communities also emphasize the need to preserve the context of current research: in the near-term, to support data sharing and reuse, and in the long-term, to document the record of scientific knowledge, discovery, and innovation, changes in scientific and scholarly communication, and public understandings of science and science policy. What kinds of documentation (also in challenging and heterogenous data types) do we need to preserve alongside current data to document the broader context in which it is created, so that researchers in the future can reexamine it, reveal new stories, and make new discoveries?

Throughout this series, we will explore the many ways in which we document research and communicate about data, and what we can learn by preserving related material for context and understanding. This exploration will illuminate research as it was being undertaken, as well as subsequent discoveries that have emerged from studying the original research. And this exploration will help to reveal the important and evolving relationships between the creators of data and the work of many today—archivists, historians, librarians, data scientists, and others—who are actively and proactively taking collective responsibility for the long-term preservation and curation of, and access to, historical and contemporary data for tomorrow.

REVEALING DATA: LONDON'S DEADLY VISITATION

https://circulatingnow.nlm.nih.gov/2017/09/27/revealing-data-londons-deadly-visitation/

September 27, 2017 • Rare Books & Journals, Revealing Data, Guests

KRISTIN HEITMAN

Circulating Now *welcomes guest blogger Kristin Heitman, PhD, who shares her insights on seventeenth-century data collection and analysis as part of our Revealing Data series. Dr. Heitman is an independent scholar living in Bethesda, Maryland. She and Professor Vanessa Harding of Birkbeck College, University of London, will convene a symposium on the London Bills of Mortality as part of the 2017–2018 program of the Folger Institute in Washington, DC.*

• • •

London's Dreadful Visitation, 1665–66 is often presented as a Bill of Mortality from the Great Plague, in which an estimated 25 percent of Londoners died. The work is actually a collection of reprints of fifty-two weekly bills plus an annual summary. Its title page declares it a *memento mori*—a reminder of the imminence of death—while the introduction, written by the printer E. Cotes, argues that perusing the bills plus a bit of careful thought would show that God did not furiously dole out the wages of sin but mercifully spared the survivors, who then had more time to repent.

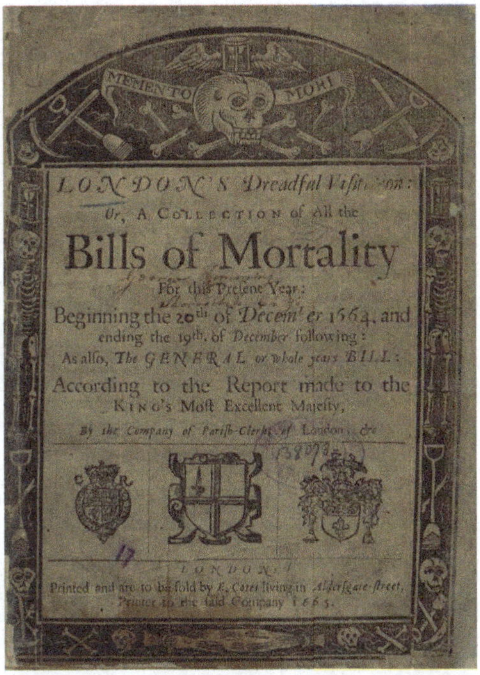
MEMENTO MORI
LONDON'S Dreadful Visit[illegible]on:
Or, A COLLECTION of All the
Bills of Mortality
For this Present Year:
Beginning the 20th of December 1664. and ending the 19th. of December following:
As also, The GENERAL or whole years BILL:
According to the Report made to the KING's Most Excellent Majesty,
By the Company of Parish-Clerks of London, &c.
LONDON,
Printed and are to be sold by E. Cotes living in Aldersgate-street, Printer to the said Company 1665.

London's Dreadful Visitation, 1665–1666 • *National Library of Medicine #2378023R*

It is a peculiar document on many counts. First, apart from the striking title page and brief introduction, Cotes provided only a series of numerical tables. The London Bills of Mortality were neither medical records nor a way to document the deaths of individuals. They were tabulated, parish-by-parish counts of burials as compiled each week by the Company of Parish Clerks, a London guild. The original surveillance program, ordered by the English Crown during the plague of 1519, was executed by London's merchant-aldermen. While other European cities kept plague *rolls*—rosters in which designated local physicians recorded each plague victim's name and social status—London recorded only counts.

Second, the Bills included weekly counts of baptisms, and of mortalities not just of plague but of causes such as old age, childbirth, accidents and suicides, smallpox, and scurvy. The Parish Clerks had conducted comprehensive mortality counts for London's aldermen since the mid-1550s, with baptisms added by the mid-1560s. Cause of death was determined by the local clerk until that duty passed to parish women appointed and trained as inspectors ("searchers") of the dead, apparently during the plague of 1592–23. These regular, comprehensive reports went only to London's aldermen, although the Crown and Chancellor began to receive next-day copies after a formal request from William Cecil, Chancellor to Elizabeth I. Publication began at the turn of the century, in step with the rising numeracy of London's population. During the plagues of 1596–97 and 1601–02, the City's printer nailed up official broadsides displaying the week's parish-by-parish counts of baptisms, plague deaths, and total burials. In 1626–67, the Parish Clerks began to print their own two-sided weekly handbills with data from the broader program instituted in the

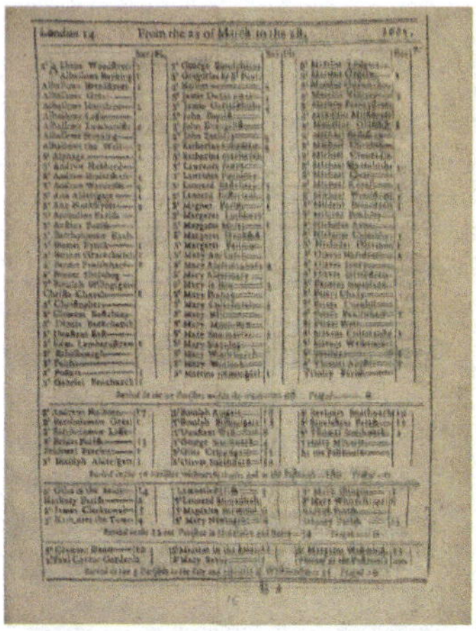

March 21–28, 1665 • *National Library of Medicine #2378023R*

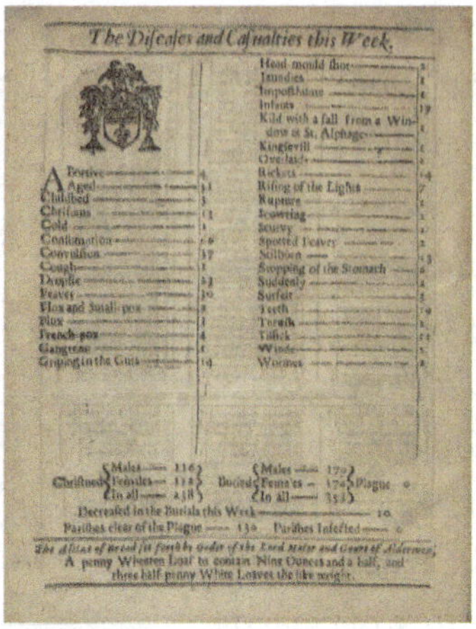

Parishes clear of plague—130 • *National Library of Medicine #2378023R*

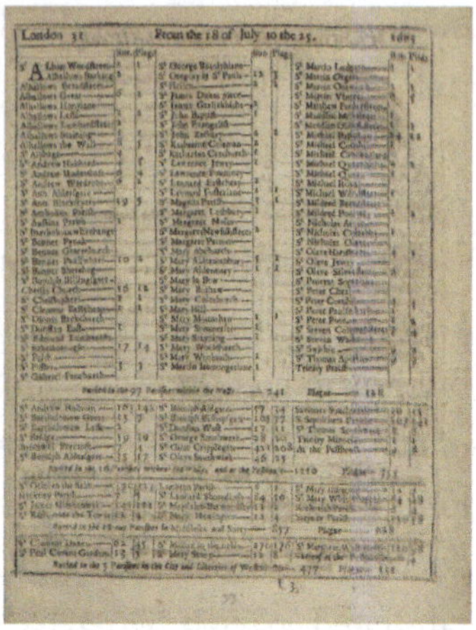

July 18–25, 1665 • *National Library of Medicine #2378023R*

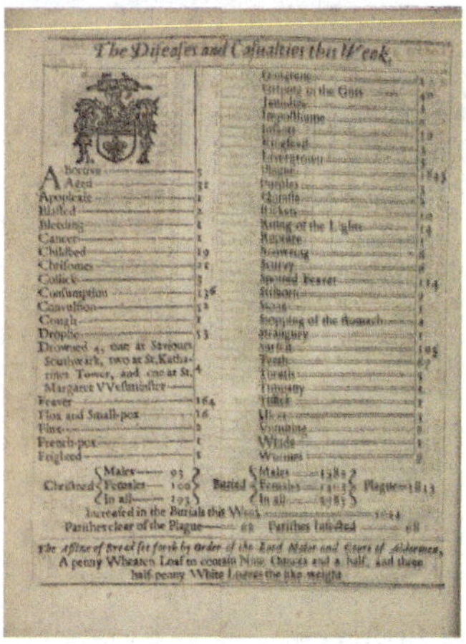

Parishes clear of plague—62 • *National Library of Medicine #2378023*

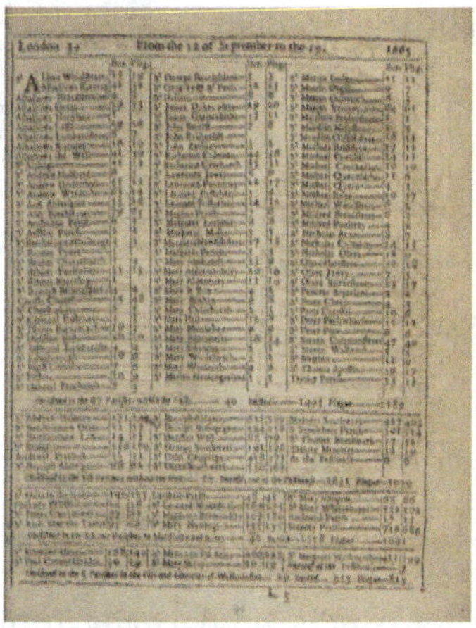

September 12–19, 1665 • *National Library of Medicine #2378023R*

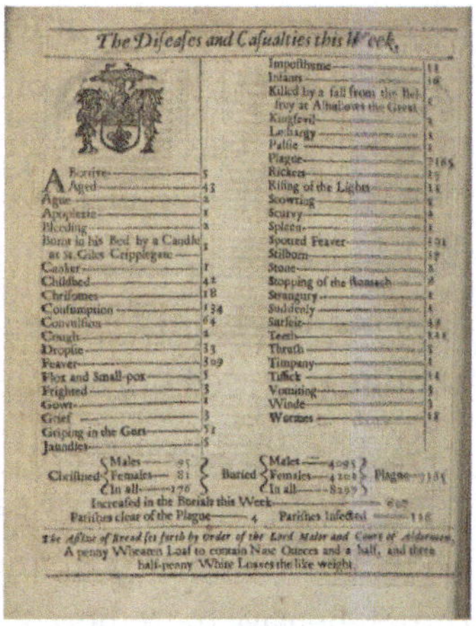

Parishes clear of plague—4 • *National Library of Medicine #2378023R*

1550s, plus an annual summary bill at Christmas. *London's Dreadful Visitation* reproduces 1665's bills in full.

Why would anyone buy a whole year's worth of outdated handbills? So many of these bills have survived to the present that historians believe they must have sold quite well. Yet they were ephemera, their information outdated from week to week. Cotes framed her work simply as a spiritual exercise, but the official Bills had already gained new interest with John Graunt's ground-breaking *Natural and Political Observations... Made Upon the Bills of Mortality*, 1662. Graunt proposed the basic methods of

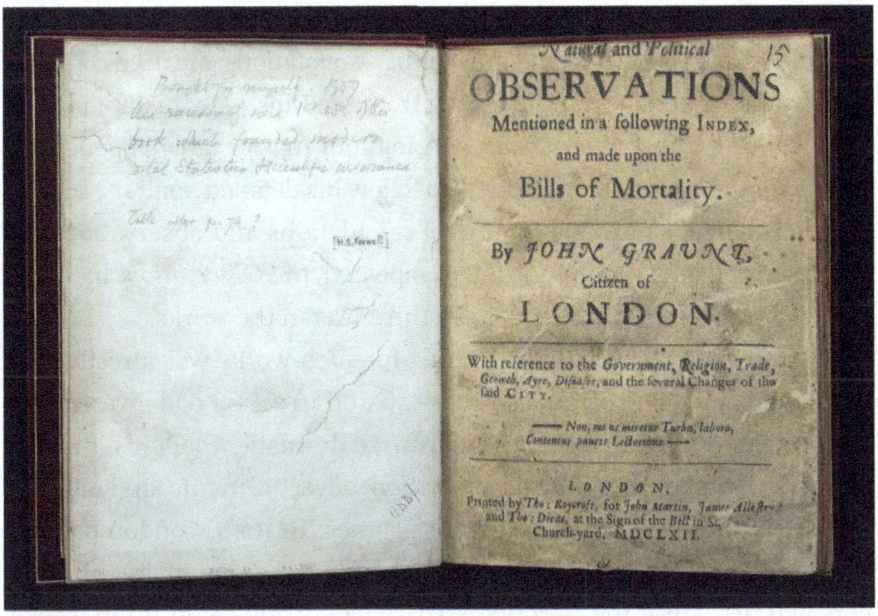

Title page, in *Natural and Political Observations Mentioned in a Following Index, and Made Upon the Bills of Mortality . . .* by John Graunt, 1662. • *National Library of Medicine #2356014R*

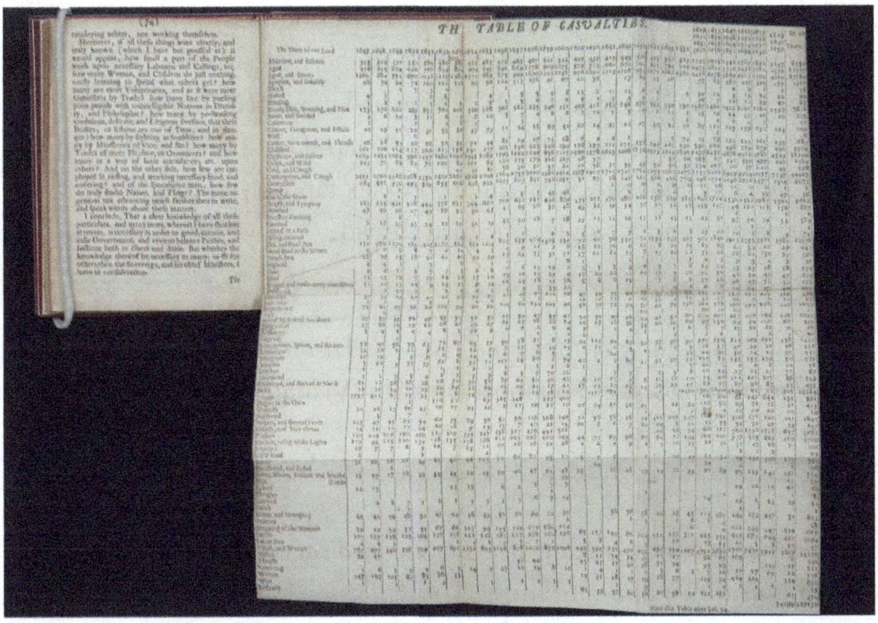

Table of Casualties, in *Natural and Political Observations Mentioned in a Following Index, and Made Upon the Bills of Mortality . . .* by John Graunt, 1662. • *National Library of Medicine #2356014R*

population-data science using only common experience and the "shop arithmetic" of proportions and the four basic operations. He used counts of both baptisms and mortalities drawn from the Bills—not just for plague, but also for more ordinary causes. A fold-out master table appended to the end of the book allowed readers to follow his detailed analysis, acquire the techniques, and make their own calculations and observations. By the time *London's Dreadful Visitation* appeared, the *Observations* had gone through two sold-out editions and a third was in the works.

Even in 1662, however, the market for such works was already both deep and broad. The plagues of 1625–26 and 1636–67 had given rise to "commemorative" broadsides that featured dramatic woodcuts, medical advice, prayers for the sick and the nation, advertisements, and tables of weekly mortality counts for previous plagues. In 1636, London printers began to sell "composite" bills, similar in layout and content but likely for personal use, since they left blank space where one could fill in weekly counts as the epidemic unfolded. Still, *London's Dreadful Visitation* differs from commemorative and composite bills as well, for it provides neither medical advice nor prayers nor even advertisements—just the reprints of the year's official Bills.

Many later assumed that Graunt himself produced *London's Dreadful Visitation* as a sort of companion piece to the *Observations*. We have no evidence for that belief; yet for those who had mastered Graunt's methods, Cotes' reprinted tables could reveal God's hand not striking suddenly in wrath but methodically weaving a complex tapestry of deaths in which plague formed but a single, dreadful thread.

• • •

The National Library of Medicine (NLM)'s History of Medicine Division's collection holds copies of London's Dreadful Visitation *and all five editions of Graunt's* Observations.

• • •

We hear about data every day. In historical medical collections, data abounds, both quantitative and qualitative. In its format, scope, and biases, data inherently contains more information than its face value. This series, Revealing Data, explores how, by preserving the research data of the past and making it publicly available, the National Library of Medicine helps to ensure that generations of researchers can reexamine it, reveal new stories, and make new discoveries. As the NLM becomes the new home of data science at the National Institutes of Health (NIH), Circulating Now *explores what researchers from a variety of disciplines are learning from centuries of preserved data, and how their work can help us think about the future preservation and uses of the data we collect today.*

Reflection

I wrote "Revealing Data: London's Deadly Visitation," as part of the lead-up to a 2018 Folger Research Institute seminar on the London Bills of Mortality, which I co-organized with Vanessa Harding. At the time, I was most interested in why and how the collection of non-plague mortality data was established. Only in assembling that story in a formal article did I begin to appreciate the challenges that a limited government must face in pursuing political and economic stability, including the maintenance of basic social functions.

From the Folger seminar came *Death by Numbers,* a project led by Jessica Otis that aims to collect and transcribe data from surviving London Bills through 1752. Funded by the National Science Foundation, it will publish its results via a searchable website, API, and downloadable CSVs. I am most interested in the correlations between this dataset and its seventeenth-century ancestor, the tables of John Graunt's *Natural and Political Observations on the Bills of Mortality* (1662 et seq.).

In the spring of 2020, Erica Charters and I assembled a multidisciplinary, multinational project called *How Epidemics End*, along with an essay in which we urged historians to reframe the way they think about epidemics. The pattern I found most striking was how quickly humans expect an epidemic to be over. This tendency is not just recent, urban, Western, or elite. Although our reasons may vary, we all crave a hopeful, sense-making narrative to protect and even amplify our deep-rooted belief in an imminent return to normalcy, often despite the data. —Kristin Heitman, 2023

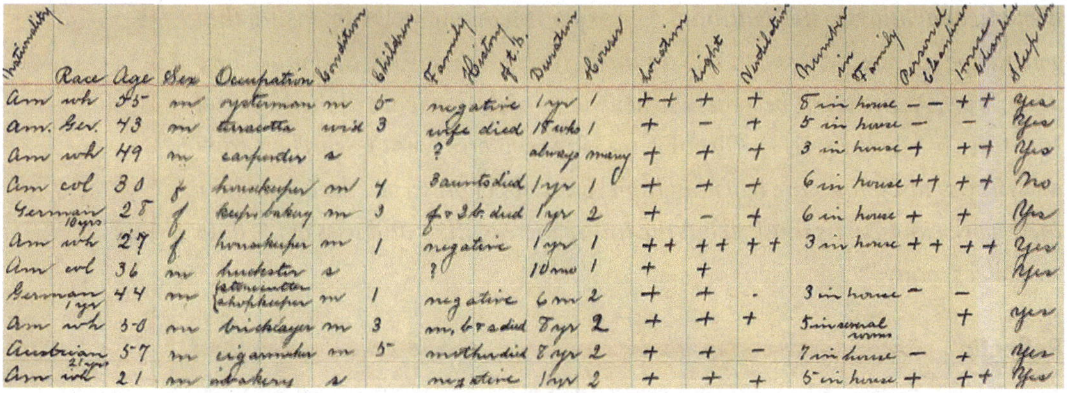

Nationality	Race	Age	Sex	Occupation	Condition	Children	Family History of t.b.	Duration	Houses	Location	Light	Ventilation	Number in Family	Personal Cleanliness	House Cleanliness	Sleep alone
Am	wh	45	m	oysterman	m	5	negative	1 yr	1	++	+	+	8 in house	--	++	yes
Am.	Ger.	43	m	terracotta	wid	3	wife died	18 wks	1	+	-	+	5 in house	-	-	yes
Am	wh	49	m	carpenter	s		?	always	many	+	+	+	3 in house	+	++	yes
Am	col	30	f	housekeeper	m	4	3 aunts died	1 yr	1	+	+	+	6 in house	++	++	no
German 10 yrs		28	f	keeps bakery	m	3	f & 3 b. died	1 yr	2	+	-	+	6 in house	+	+	yes
Am	wh	27	f	housekeeper	m	1	negative	1 yr	1	++	++	++	3 in house	++	++	yes
Am	col	36	m	huckster	s		?	10 mo	1	+	+					yes
German 1 yr		44	m	stonecutter shopkeeper	m	1	negative	6 m	2	+	+	.	3 in house	-	-	yes
Am	wh	50	m	bricklayer	m	3	m, b & s died	3 yr	2	+	+	+	5 in several rooms		+	yes
Austrian 21 yrs		57	m	cigarmaker	m	5	mother died	8 yr	2	+	+	-	7 in house	-	+	yes
Am	wh	21	m	in bakery	s		negative	1 yr	2	+	+	+	5 in house	+	++	yes

REVEALING DATA: COLLECTING DATA ABOUT TB, CA. 1900

https://circulatingnow.nlm.nih.gov/2018/01/31/collecting-data-about-tuberculosis-ca-1900/

January 31, 2018 • Archives & Manuscripts, Revealing Data

SUSAN L. SPEAKER

In the summer of 1901, Elizabeth Blauvelt, a Johns Hopkins medical student, prepared a summary of data ("Report on Data Obtained in Visits to Tuberculosis Patients. . . .") she had collected on 116 tuberculosis (TB) patients between January and June of that year.

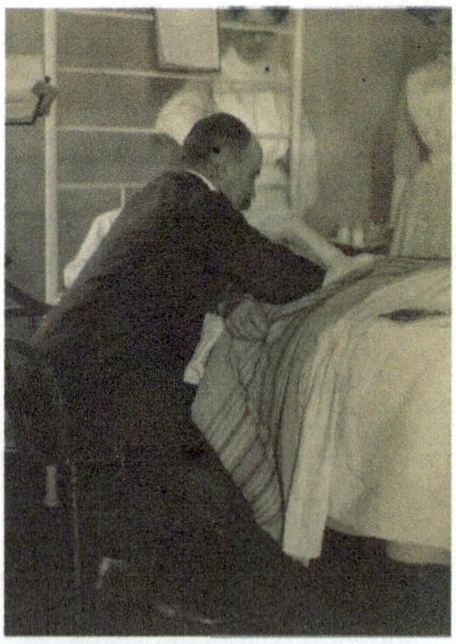

Osler at the bedside, 1903 • *William Osler Papers*, Profiles in Science, *National Library of Medicine*

The patients, too poor to afford a private physician, had been seen at the Johns Hopkins Hospital outpatient dispensary. Blauvelt and three other women medical students—Adelaide Dutcher, Blanche Epler, and Esther Rosencrantz—were part of a project begun by Dr. William Osler to provide follow-up care via home visits. The program had several related purposes: to check the patients' health status; to educate them about their disease and how to avoid spreading it; and to gather information about the patients' living conditions and how those conditions might encourage and spread the illness.

Tuberculosis of the lungs (aka "consumption" or "phthisis") was one of the two leading causes of death in the early 1900s (the other was pneumonia). It often killed slowly, and patients might be coughing up infected sputum for years, as the disease gradually destroyed their lungs and wasted their bodies. It became an especially pressing public health issue in the late nineteenth century, as millions of immigrants poured into America's larger cities. The crowded, dirty tenements where many were forced to live provided ideal conditions for the transmission of TB and other illnesses, as did some of the workplaces, such as garment sweatshops, where immigrants often found jobs. Though mortality rates for TB had been declining overall by the late 1800s, incidence among the poor was still high, and more affluent citizens worried about the reservoirs of infection present in the urban slums. With early diagnosis, adequate diet, rest, and fresh air—at a TB sanitarium, for example—some victims could recover, or at least have a remission, but such care wasn't an option for the poor. Osler's students, along with visiting nurses, advised their patients about basic "containment" measures, particularly disposing of sputum properly, and sleeping alone, so others in the household would be less exposed. They also encouraged families to spend a little more on nourishing food (eggs, milk, etc.) for the patients if they could.

The students were also gathering data as they cared for patients, and the types of data included in their published reports and in Ms. Blauvelt's

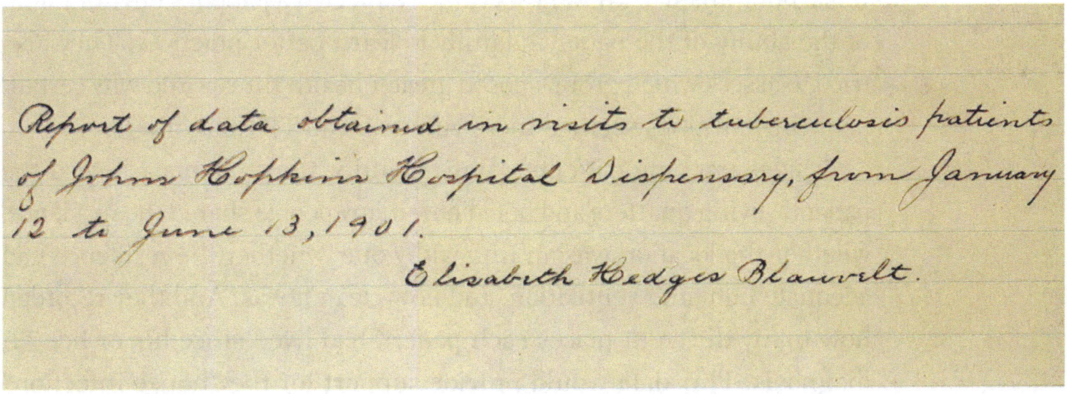
Report of data obtained in visits to tuberculosis patients of Johns Hopkins Hospital Dispensary, from January 12 to June 13, 1901.
Elisabeth Hedges Blauvelt.

Elizabeth Blauvelt's handwritten record, 1901 • *William Osler Papers*, Profiles in Science, *National Library of Medicine*

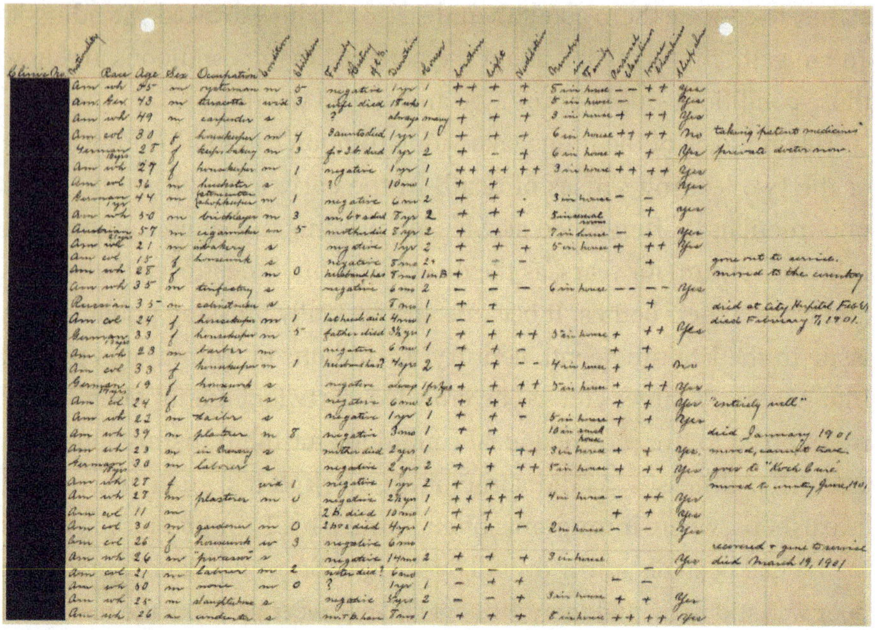

Elizabeth Blauvelt's handwritten record, 1901 • *William Osler Papers*, Profiles in Science, *National Library of Medicine*

handwritten record show how some physicians of this era approached TB prevention and control. Along with basic demographic data (age, gender, marital status, number of children, and occupation), they also noted ethnicity (was the patient White, native-born, German, Italian, Russian, or Black?), because ethnic groups in the cities were also small homogenous communities occupying specific geographic spaces. Public health workers already understood that poverty fostered illness and vice-versa, but wanted to know how ethnicity affected a patient's environment, or the ability of the patient's family to learn better practices. They also tried to assess which groups posed greater health threats and why certain poor communities seemed more vulnerable to TB than others.

Besides tracking patients' ethnic identity, the students assessed the patients' living quarters and noted how many people shared the residence, whether the location was an unhealthy one, whether the residence had adequate light and ventilation, and how clean it was. And they recorded how many different places each patient had lived since his or her TB diagnosis. This data would provide support for the "house infection" concept introduced by Philadelphia TB expert Lawrence Flick in 1888.

Flick's research had shown that TB bacteria could persist in rooms even after TB patients had moved out; as most landlords wouldn't disinfect apartments between tenants, the next occupants might contract the disease, too. Flick recommended that cities require physicians to register all TB cases, and arrange to have all TB patient residences disinfected by either landlords or city health departments. He and others, including Osler, also advocated building public sanitaria and sending patients there so that they couldn't spread infection and might be cured.

Mandatory registration and other measures were not as effective in controlling TB as advocates had hoped. Private physicians resisted reporting cases, as they didn't wish to expose their patients' medical condition in public records, or subject their homes to bureaucratic regulation. Thus, though many large cities enacted TB registration ordinances between 1890 and 1915, some made reporting optional for private physicians. Health departments also were often overwhelmed by the record-keeping

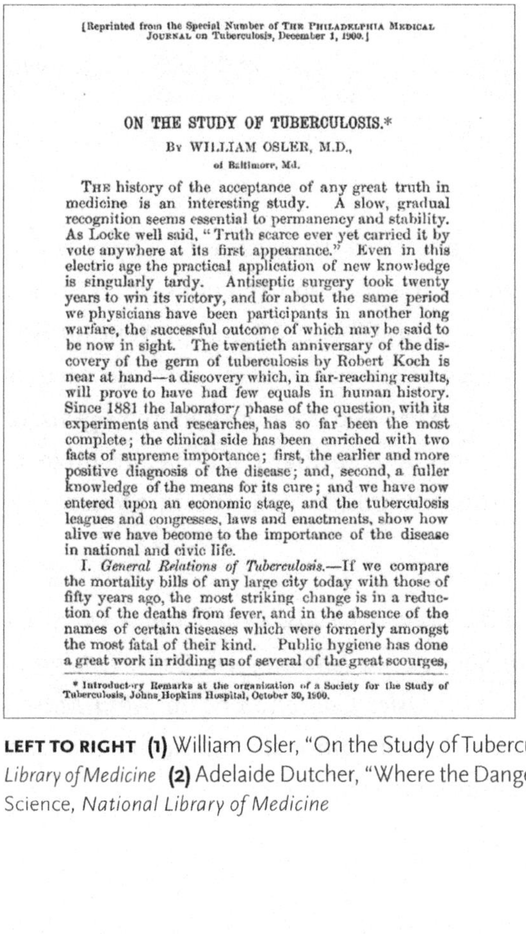

[Reprinted from the Special Number of THE PHILADELPHIA MEDICAL JOURNAL on Tuberculosis, December 1, 1900.]

ON THE STUDY OF TUBERCULOSIS.*

BY WILLIAM OSLER, M.D.,
of Baltimore, Md.

THE history of the acceptance of any great truth in medicine is an interesting study. A slow, gradual recognition seems essential to permanency and stability. As Locke well said, "Truth scarce ever yet carried it by vote anywhere at its first appearance." Even in this electric age the practical application of new knowledge is singularly tardy. Antiseptic surgery took twenty years to win its victory, and for about the same period we physicians have been participants in another long warfare, the successful outcome of which may be said to be now in sight. The twentieth anniversary of the discovery of the germ of tuberculosis by Robert Koch is near at hand—a discovery which, in far-reaching results, will prove to have had few equals in human history. Since 1881 the laboratory phase of the question, with its experiments and researches, has so far been the most complete; the clinical side has been enriched with two facts of supreme importance; first, the earlier and more positive diagnosis of the disease; and, second, a fuller knowledge of the means for its cure; and we have now entered upon an economic stage, and the tuberculosis leagues and congresses, laws and enactments, show how alive we have become to the importance of the disease in national and civic life.

I. *General Relations of Tuberculosis.*—If we compare the mortality bills of any large city today with those of fifty years ago, the most striking change is in a reduction of the deaths from fever, and in the absence of the names of certain diseases which were formerly amongst the most fatal of their kind. Public hygiene has done a great work in ridding us of several of the great scourges,

* Introductory Remarks at the organization of a Society for the Study of Tuberculosis, Johns Hopkins Hospital, October 30, 1900.

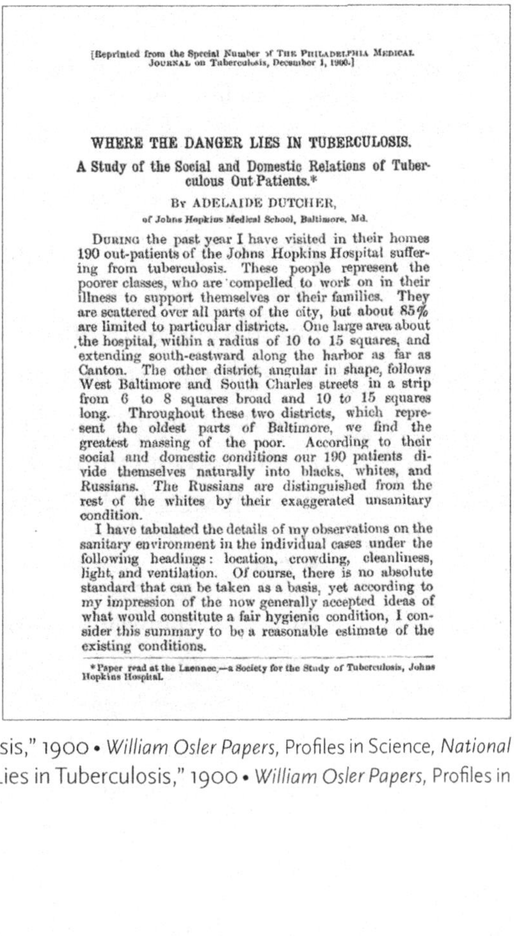

[Reprinted from the Special Number of THE PHILADELPHIA MEDICAL JOURNAL on Tuberculosis, December 1, 1900.]

WHERE THE DANGER LIES IN TUBERCULOSIS.

A Study of the Social and Domestic Relations of Tuberculous Out-Patients.*

BY ADELAIDE DUTCHER,
of Johns Hopkins Medical School, Baltimore, Md.

DURING the past year I have visited in their homes 190 out-patients of the Johns Hopkins Hospital suffering from tuberculosis. These people represent the poorer classes, who are compelled to work on in their illness to support themselves or their families. They are scattered over all parts of the city, but about 85% are limited to particular districts. One large area about the hospital, within a radius of 10 to 15 squares, and extending south-eastward along the harbor as far as Canton. The other district, angular in shape, follows West Baltimore and South Charles streets in a strip from 6 to 8 squares broad and 10 to 15 squares long. Throughout these two districts, which represent the oldest parts of Baltimore, we find the greatest massing of the poor. According to their social and domestic conditions our 190 patients divide themselves naturally into blacks, whites, and Russians. The Russians are distinguished from the rest of the whites by their exaggerated unsanitary condition.

I have tabulated the details of my observations on the sanitary environment in the individual cases under the following headings: location, crowding, cleanliness, light, and ventilation. Of course, there is no absolute standard that can be taken as a basis, yet according to my impression of the now generally accepted ideas of what would constitute a fair hygienic condition, I consider this summary to be a reasonable estimate of the existing conditions.

* Paper read at the Laennec,—a Society for the Study of Tuberculosis, Johns Hopkins Hospital.

LEFT TO RIGHT (1) William Osler, "On the Study of Tuberculosis," 1900 • *William Osler Papers,* Profiles in Science, *National Library of Medicine* **(2)** Adelaide Dutcher, "Where the Danger Lies in Tuberculosis," 1900 • *William Osler Papers,* Profiles in Science, *National Library of Medicine*

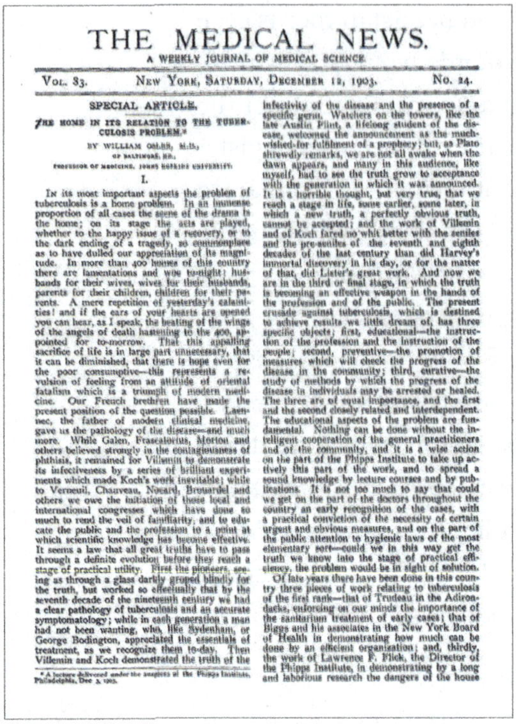

THE MEDICAL NEWS.

A WEEKLY JOURNAL OF MEDICAL SCIENCE

VOL. 83. NEW YORK, SATURDAY, DECEMBER 12, 1903. NO. 24.

SPECIAL ARTICLE.

THE HOME IN ITS RELATION TO THE TUBERCULOSIS PROBLEM.*

BY WILLIAM OSLER, M.D.,
OF BALTIMORE, MD.,
PROFESSOR OF MEDICINE, JOHNS HOPKINS UNIVERSITY.

I.

IN its most important aspects the problem of tuberculosis is a home problem. In an immense proportion of all cases the scene of the drama is the home; on its stage the acts are played, whether to the happy issue of a recovery, or to the dark ending of a tragedy, so commonplace as to have dulled our appreciation of its magnitude. In more than 400 homes of this country there are lamentations and woe to-night: husbands for their wives, wives for their husbands, parents for their children, children for their parents. A mere repetition of yesterday's calamities! and if the ears of your hearts are opened you can hear, as I speak, the beating of the wings of the angels of death hastening to the 400, appointed for to-morrow. That this appalling sacrifice of life is in large part unnecessary, that it can be diminished, that there is hope even for the poor consumptive—this represents a revulsion of feeling from an attitude of oriental fatalism which is a triumph of modern medicine. Our French brethren have made the present position of the question possible. Laennec, the father of modern clinical medicine, gave us the pathology of the disease—and much more. While Galen, Frascatorius, Morton and others believed strongly in the contagiousness of phthisis, it remained for Villemin to demonstrate its infectiveness by a series of brilliant experiments which made Koch's work inevitable; while to Verneuil, Chauveau, Nocard, Brouardel and others we owe the initiation of these local and international congresses which have done so much to rend the veil of familiarity, and to educate the public and the profession to a point at which scientific knowledge has become effective. It seems a law that all great truths have to pass through a definite evolution before they reach a stage of practical utility. First the pioneers, seeing as through a glass darkly groped blindly for the truth, but worked so effectually that by the seventh decade of the nineteenth century we had a clear pathology of tuberculosis and an accurate symptomatology; while in each generation a man had not been wanting, who, like Sydenham, or George Bodington, appreciated the essentials of treatment, as we recognize them to-day. Then Villemin and Koch demonstrated the truth of the infectivity of the disease and the presence of a specific germ. Watchers on the towers, like the late Austin Flint, a lifelong student of the disease, welcomed the announcement as the much-wished-for fulfilment of a prophecy; but, as Plato shrewdly remarks, we are not all awake when the dawn appears, and many in this audience, like myself, had to see the truth grow to acceptance with the generation in which it was announced. It is a horrible thought, but very true, that we reach a stage in life, some earlier, some later, in which a new truth, a perfectly obvious truth, cannot be accepted; and the work of Villemin and of Koch fared no whit better with the seniles and the pre-seniles of the seventh and eighth decades of the last century than did Harvey's immortal discovery in his day, or for the matter of that, did Lister's great work. And now we are in the third or final stage, in which the truth is becoming an effective weapon in the hands of the profession and of the public. The present crusade against tuberculosis, which is destined to achieve results we little dream of, has three specific objects; first, educational—the instruction of the profession and the instruction of the people; second, preventive—the promotion of measures which will check the progress of the disease in the community; third, curative—the study of methods by which the progress of the disease in individuals may be arrested or healed. The three are of equal importance, and the first and the second closely related and interdependent. The educational aspects of the problem are fundamental. Nothing can be done without the intelligent cooperation of the general practitioners and of the community, and it is a wise action on the part of the Phipps Institute to take up actively this part of the work, and to spread a sound knowledge by lecture courses and by publications. It is not too much to say that could we get on the part of the doctors throughout the country an early recognition of the cases, with a practical conviction of the necessity of certain urgent and obvious measures, and on the part of the public attention to hygienic laws of the most elementary sort—could we in this way get the truth we know into the stage of practical efficiency, the problem would be in sight of solution.

Of late years there have been done in this country three pieces of work relating to tuberculosis of the first rank—that of Trudeau in the Adirondacks, enforcing on our minds the importance of the sanitarium treatment of early cases; that of Biggs and his associates in the New York Board of Health in demonstrating how much can be done by an efficient organization; and, thirdly, the work of Lawrence F. Flick, the Director of the Phipps Institute, in demonstrating by a long and laborious research the dangers of the house

* A lecture delivered under the auspices of the Phipps Institute, Philadelphia, Dec. 3, 1903.

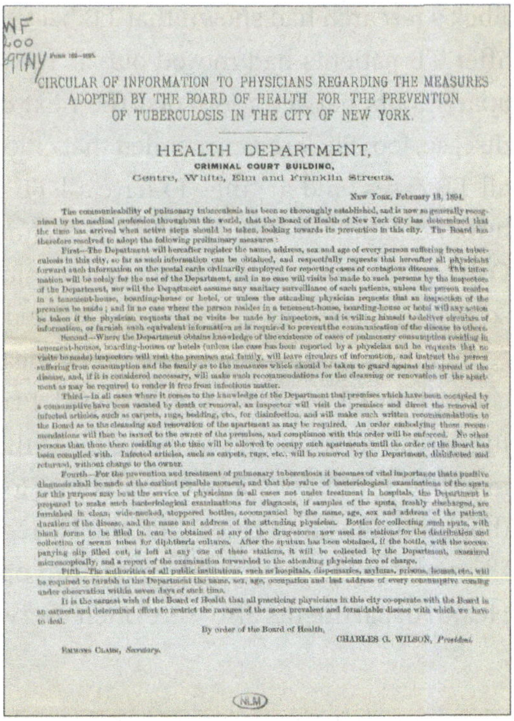

CIRCULAR OF INFORMATION TO PHYSICIANS REGARDING THE MEASURES ADOPTED BY THE BOARD OF HEALTH FOR THE PREVENTION OF TUBERCULOSIS IN THE CITY OF NEW YORK.

HEALTH DEPARTMENT,
CRIMINAL COURT BUILDING,
Centre, White, Elm and Franklin Streets.

New York, February 13, 1894.

The communicability of pulmonary tuberculosis has been so thoroughly established, and is now so generally recognized by the medical profession throughout the world, that the Board of Health of New York City has determined that the time has arrived when active steps should be taken, looking towards its prevention in this city. The Board has therefore resolved to adopt the following preliminary measures:

First—The Department will hereafter register the name, address, sex and age of every person suffering from tuberculosis in this city, so far as such information can be obtained, and respectfully requests that hereafter all physicians forward such information on the postal cards ordinarily employed for reporting cases of contagious diseases. This information will be solely for the use of the Department, and in no case will visits be made to such persons by the inspectors of the Department, nor will the Department assume any sanitary surveillance of such patients, unless the person resides in a tenement-house, boarding-house or hotel, or unless the attending physician requests that an inspection of the premises be made; and in no case where the person resides in a tenement-house, boarding-house or hotel will any action be taken if the physician requests that no visits be made by inspectors, and is willing himself to deliver circulars of information, or furnish such equivalent information as is required to prevent the communication of the disease to others.

Second—Where the Department obtains knowledge of the existence of cases of pulmonary consumption residing in tenement-houses, boarding-houses or hotels (unless the case has been reported by a physician and he requests that no visits be made) inspectors will visit the premises and family, will leave circulars of information, and instruct the person suffering from consumption and the family as to the measures which should be taken to guard against the spread of the disease, and, if it is considered necessary, will make such recommendations for the cleansing or renovation of the apartment as may be required to render it free from infectious matter.

Third—In all cases where it comes to the knowledge of the Department that premises which have been occupied by a consumptive have been vacated by death or removal, an inspector will visit the premises and direct the removal of infected articles, such as carpets, rugs, bedding, etc., for disinfection, and will make such written recommendations to the Board as to the cleansing and renovation of the apartment as may be required. An order embodying these recommendations will then be issued to the owner of the premises, and compliance with this order will be enforced. No other persons than those there residing at the time will be allowed to occupy such apartments until the order of the Board has been complied with. Infected articles, such as carpets, rugs, etc., will be removed by the Department, disinfected and returned, without charge to the owner.

Fourth—For the prevention and treatment of pulmonary tuberculosis it becomes of vital importance that a positive diagnosis shall be made at the earliest possible moment, and that the value of bacteriological examinations of the sputa for this purpose may be at the service of physicians in all cases not under treatment in hospitals, the Department is prepared to make such bacteriological examinations for diagnosis, if samples of the sputa, freshly discharged, are furnished in clean, wide-necked, stoppered bottles, accompanied by the name, age, sex and address of the patient, duration of the disease, and the name and address of the attending physician. Bottles for collecting such sputa, with blank forms to be filled in, can be obtained at any of the drug-stores now used as stations for the distribution and collection of serum tubes for diphtheria cultures. After the sputum has been obtained, if the bottle, with the accompanying slip filled out, is left at any one of these stations, it will be collected by the Department, examined microscopically, and a report of the examination forwarded to the attending physician free of charge.

Fifth—The authorities of all public institutions, such as hospitals, dispensaries, asylums, prisons, homes, etc., will be required to furnish to the Department the name, sex, age, occupation and last address of every consumptive coming under observation within seven days of such time.

It is the earnest wish of the Board of Health that all practicing physicians in this city co-operate with the Board in an earnest and determined effort to restrict the ravages of the most prevalent and formidable disease with which we have to deal.

By order of the Board of Health,

CHARLES G. WILSON, *President.*

EMMONS CLARK, *Secretary.*

LEFT TO RIGHT **(1)** William Osler, "The Home in Relation to the Tuberculosis Problem," 1903 • *William Osler Papers,* Profiles in Science, *National Library of Medicine* **(2)** *Circular of Information to Physicians Regarding the Measures Adopted by the Board of Health for the Prevention of Tuberculosis in the City of New York* • New York City Health Department notice, 1894 • *National Library of Medicine #101600551*

process, though efforts to track TB and other diseases eventually provided data needed to justify improvements in sanitation and housing. It turned out that the most effective strategy for TB control and prevention was to make patients and communities active participants through various education campaigns. By the early 1920s, the home visitation program of the Johns Hopkins medical students, and similar public health projects that followed, had achieved significant reductions in TB incidence.

• • •

Note: Ms. Blauvelt's report and the articles by Ms. Dutcher and Dr. Osler appear on the NLM's Profiles in Science *site featuring Dr. Osler. The handwritten report is part of the William Osler Collection at the Alan Mason Chesney Medical Archives at Johns Hopkins University. Clinic case numbers have been redacted as protected health information.*

We hear about data every day. In historical medical collections, data abounds, both quantitative and qualitative. In its format, scope, and biases, data inherently contains more information than its face value. This series, Revealing Data, explores how, by preserving the research data of the past and making it publicly available, the National Library of Medicine (NLM) helps to ensure that generations of researchers can reexamine it, reveal new stories, and make new discoveries. As the NLM becomes the new home of data science at the National Institutes of Health (NIH), Circulating Now *explores what researchers from a variety of disciplines are learning from centuries of preserved data, and how their work can help us think about the future preservation and uses of the data we collect today.*

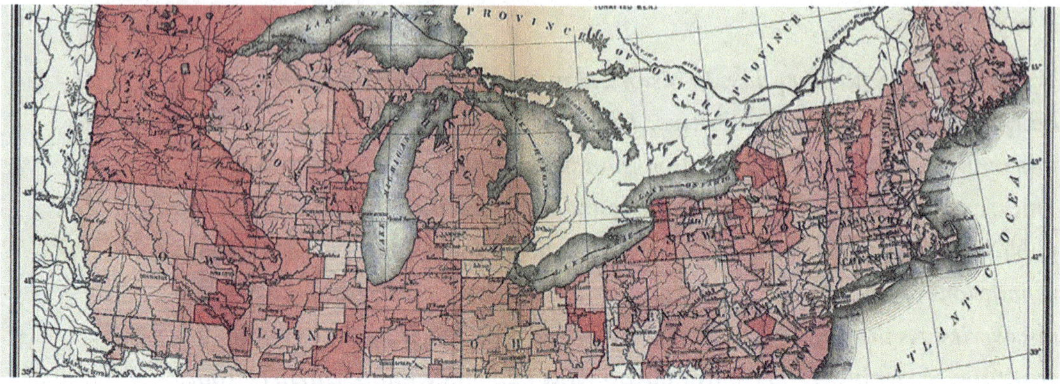

REVEALING DATA: THE COLOR OF THEIR EYES

https://circulatingnow.nlm.nih.gov/2017/11/02/revealing-data-the-color-of-their-eyes/

November 2, 2017 • Rare Books & Journals, Revealing Data, Guests

DAN BOUK

Circulating Now *welcomes guest blogger* *Dan Bouk, PhD who shares his insights on nineteenth-century government data collection and analysis as part of our* *Revealing Data* *series. Dr. Bouk is Associate Professor of History at Colgate University.*

• • •

By popular legend, although attributions are slippery, the American Revolution brought with it the warning that soldiers ought not fire until they could see the white of the enemy's eyes. But as a gorgeous book held in the history of medicine collections proves, by the time of the American Civil War, doctors and surgeons concerned themselves not with the whites, but with the color of potential soldiers' eyes. They looked at each set of brown, blue, black, gray, or hazel eyes and noted down what they found on a "blank" form.

That blank form demanded further observations that may have struck some of those making them as odd or beside the point: hair color, girth of chest, "nativity," occupation. The point is not that these categories had nothing to do with health or medicine. Various nineteenth-century medical theories made the surface of the body (including eye color) a possible guide to its interior and made heredity or occupation into potential predictors of longevity or character. Still, doctors drawn into this nation-spanning project could be forgiven for wondering what such questions had to do with the most important question (number 17) on the blank: should the examined man be accepted or rejected for service in the union army?

One Pennsylvania surgeon groused about all the paperwork. He wrote: "the filling-up of the blanks for the examination of recruits, which has been recently required with each recruit, consumes so much time that, without assistance, the surgeon cannot examine a much greater number than of drafted men." He may have been angling for clerical help, or he may have been pushing back against being made into a clerk himself—a fate feared in coming years by doctors who supplemented their incomes by conducting examinations for booming life insurance corporations.

The surgeon likely understood, as did many of the doctors and surgeons involved, why these blanks and their odd questions had so suddenly appeared. The blanks served the ambitions of Jedediah Hyde Baxter, the Chief Medical Officer of the Provost-Marshal-General Bureau, who saw an opportunity for science to benefit from the sprawling bureaucracy being built to direct one of the world's first industrial wars. When the Belgian Adolphe Quetelet first reported in 1846 that measurements of chest girths of soldiers produced not only a national average but a bell curve or binomial distribution, his findings inspired statistical fever. Baxter burned with it, as did many doctors who joined him enthusiastically. One surgeon, for example, wrote Baxter not to complain about the length of the blanks, but instead to beg for more "specificness in the description of diseases."

Having gathered data from a half million examinations, Baxter possessed the nineteenth-century equivalent of "Big Data." He did not, however, entirely trust it, because he knew how politics pulsed through his measurements. Historian Ted Porter has a good name for the way that the process of quantification can go awry when the stakes are high: "funny numbers." Civil War data often proved to be funny. Surgeons—already

LXXX INTRODUCTORY.

Comparison of actual and calculated circumference of chest, 5,738 men.—(*Sir. J. F. W. Herschel and M. Quetelet.*)

Circumference of chest.		Number of men at each circumference.	Sir J. F. W. Herschel.		M. Quetelet.	
English inches.	Centimetres.		Calculated.	Difference.	Calculated.	Difference.
33	83.82	3	6	− 3	4	− 1
34	86.36	18	21	− 3	17	+ 1
35	88.90	81	72	+ 9	63	+ 18
36	91.44	185	200	− 15	186	− 1
37	93.98	420	433	− 13	420	0
38	96.52	749	746	+ 3	765	− 16
39	99.06	1,073	1,024	+ 49	1,056	+ 17
40	101.60	1,079	1,103	− 24	1,139	− 60
41	104.14	934	943	− 9	961	− 27
42	106.68	658	639	+ 19	628	+ 30
43	109.22	370	341	+ 29	321	+ 49
44	111.76	92	145	− 53	126	− 34
45	114.30	50	50	0	40	+ 10
46	116.84	21	12	+ 9	9	+ 12
47	119.38	4	2	+ 2	2	+ 2
48	121.92	1	1	0	1	0
Total......	....	5,738	5,738	−120 +120	5,738	−139 +139

Comparison of actual and calculated height.—(*E. B. Elliott.*)

Height.		Number of men at each height.	Proportion per thousand at each height.		
English inches.	Centimetres.		Actual measure.	Calculated.	Difference.
55 and under.	140 and under.	4			
56	142	1			
57	145	3	1	2	− 1
58	147	7			
59	150	6			
60	152	10			
61	155	15	1	3	− 2
62	158	50	2	9	− 7
63	160	526	20	21	− 1
64	163	1,237	48	42	+ 6
65	165	1,947	75	72	+ 3
66	168	3,019	117	107	+10
67	170	3,475	134	137	− 3
68	173	4,054	157	153	+ 4
69	175	3,631	140	146	− 6
70	178	3,133	121	121	0
71	180	2,075	80	86	− 6
72	183	1,485	57	53	+ 4
73	185	680	26	28	− 2
74	188	348	13	13	0
75	191	118	5	5	0
76	193	42	2	2	0
77	196	9			
78	198	6	1	0	+ 1
79	201	2			
Total......	....	25,878	1,000	1,000	−28 +28

Circumference of Chest in 5,378 Men, in *Statistics, Medical and Anthropological, of the Provost-Marshal-General's Bureau, Derived from Records of the Examination for Military Service in the Armies of the United States during the Late War of the Rebellion*. . . . Comp. under direction of the Secretary of War, by J.H. Baxter, 1875. • *National Library of Medicine #62430820R*

peeved by the frequency with which boards of examiners ignored their recommendations on whether to take a man or not—fumed about ongoing scams by which a "sound" individual would be allowed to disingenuously substitute himself during the examination in place of a volunteer plagued by some defect. They did not find the scam funny, but it could make their numbers hilarious.

No data were funnier, however, than hernia data. Baxter explained how President Lincoln's efforts to round up fresh soldiers also gathered the herniated. The U.S. government assigned recruiting quotas to each district according to the number of eligible men in each. Savvy politicians realized that the quickest way to fill a quota was to lower it, and they could lower the quota by declaring more citizens unfit for duty. Hernias became a favored excuse, and local officials and doctors rounded up all those with hernia to ensure their names were stricken from the rolls to a degree they did not for other diseases. Baxter stopped short of claiming that some of these hernias might have been dreamed up from whole cloth and yet that too seems at least possible—those doctors working for life insurers (with lower stakes) sometimes committed such frauds or much worse.

Baxter's lithographer (who designed and printed the maps), Julius Bien, chose not to capture any humor in the hernia or other data. His breathtaking maps hint at no uncertainties, at no challenges. They evoke objectivity. They filled massive scientific volumes meant to express the

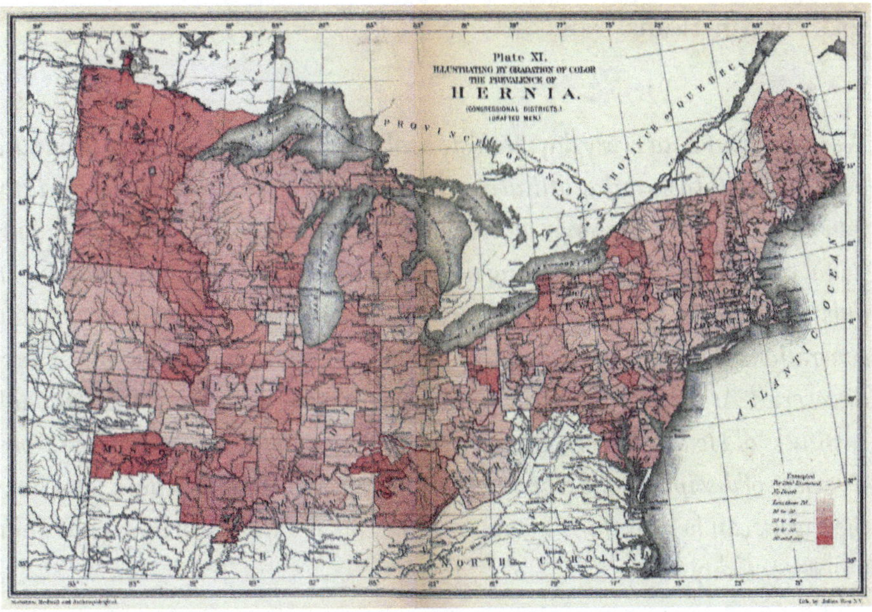

Prevalence of Hernia in Drafted Men, in *Statistics, Medical and Anthropological, of the Provost-Marshal-General's Bureau, Derived from Records of the Examination for Military Service in the Armies of the United States during the Late War of the Rebellion* . . . Comp. under direction of the Secretary of War, by J.H. Baxter, 1875. • *National Library of Medicine #62430820R*

American nation's scientific capacity, destined for exchange among the world's statistical experts and for popular viewing at then frequent global expositions, forerunners to the world's fairs.

They represented, at a glance, the nation. Yet as is often the case in Big Data projects today too, these statistical depictions had their limits and blindspots. They were organized around congressional districts, a category with no obvious medical significance, but one dictated by the needs of the draft. They extended no farther south than Missouri and excluded all women and many men (who were either too old or too young). While the data included people of color and men born in many different countries, Baxter used that data to establish racial and national differences. In fact, to bring us back to where we began, it was Baxter's desire to tease out the differences between "complexion" and race that made the reporting of superficial characteristics so important. Before he could assert the superiority of "blonde races," (unsurprisingly for a moment when many were turning science to the project of justifying racism and exploitation) Baxter charged his small army of doctors and surgeons to inventory the colors of Americans' eyes.

• • •

We hear about data every day. In historical medical collections, data abounds, both quantitative and qualitative. In its format, scope, and biases, data inherently contains more information than its face value. This series, Revealing Data, explores how, by preserving the research data of the past and making it publicly available, the National Library of Medicine (NLM) helps to ensure that generations of researchers can reexamine it, reveal new stories, and make new discoveries. As the NLM becomes the new home of data science at the National Institutes of Health (NIH), Circulating Now *explores what researchers from a variety of disciplines are learning from centuries of preserved data, and how their work can help us think about the future preservation and uses of the data we collect today.*

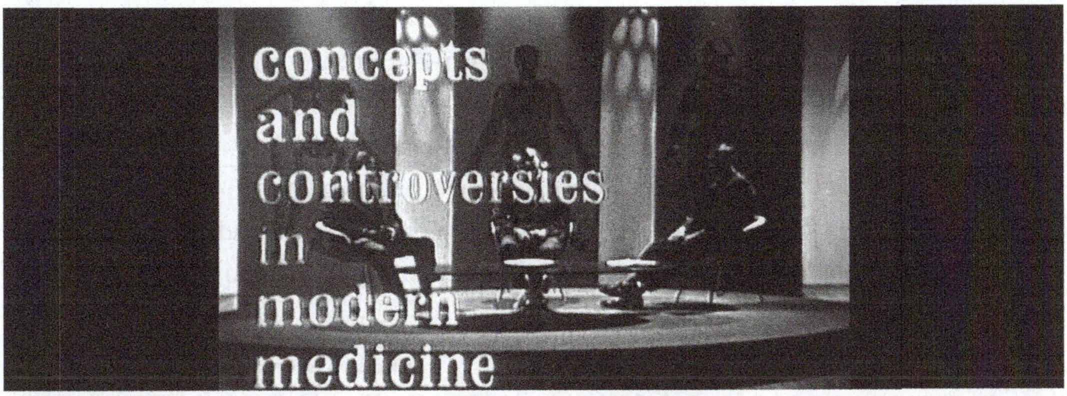

REVEALING DATA: CONCEPTS AND CONTROVERSIES IN MODERN MEDICINE, 1969–70

https://circulatingnow.nlm.nih.gov/2018/07/26/revealing-data-concepts-and-controversies-in-modern-medicine-1969-70/

July 26, 2018 • Films & Videos, Revealing Data

SARAH EILERS

A host emerges from the shadows of a video production set. In measured tones, he introduces the viewer to a series of energetic but respectful debates on medical topics.

> Welcome to the exploration of Concepts and Controversies in Modern Medicine, one of a series of programs dedicated to examining the uncertain, candidly recognizing that much of today's teaching is necessarily based upon opinion, and that the opinions of eminent physicians in a given field vary widely. The National Medical Audiovisual Center [NMAC] believes that openly airing such opposing views is a basic responsibility of medical communications.

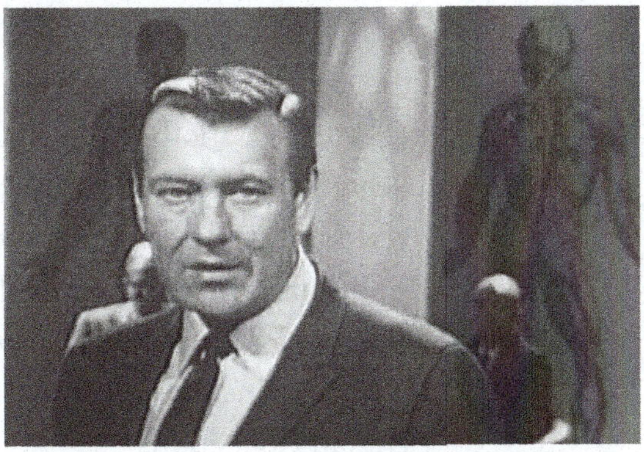

Concepts and Controversies in Modern Medicine, 1969 • *National Library of Medicine #8600254A*

The NMAC became part of the National Library of Medicine (NLM) in 1967, having been transferred from the Communicable Disease Center (now the Centers for Disease Control). The center was predecessor to the Library's current Audiovisual Program and Development Branch. *Concepts and Controversies in Modern Medicine*, produced in 1969–70, comprised a set of moderated, videotaped discussions on health and medical concerns about which reasonable people could disagree. And did.

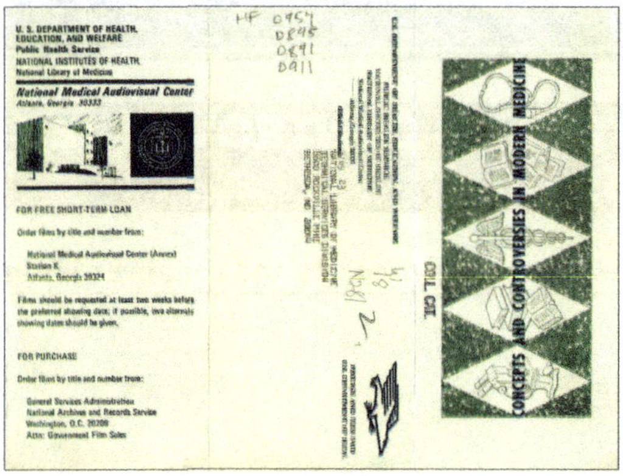

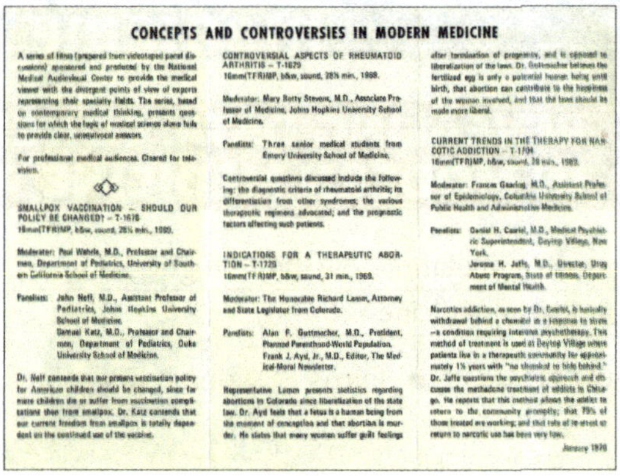

LEFT Cover of a brochure advertising *Concepts and Controversies in Modern Medicine*, 1970
RIGHT Inside of a brochure advertising *Concepts and Controversies in Modern Medicine*, 1970

Face-Off

Live debates with broadcast audiences were relatively new to the political and cultural landscape at the time. The 1960 Kennedy-Nixon debate was the first televised presidential one, and its optics were thought to have resulted in votes for Kennedy; he looked calmer, taller, handsomer than his opponent. In 1965, James Baldwin debated William F. Buckley at Cambridge University on the topic of whether or not "The American dream is at the expense of the Negro." Besides the 700 students in the debate hall, another 500 watched via closed-circuit TV, and the recorded debate was eventually released in both the U.K. and the U.S. Other televised political debates followed in the latter half of the 1960s.

In this environment, the National Library of Medicine developed *Concepts and Controversies in Modern Medicine*. The historical audiovisuals collection includes nine *Concepts* titles, five of which are available in NLM Digital Collections.

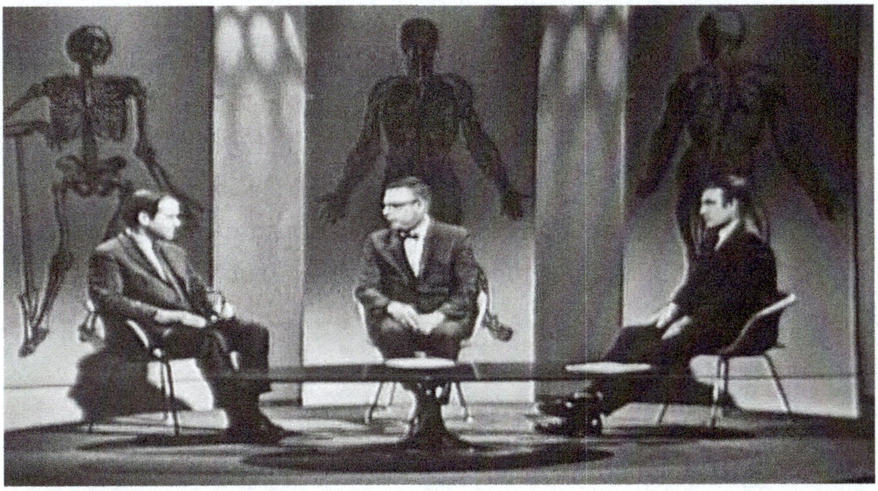

"Diet and Atherosclerotic Disease: Are They Related," 1969 • *National Library of Medicine #8600254A*

Presenting a mix of data, clinical observation, anecdote, and opinion to support their conclusions, each *Concepts* panel of doctors is guided by a moderator who is usually a physician as well. The participants argue issues including vaccination policies, narcotic addiction treatments, women's use of oral contraceptives, and involuntary hospitalization of people with psychiatric illnesses. Designed for a professional medical audience, the series featured a plain set—a few chairs, a small coffee table, and a backdrop of life-sized anatomical drawings.

The videos were available for loan to medical educators for many years, but we don't know how often they were requested or in what context they were used. We do know that some segments were cited in later research. For example, *The Psychiatrist in the Courtroom: Selected Papers of Bernard L. Diamond*, 1994, cites the *Concepts* episode titled "Psychiatry and Law: How are they Related?"

The Sharpest Minds on Opposite Sides

One of the panelists in the "Psychiatry and Law" episode, Dr. Thomas Szasz, also appears in "Involuntary Hospitalization of the Psychiatric Patient: Should it be Abolished?" Dr. Szasz, who died in 2012, was deeply influential in the field of mental health, though his foundational arguments sound extreme today. Szasz never wavered in his belief that mental illness is a myth, and that a medical, neuro-diagnostic model is not useful for understanding the human struggle. In the early years of his career, Dr. Szasz stated that the psychiatric discipline, of which he was a member, belonged "in the company of alchemy and astrology." Opposing Dr. Szasz in the "Psychiatry and Law" debate was Dr. Bernard Diamond, mentioned above, who developed the "diminished capacity" legal defense. Diamond testified on behalf of Sirhan Sirhan during his trial for the assassination of Senator Robert F. Kennedy.

Evidence and opinion on . . .

Heart disease

The debates clearly illustrate that people, even experts in their fields, can take the same set of data or circumstances and reach different conclusions about what it all means, or which elements should receive the most attention.

Here's how a typical discussion begins—in this case, about the causes of heart disease.

> [Dr. Jeremiah Stamler, Associate Professor, Department of Medicine, Northwestern University Medical School:] I'm convinced that a mass of evidence exists demonstrating that diet is one of the key factors responsible for the current epidemic of severe premature atherosclerotic disease in the United States population, and accounting for the very high incidence of heart attacks in the middle decades of life. . . .
>
> [Dr. Mark Altschule, Assistant Professor, Harvard Medical School:] I'm convinced that diet cannot have a primary role in . . . atherosclerosis.

Dr. Stamler argues his position first, citing numerous and varied datasets.

> Now, study after study of these international differences, both analyses of United Nations data, World Health Organization data, the very important International Autopsy Study done by our colleagues at the Louisiana State University Medical School, together with the very important field studies of Dr. Keys and his group in

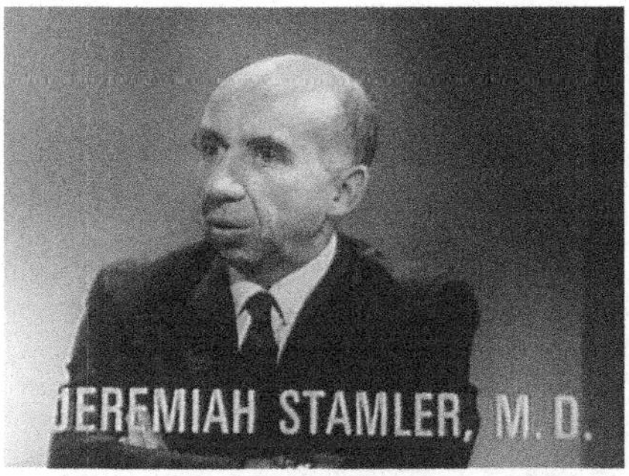

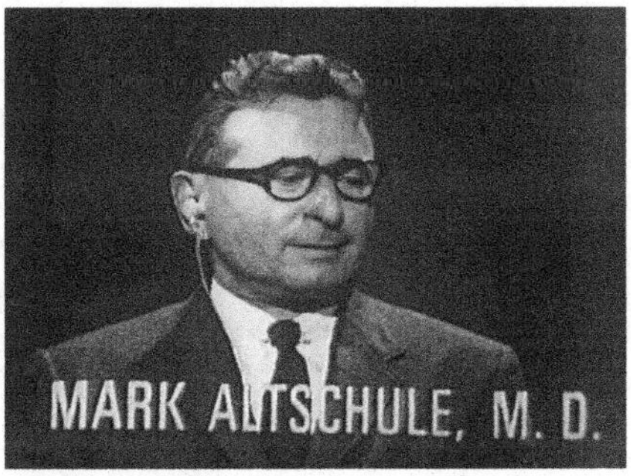

LEFT TO RIGHT (1) Jeremiah Stamler, MD. "Diet and Atherosclerotic Disease: Are They Related," 1969 • *National Library of Medicine #8600254A* **(2)** Mark Altschule, MD. "Diet and Atherosclerotic Disease: Are They Related," 1969 • *National Library of Medicine #8600254A*

> twelve different populations of Europe plus the Japanese, all show a very close correlation among the pattern of a diet, particularly the saturated fat intake, the dietary cholesterol intake, the serum lipids of the populations under study, and the incidence and mortality rates as well as the prevalence rates of coronary heart disease.

Dr. Altschule counters.

> The authors of the report of the Helsinki study and the Los Angeles study, in their own reports, said that their groups were not matched. The one from Los Angeles, in particular, referred to the fact that one of their groups smoked more than the other and they hadn't taken that into account before starting it. They said they didn't think it made any difference, I don't know on what basis.

Smallpox

In another session, debating the utility of continued routine smallpox vaccination, Dr. John M. Neff, Assistant Professor of Pediatrics at Johns Hopkins University, and Dr. Samuel Lawrence Katz, Professor and Chairman of the Department of Pediatrics at Duke University, cite national and international vaccination statistics and mortality figures as they argue their cases. Neff describes the smallpox shot as "a very poor vaccine," whose effectiveness is short in duration, with "a significant amount of mortality." Katz is squarely on the other side. "I believe that our nation's freedom from smallpox rests upon the widespread use of

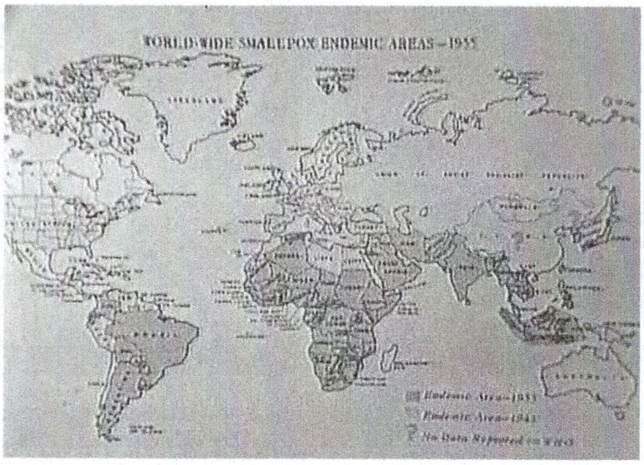

World Wide Smallpox Endemic Areas—1955 • "Smallpox Vaccination: Should our Policy be Changed?," 1969 • *National Library of Medicine #8601126A*

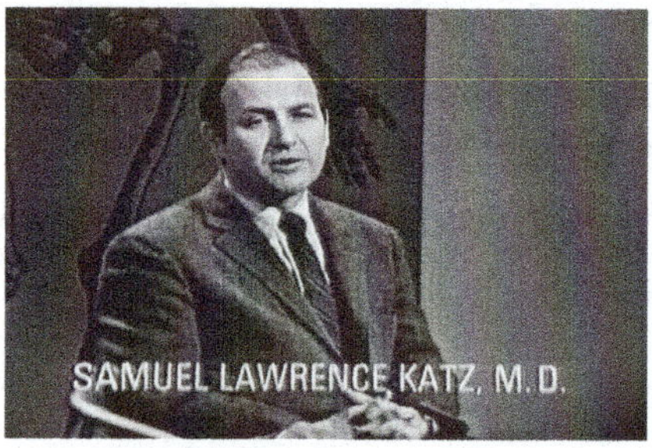

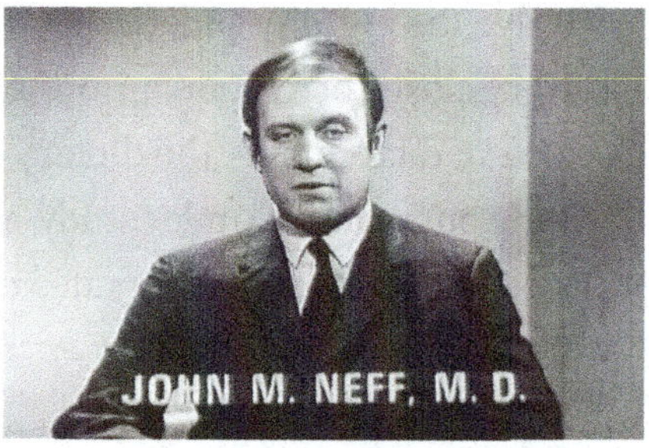

LEFT TO RIGHT **(1)** Samuel Lawrence Katz, MD. "Smallpox Vaccination: Should our Policy be Changed?," 1969 • *National Library of Medicine #8601126A* **(2)** John M. Neff, MD. "Smallpox Vaccination: Should our Policy be Changed?," 1969 • *National Library of Medicine #8601126A*

smallpox vaccine." They agreed, at least, on this graphic that shows regions of the world where smallpox was endemic in 1955.

In other presentations, doctors considered the most effective treatment for narcotic addicts (intensive inpatient therapies vs. reliance on methadone), as well as access to birth control pills. In "The Oral Contraceptives," the debate was mostly about side effects, and how tightly access to the pill should be controlled by the medical establishment. Just four years before, in 1965's Griswold v. Connecticut, the U.S. Supreme Court had struck down a state law banning the use of contraceptives by married women. Individual states could still prevent unmarried females' access to contraception, and many did. In the *Concepts* segments, the question of who should have access and under what circumstances arises. Dr. Louis Lasagna argued that many women don't want or need 100 percent effectiveness in birth control, and the possible complications are therefore not worth the health risks when safer, almost as effective methods are available.

Preserving Data

The *Concepts* debates, informed and thought-provoking, were possible because data were collected, disseminated, and analyzed. Continued interpretations and criticisms of those studies are possible today because, just as critically, the data were preserved. A PubMed search reveals forty-one articles that interpret or re-interpret data from Ancel Keys' Seven Countries Study (cited by Dr. Stamler), including this one from 2015 about the impact of the study on the Mediterranean diet concept.

• • •

We hear about data every day. In historical medical collections, data abounds, both quantitative and qualitative. In its format, scope, and biases, data inherently contains more information than its face value. This series, Revealing Data, explores how, by preserving the research data of the past and making it publicly available, the National Library of Medicine helps to ensure that generations of researchers can reexamine it, reveal new stories, and make new discoveries. As the NLM becomes the new home of data science at the National Institutes of Health (NIH), Circulating Now *explores what researchers from a variety of disciplines are learning from centuries of preserved data, and how their work can help us think about the future preservation and uses of the data we collect today.*

• • •

Learn more about the NLM's world-renowned historical audiovisuals collection.

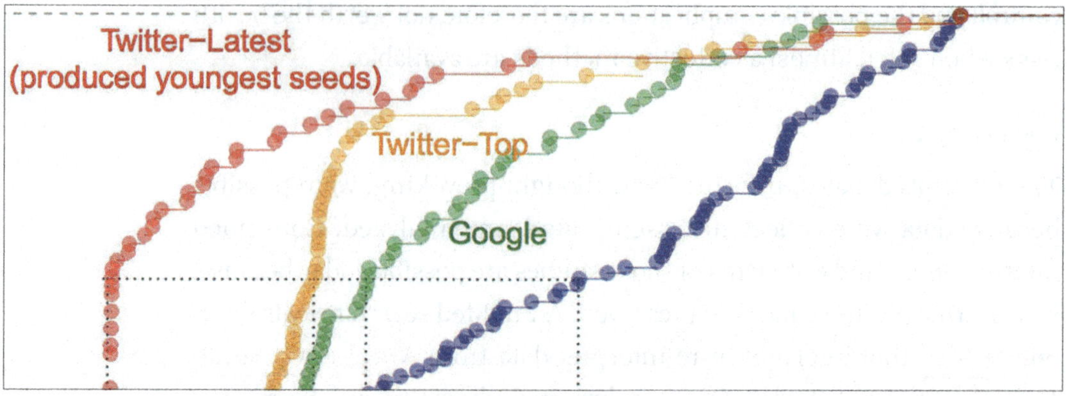

REVEALING DATA: WHY WE NEED HUMANS TO CURATE WEB COLLECTIONS

https://circulatingnow.nlm.nih.gov/2018/08/14/revealing-data-why-we-need-humans-to-curate-web-collections/

August 14, 2018 • Archives & Manuscripts, Revealing Data, Guests

ALEXANDER NWALA

In this Revealing Data series we explore data in historical medical collections, and how preserving this data helps to ensure that generations of researchers can reexamine it, reveal new stories, and make new discoveries. Future researchers will likely want to examine the data of the web archive collections, collected and preserved by libraries, archives, and others, using a wide range of approaches, to document unfolding events. Today Circulating Now *welcomes guest blogger Alexander Nwala (@acnwala), writing on his research using the National Library of Medicine (NLM) web archive collections to compare different methods of selecting web content, and some of the difficulties encountered in generating seeds automatically.*

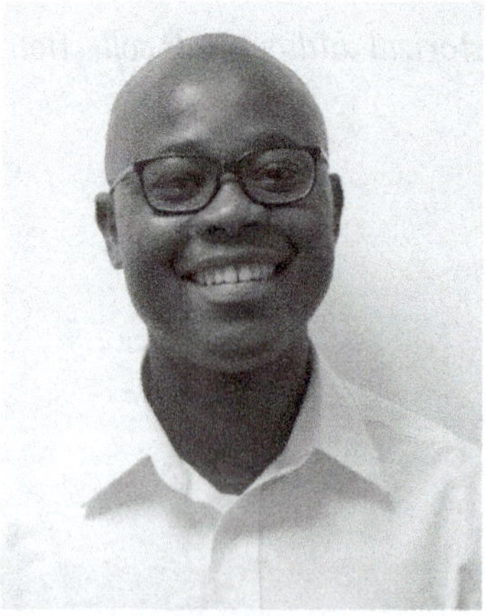

Alexander Nwala

• • •

I am a computer science PhD student and member of the Web Science and Digital Libraries Research Group at Old Dominion University, Norfolk Virginia. For the past three years, I have been researching generating collections for stories and events under the supervision of Dr. Michael Nelson and Dr. Michele Weigle. There is a shortage of curators to build web archive collections in a world of rapidly unfolding events. A primary objective of my research is investigating how to automatically generate seeds (in the absence of domain knowledge) to create or augment web archive collections.

In the past four years there have been three outbreaks of Ebola virus in Western and Central Africa. Between March 2014 and June 2016, Guinea, Liberia, and Sierra Leone experienced the largest Ebola epidemic in history with over 11,000 deaths. More recently (2017–2018), the Democratic Republic of Congo in Central Africa has been grappling with another Ebola outbreak.

Two months after the World Health Organization declared the 2014 Ebola outbreak a Public Health Emergency of International Concern (PHEIC), the NLM Web Collecting and Archiving Working Group started collecting website URLs as part of the NLM Global Health Events web archive collection. The NLM Ebola virus web archive collection includes websites of organizations, journalists, healthcare workers, and scientists related to the 2014 Ebola virus discourse. More recently as part of a new web archiving initiative, historian Christine Wenc and archivist Erin Mashni collaborated with the NLM to collect URLs for the HIV/AIDS web archive collection. This collection consists of websites and social media archived to document HIV/AIDS in the early twenty-first century.

Anyone who has ever clicked a link and was presented with a disappointing 404 response indicating the absence of a resource understands the impermanence of web resources. You've probably seen many 404 pages from the conventional (CNN) to the creative (Pixar).

This decay of web links over time is known as *link rot*. Consequently, the preservation of elements of our collective digital heritage, ranging from disease outbreaks to elections is critical, and this is a primary purpose of web archive collections such as the NLM Ebola virus and HIV/AIDS collections.

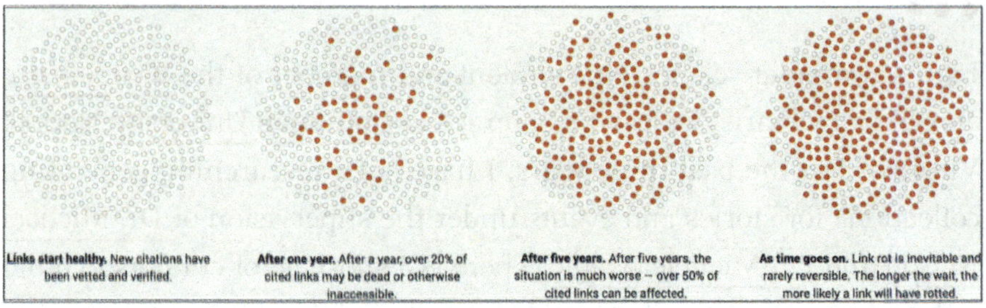

Link Rot over Time • An illustration from Perma.cc showing how links rot (orange circles) over time, August 10, 2018

Web archive collections consist of groups of web pages that are copied into an archive so as to resist link rot on the live web. These collections share a common topic e.g., "Ebola virus" or "2018 Winter Olympics", and begin with an initial selection of website URLs called *seeds*. For example, below is a sample of five seeds selected by the NLM for the Archive-It Ebola virus collection:

1. http://www.niaid.nih.gov/topics/ebolaMarburg/understandingEbola/
2. http://www.cdc.gov/vhf/ebola/pdf/facts-about-ebola-french.pdf
3. http://nypost.com/2014/10/29/ebola-doctor-lied-about-his-nyc-travels-police/
4. http://blogs.plos.org/dnascience/2014/11/06/eman-reports-ebola-ground-zero/
5. http://blogs.plos.org/speakingofmedicine/2014/10/22/ebola-taught-us-crucial-lesson-views-irrational-health-behaviors/

Quality seeds lead to quality archive collections. A collection of seeds with variations of "buy cheap Rolex watches" or "we sell gold nuggets" is not expected to yield a good web archive collection for the "2009 Swine Flu outbreak." This is where curators come into the picture. Curators must ensure they select seeds that are relevant for the collection topic. This means curators such as those at the NLM not only have the responsibility of searching for URLs to populate the seed list, but they also serve as filters to remove irrelevant URLs. This is a time consuming process because it is mostly done manually. For example, it took several months to collect the NLM Ebola virus seeds. A natural question is: can we automate the seed generation process? In other words, to what extent can a computer program replicate creating seeds for web archive collection?

See: "Bootstrapping Web Archive Collections from Social Media," for more details about automating the seed generation process.

Can We Automate the Seed Generation Process?

To answer this question I compared seed URLs from the NLM HIV/AIDS collection to those generated automatically on June 18, 2018 from search results on Google and Twitter.

TL;DR

Automating seed selection is hard. It is difficult to encode the various nuanced objectives of collections with a narrow scope, consequently, machine-generated seeds are not well-suited for collections with a narrow scope. But machine-generated seeds are suitable for collections with a broad scope especially when off-topic seeds are removed.

Generating seeds automatically from Google and Twitter

The Google seeds were generated automatically by issuing the query "hiv aids" to Google and extracting 115 links from the first five pages. Two sets of seeds (Twitter-Top and Twitter-Latest) were generated automatically by extracting URLs from tweets with the hashtag #hivaids from the Top (157 URLs) and Latest (146 URLs) Twitter search results. These automatically generated URLs constitute the seeds for the Google, Twitter-Top, and Twitter-Latest collections, in comparison with the human selected seeds of the NLM collection, for the purposes of this study.

Seed comparison: human curated NLM HIV/AIDS vs. Google and Twitter generated HIV/AIDS seeds

The NLM seeds were compared to the seeds from Google and Twitter across four dimensions: precision, percentage of top-level sites, age distribution, and topical coverage.

Precision

A precision score of 0 indicates that no URL is relevant to HIV/AIDS, while a precision score of 1 indicates that all URLs under consideration are relevant. To measure precision, all URLs in the Google and Twitter collections were manually inspected and assigned a relevance score of 0, 0.5, or 1. A 0 was assigned to URLs irrelevant to the HIV/AIDS topic, 0.5—somewhat related, and 1—primarily related. Subsequently, the sum of all the relevance scores of each URL divided by the seed list size produced the precision.

Unsurprisingly, URLs from Google (0.98) outranked URLs from Twitter (0.70–0.77) in the precision ranking (Fig. 1). Also, more relevant URLs were included in tweets from Twitter's Top (0.77) than the Latest (0.70) search results—popularity may be correlated to quality.

These precision results show that we cannot blindly include URLs generated automatically in a seed list without inspection, especially if the URLs are from tweets, since hashtags are frequently used by spammers. However, Twitter and Google still offer an opportunity for generating good seeds, but URLs extracted from these sources should be screened to remove off-topic URLs.

Percentage of top-level sites

Almost half (47 percent) of the URLs in the NLM HIV/AIDS seed list are top-level sites (e.g., https://hiv-age.org/) (Fig. 2). This is in contrast to Twitter and Google, which tend to give deep links (e.g., http://hiv-age.org/2018/04/06/75-deaths-older-adults-non-hiv/), which typically correspond to a narrow topic or specific story.

Age distribution

The date a web page was created can be used to rule out the kinds of topics it discusses. For example, web pages created before January 2017 are not expected to discuss the policies President Trump implemented to combat HIV/AIDS, since the Trump administration began in January 2017 (of course, a page created in October 2016 could speculate about future events [2017] or review past events [1987], but we focus only on the date the page was created [2016]). This means that without analyzing the content of seeds, we may be able to use the creation dates of the URLs to predict the topics to expect. As a result, we expect the creation dates of the NLM seeds to cover a broad range, providing a twenty-first-century perspective on HIV/AIDS. The age distribution confirms this expectation—the NLM seeds produced the oldest documents.

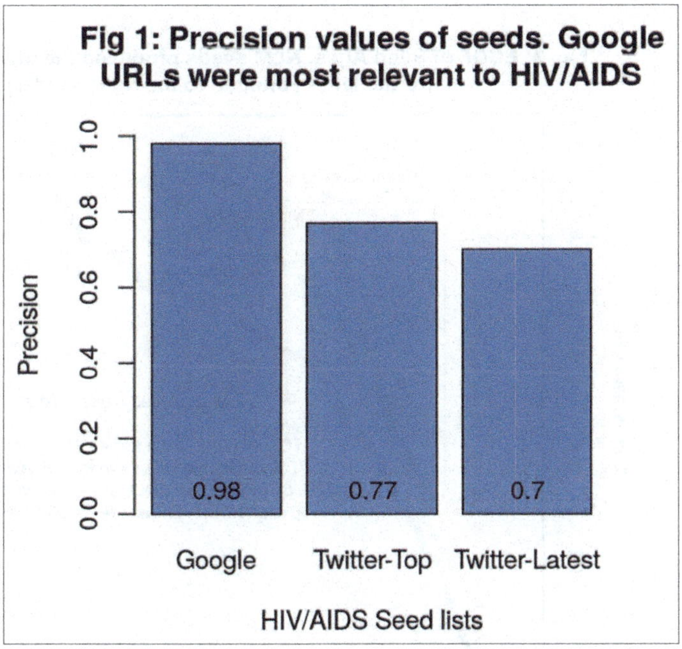

Precision values of seeds

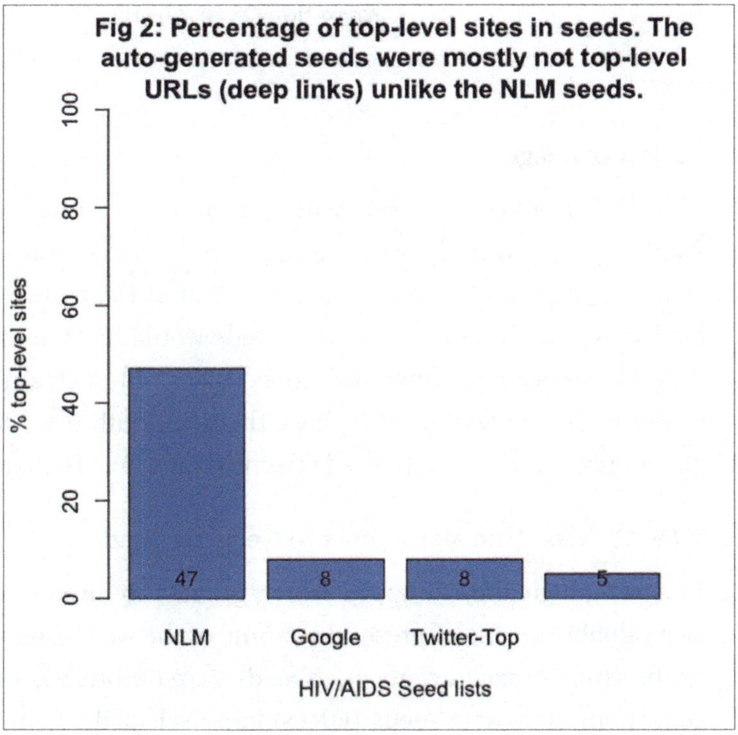

Percentage of seeds that are top-level sites

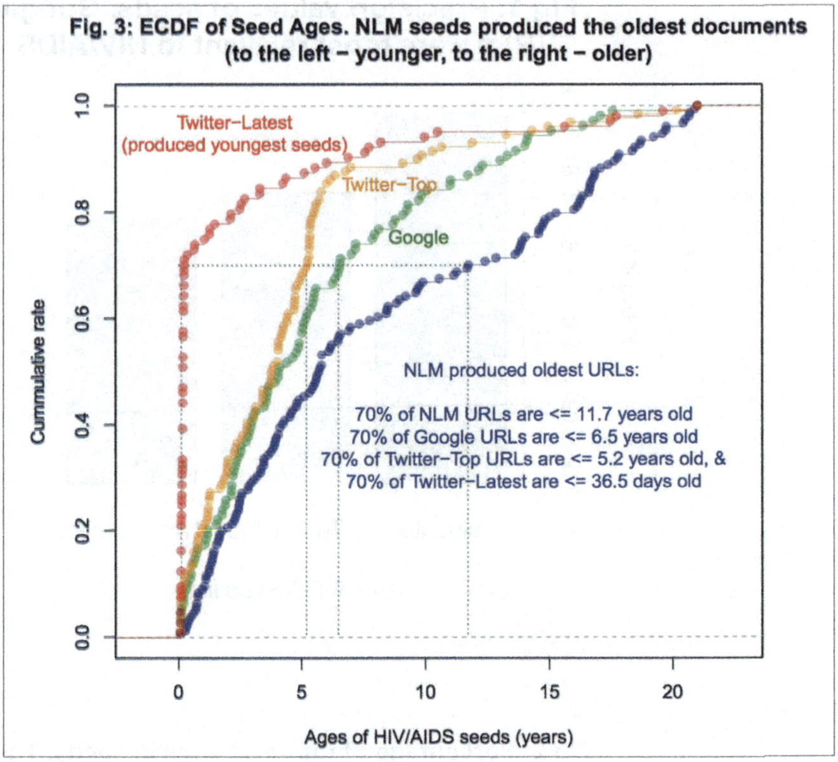

Empirical Cumulative Distribution Function (ECDF) of Seed Ages • NLM seeds produced the oldest documents.

Topical coverage

The seeds from Google and Twitter are a mix of various topics on HIV/AIDS ranging from the worsening AIDS epidemic in Russia to a tweet encouraging men to get tested. The intent of the NLM HIV/AIDS collection is broadly scoped, so these seeds would be at home in the NLM collection. But a more narrowly scoped collection, such as the 2018 Ebola outbreak vs. the 2016 outbreak vs. the 2014 outbreak, would be more challenging to create with seeds from Google and Twitter.

Why We Need Human Curators to Generate Seeds

In a web plagued by disappearing resources, archived collections stand as a valuable means of preserving some of the web resources important to the study of past events such as disease outbreaks. These archived collections start with seeds (URLs) hand selected by curators. Human curators produce high-quality seeds by removing irrelevant URLs, adding

URLs from credible and authoritative sources, but most importantly, they include only URLs that meet the collecting policy of the collection. The collecting policy could be broad (e.g., HIV/AIDS in the twenty-first century) or narrow (e.g., 2017 Opioid epidemic in Pennsylvania) and the curator has the ability to adapt to the multiple objectives of a collection. But this ability comes at a cost: it is time consuming to collect these seeds.

Machines, on the other hand, are fast and can discover a lot of seeds quickly, but even if content analysis is applied to filter non-relevant URLs, it is still hard to seamlessly adapt specific collecting policies (broad or narrow scope). Although search engines and social media can be used to generate seeds for collections with a broad scope, collections with nuance and subtlety are harder to automate. This is a primary objective of my research: to leverage the collective domain expertise of users on social media by extracting seeds from their social media "micro-collections" instead of simply using search engines and social media directly.

The web archive community has invested significant effort in building collections for specific topics through focused-crawling. But not much research effort addresses the discovery of seeds needed by focused-crawlers. My research addresses automating the seed generation stage of building web archive collections.

• • •

Learn more about Web Collecting at the NLM.

• • •

We hear about data every day. In historical medical collections, data abounds, both quantitative and qualitative. In its format, scope, and biases, data inherently contains more information than its face value. This series, Revealing Data, explores how, by preserving the research data of the past and making it publicly available, the National Library of Medicine helps to ensure that generations of researchers can reexamine it, reveal new stories, and make new discoveries. As the NLM becomes the new home of data science at the National Institutes of Health (NIH), Circulating Now *explores what researchers from a variety of disciplines are learning from centuries of preserved data, and how their work can help us think about the future preservation and uses of the data we collect today.*

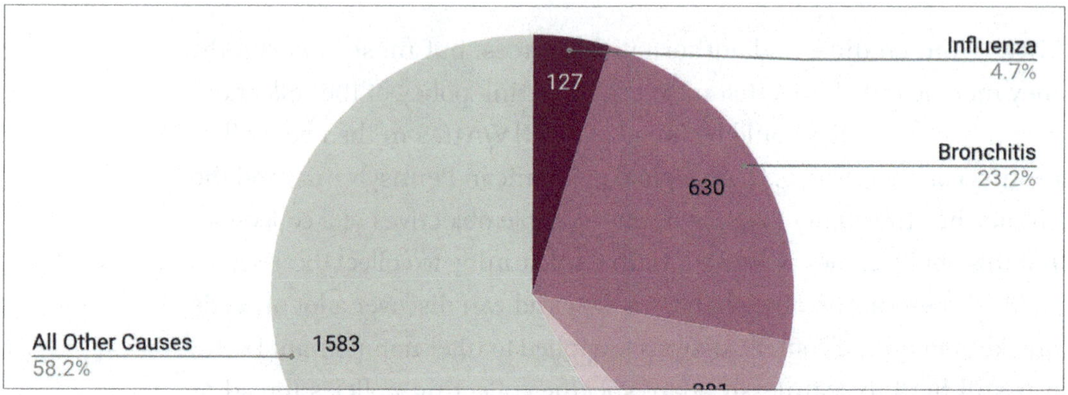

REVEALING DATA: MEASURING MORTALITY DURING AN EPIDEMIC

https://circulatingnow.nlm.nih.gov/2018/11/15/revealing-data-measuring-mortality-during-an-epidemic/

November 15, 2018 • Rare Books & Journals, Revealing Data, Guests

E. THOMAS EWING, IAN HARGREAVES, JESSICA KING, ANDREW PREGNALL, AND TYLER TALNAGI

Historical medical journals provide unique perspectives on the development of expert understanding of transmission, morbidity, and impact during an epidemic. Examining the ways that medical journals contributed to the spread of information, evaluation of interpretations, and creation of new knowledge in a specific historical process can contribute to current discussions about the relationship between expert perspectives and public understanding. Information on the Russian Influenza (1889–1890) in the British Medical Journal *offers an excellent case study for evaluating historical significance and contemporary relevance.* Circulating Now *welcomes guest bloggers E. Thomas Ewing, Ian Hargreaves, Jessica King, Andrew Pregnall, and Tyler Talnagi who examine different dimensions of the role of medical journals in collecting, presenting, and interpreting knowledge of a disease outbreak in this second of three posts for our ongoing Revealing Data series.*

• • •

The January 1890 issues of the *British Medical Journal* included several reports on the Russian influenza epidemic in European and British locations that combined summary analysis of the spread of the disease, first-hand accounts from physicians, and statistics on cases and deaths. This post examines the quantitative evidence presented in three *British Medical Journal* issues as a case study of how a medical journal revealed data about influenza deaths as a means of communicating information about this epidemic while it was occurring.

The statistical information included several reporting categories as well as methods of calculating and reporting changes. These statistics primarily deal with mortality, meaning the number of deaths associated with the epidemic, and include four main categories: total number of dead, number of deaths from diseases associated with influenza, death rate per 1,000 of the population, and deaths reported on a weekly basis. These methods were designed to address key issues recognized as critical for measuring the impact of an epidemic, including influenza as a primary or secondary cause of death, identifying unusual levels of mortality associated with influenza, and defining periods of time long enough to allow for variation yet short enough to make comparisons. Reporting on the number of deaths during a week, for example, overcomes potentially misleading fluctuations when deaths are reported daily, yet also allows for meaningful comparisons that show significant change over time. Reporting deaths per 1,000 people makes it possible to compare the impact of the epidemic in different geographical regions in ways that would be obscured by measuring total deaths, while also allowing for comparisons to average death rates over a period of time to document change. Comparing the number of deaths from influenza to other related diseases, including respiratory diseases more generally as well as specific diseases such as pneumonia, allows for recognition of the fact that influenza was, and still is, often a secondary cause of death, with the primary cause being a related disease that is more deadly when victims have been compromised by the influenza.

The statistics about Vienna, Paris, and London published in three successive issues of the *British Medical Journal* represent a small fraction of the total reporting of this disease, yet it shows how statistics were used to make sense of the epidemic at its peak and also as it began to decline in intensity. In these articles, the statistics were embedded in the text, which requires careful reading to distinguish quantitative data from other kinds of reporting, including identification of symptoms, discussion of how the disease spreads, and possible treatments. Converting the statistical information embedded in texts into charts makes it possible to see change over time, compare rates, and identify causation.

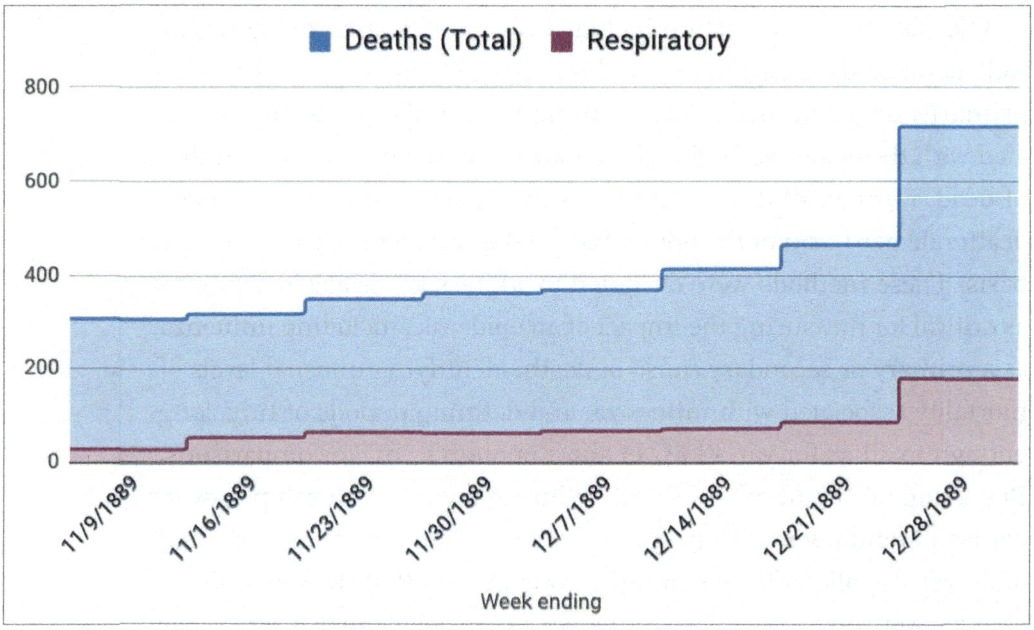

FIGURE 1 • Total deaths from all causes and from respiratory diseases, weekly, November and December 1889, Vienna, in "The Epidemic of Influenza," *British Medical Journal*, Issue 1515, Vol. 1, January 11, 1890, pp. 95–98.

Using statistics published in a report on Vienna, Figure 1 illustrates how the number of deaths from all causes and the number of deaths from respiratory diseases increased in parallel during the final eight weeks of 1889. Even though the deaths from respiratory diseases increased significantly during the week ending December 28, 1889, the number of deaths from all causes rose even more significantly, as indicated in the chart, which suggests that the epidemic contributed to a higher toll of deaths from causes other than respiratory diseases.

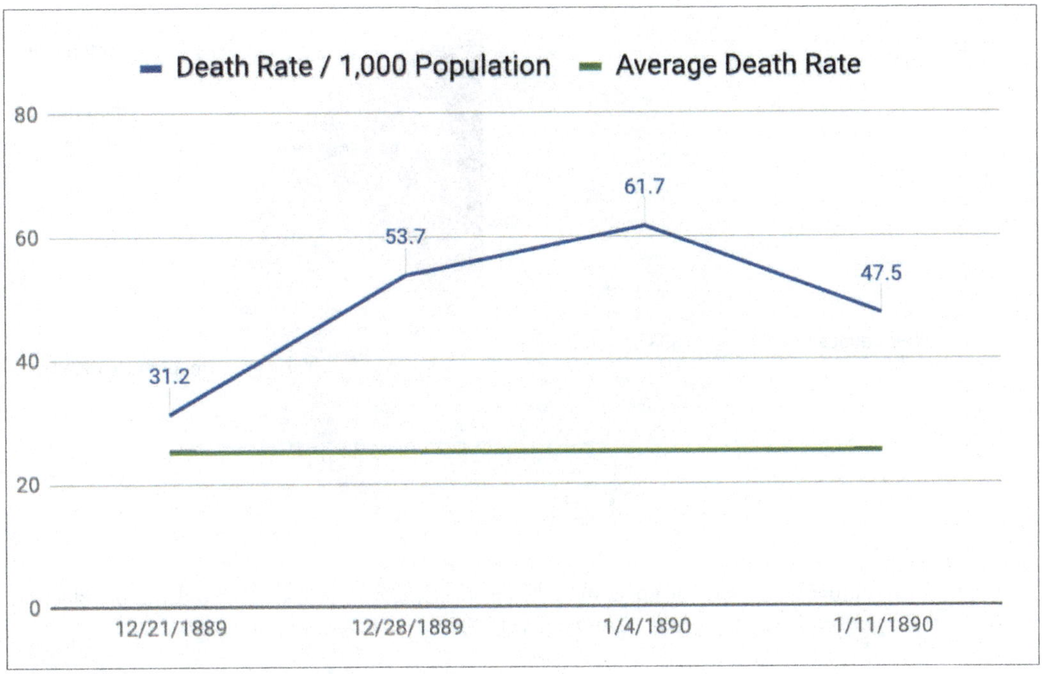

FIGURE 2 • Rate of deaths from all causes, compared to rate from similar weeks in 1889, Paris, December 1889 and January 1890, in "The Epidemic of Influenza," *British Medical Journal*, Issue 1516, Vol. 1, January 18, 1890, pp. 146–150.

In Figure 2, the average death rate for weeks in December 1888 and January 1889 is compared to the sudden increase in death rates in Paris at the height of the Russian influenza. As indicated in this chart, the death rate doubled from the third week of December to the first week of January, yet was already declining by the time this report was published in the January 18, 1890 issue of the *British Medical Journal*.

Similar changes are revealed in Figure 3, which compares the death rate from all causes with the total number of deaths from respiratory diseases for London. The significant increase in both death rates and total deaths from respiratory diseases from the last week of December through the second week of of January suggests that most of the increase in total deaths was due to higher numbers of respiratory deaths.

As these charts indicate, understanding the impact of the epidemic depended on a full understanding of the relationship between different causes of death. Figures 4 and 5 compare reports on causes of death in Paris and London during a particular week of the epidemic. Both charts

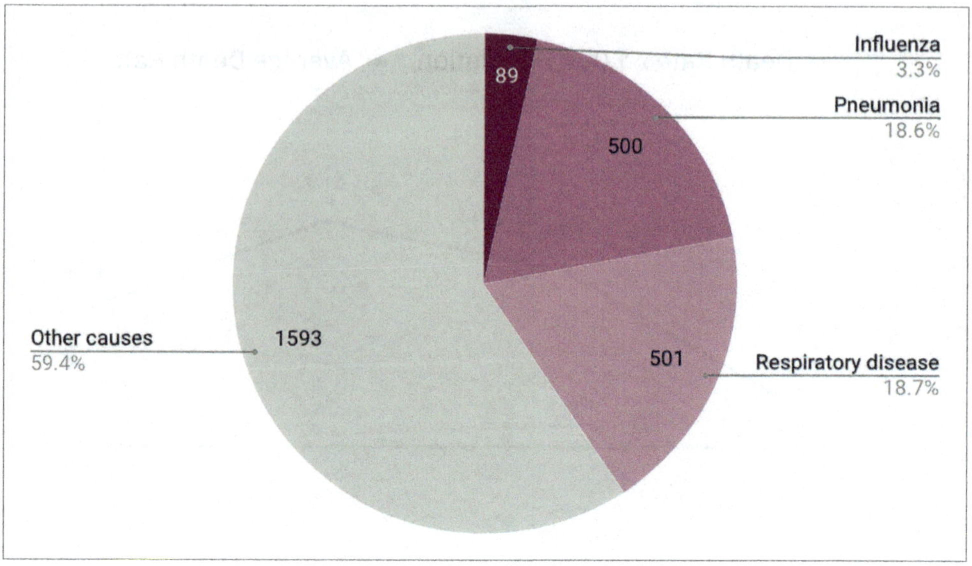

FIGURE 3 • Cause of death, week ending January 4, 1890, Paris, in "The Epidemic of Influenza," *British Medical Journal*, Issue 1516, Vol. 1, January 18, 1890, pp. 146–150.

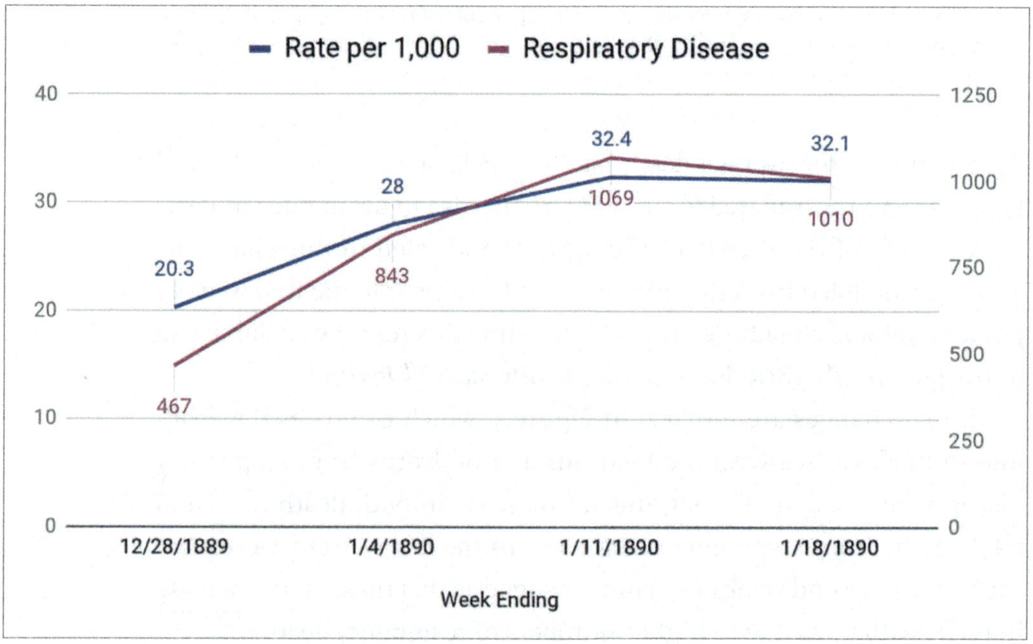

FIGURE 4 • Rate of death from all causes and total number of deaths from respiratory diseases, weekly, London, December 1889 and January 1890, in "The High Death-Rate in London and Paris," *British Medical Journal*, Issue 1517, Vol. 1, January 25, 1890, pp. 196–197.

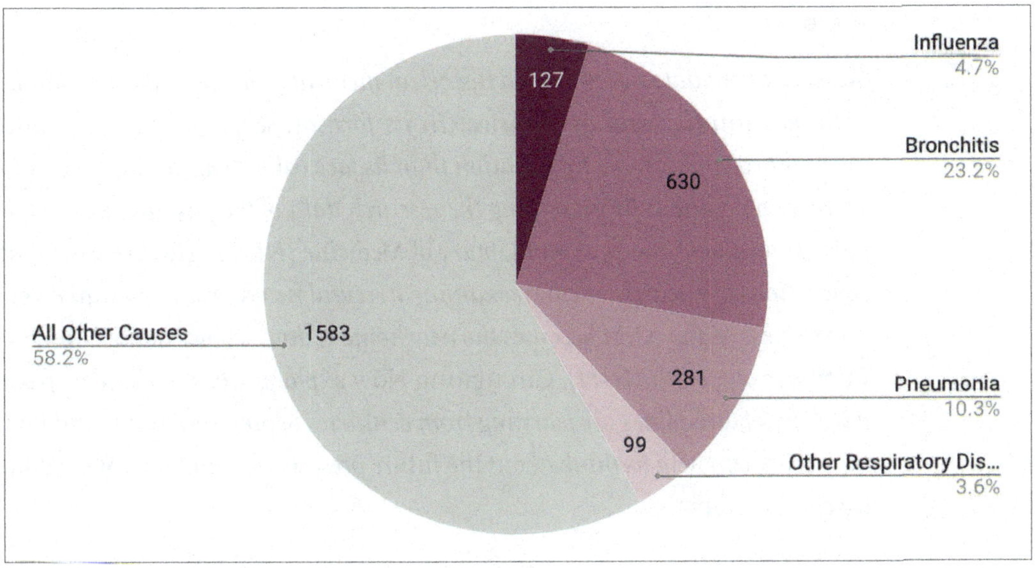

FIGURE 5 • Cause of death, week ending January 18, London, in "The High Death-Rate in London and Paris," *British Medical Journal*, Issue 1517, Vol. 1, January 25, 1890, pp. 196–197.

indicate that influenza was the direct cause of a relatively small proportion of deaths (3.3 percent in Paris and 4.7 percent in London). In both cities, much higher proportions of deaths were caused by pneumonia (18.6 percent in Paris and 10.3 percent in London) and other respiratory diseases (18.7 percent in Paris and 26.8 percent in London). Combining these categories indicates that nearly one-half of all deaths during these weeks could be attributed directly or indirectly to the influenza epidemic.

Using contemporary tools to visualize these statistics allows for new ways to use data from the past to reveal patterns of historical change and causal relationships. Yet these statistical reports and the data visualization raise questions that cannot be resolved using just this quantitative evidence. In each case, understanding how the epidemic affected the total number of deaths, the death rate, and the pattern of deaths by specific causes all requires more research on how these categories were defined, recorded, and changed over time. For the historian looking back on this evidence, as much as for the physician or epidemiologist at the time, counting victims was an important means for making sense of the epidemic of influenza.

• • •

We hear about data every day. In historical medical collections, data abounds, both quantitative and qualitative. In its format, scope, and biases, data inherently contains more information than its face value. This series, Revealing Data, explores how, by preserving the research data of the past and making it publicly available, the National Library of Medicine (NLM) helps to ensure that generations of researchers can reexamine it, reveal new stories, and make new discoveries. As the NLM becomes the new home of data science at the National Institutes of Health (NIH), Circulating Now *explores what researchers from a variety of disciplines are learning from centuries of preserved data, and how their work can help us think about the future preservation and uses of the data we collect today.*

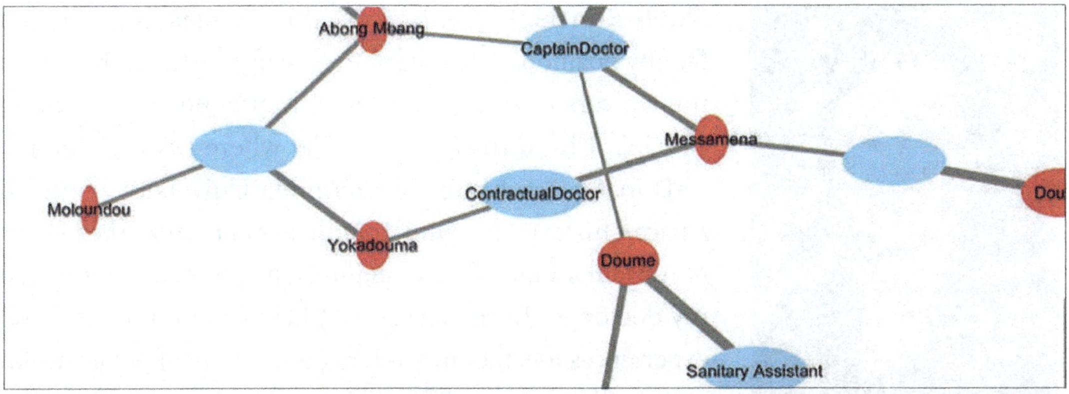

NAMING, NETWORKS, AND POWER IN HISTORIES OF MEDICINE IN AFRICA

https://circulatingnow.nlm.nih.gov/2019/04/04/naming-networks-and-power-in-histories-of-medicine-in-africa/

April 4, 2019 • Revealing Data

SARAH RUNCIE

Sarah Runcie, PhD, will speak on April 4, 2019 at 2:00 ET in the Lister Hill Auditorium at the National Library of Medicine (NLM) on "Naming, Networks, and Power in Histories of Medicine in Africa" as part of a panel. This special program "Viral Networks, Reconnected" reunites three scholars who participated in the January 2018 Viral Networks workshop at the NLM—funded by the National Endowment for the Humanities through a grant to Virginia Tech—to share the progress of their research and their thoughts about the future of the digital humanities and the history of medicine.

• • •

Circulating Now: Tell us a little about yourself. Where are you from? What do you do? What is your typical workday like?

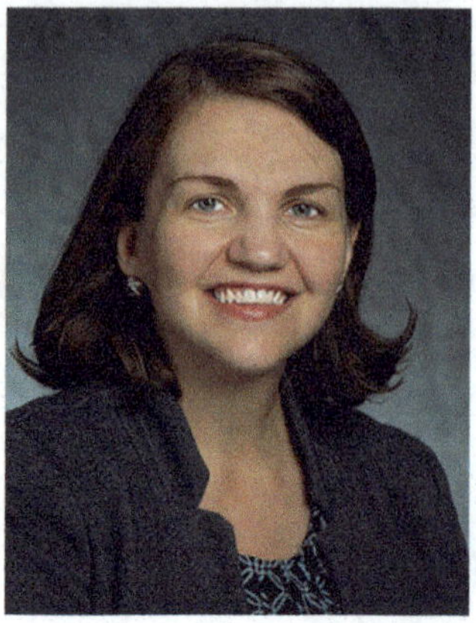

Sarah Runcie: I recently moved to Louisiana to begin a faculty position as Assistant Professor of African history at the University of Louisiana at Lafayette. Before beginning this job, I lived in New York City where I completed my PhD in African history at Columbia University. I studied African history as an undergraduate but then worked in the non-profit sector focused on public health before I pursued my doctorate. In my research, I bring these interests and experiences together by studying the history of public health and medicine in modern Africa.

In a typical workday, I'm involved in different activities related to teaching, research, and service work on campus. This spring I am teaching a survey class of world history as well as a new class I designed on Africa and World War II. I find that few students in the United States have been taught very much about African history but are eager to learn about this past. It's very satisfying to explore these new perspectives with them. When I'm not teaching or meeting with students, I can be found working on my current research and writing on the history of decolonization and global health programs in Cameroon.

CN: Your chapter in the newly released *Viral Networks* book is titled "Networks of the Unnamed and Medical Interventions in Colonial Cameroon," would you tell us a little of what you discovered about the work of mobile health teams in French colonial Cameroon?

SR: The mobile health teams in French colonial Cameroon are the basis of my ongoing research—from my doctoral dissertation to my current book manuscript. French doctors created these teams across colonies in Africa to travel to rural areas and assemble people for examination and vaccination. The teams have a complicated legacy, because many things about them were very "colonial," such as the use of coercion to make Africans comply with the medical interventions of the teams. One thing I've always been interested about with regard to the teams, however, is how French doctors really celebrated their work as a major achievement of French medicine in the colonies, but how heavily they relied on the labor of Africans whether as medical auxiliaries or porters. In my chapter for *Viral Networks*, I had the chance to think through what it means to

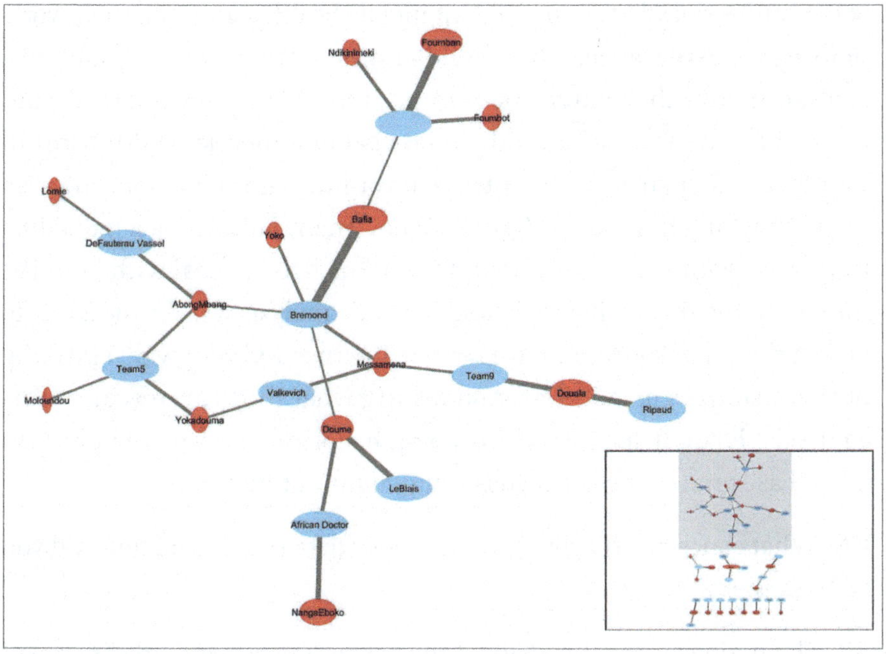

FIGURE 1.1 • Visits, 1947–1951 • Blue ovals represent the mobile health teams. Red ovals represent locations of the visits with size based on the recorded population for that location. The width of the connecting lines represents the number of patients seen at each visit.

try to visually represent this labor, given that African participants are often not counted or named in the same way as the French doctors in the archival records of the teams. One of the main questions I explored is: how can I bring my research perspectives and commitments to life with digital tools?

CN: You used network analysis in your research. What is this technique and how was it useful in this case?

SR: Network analysis is a framework to help us think in new ways about how people, places, or events are connected to one another. I was new to network analysis when I participated in the workshop that led to the publication of *Viral Networks,* but I found that it helped me think in new ways about my research. For this project I created a database on mobile health team visits using colonial medical records and then used the program Cytoscape to create a network analysis of the work of mobile health teams. This program allowed me to create different visualizations of the connections between different mobile health teams and their work. Before this experience, I have tended much more toward qualitative analysis in my scholarship. For example, I might be more drawn toward recounting the story of an individual visit of a mobile health team in Cameroon, focusing on the intricacies of human interaction, more so than crunching numbers to figure out how many villages each individual team was visiting in a given year. Historians need to deal with both the micro and the macro, however, and network analysis was for me a way to look at the same sources I have been using in a different way. Thinking of these sources as datasets, and asking what they can reveal in this aggregate form, helped me think about historical patterns in new ways as well as some of the concerns of digital humanities.

CN: What concerns did you have with your data source and how did you address them?

SR: The main concern I had about my data is a very standard concern of historians of Africa, which is that I was using colonial records produced by Europeans to try to analyze African history. The names and perspectives of Africans themselves are often absent from such records. Scholars

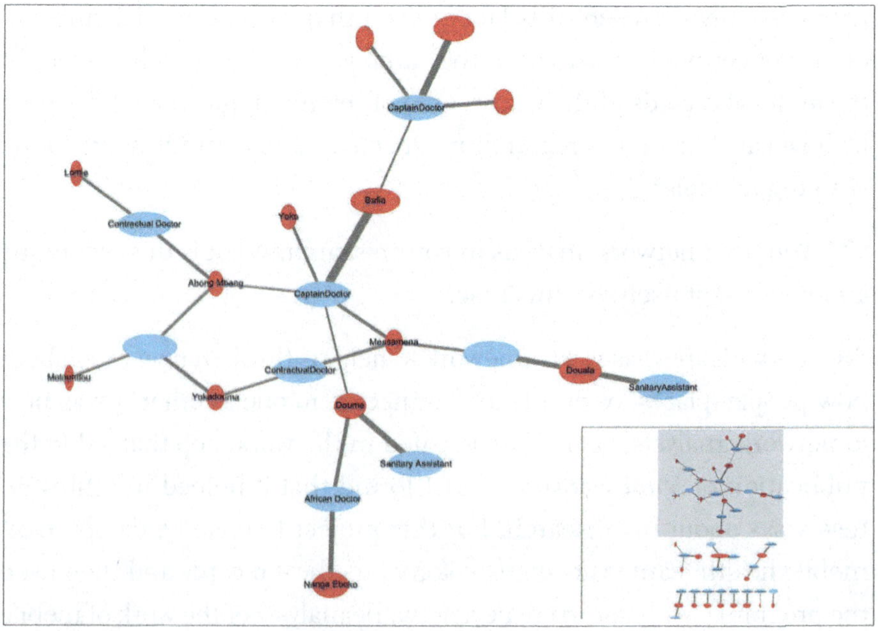

FIGURE 1.2 • Highlights the professional rank of the team head

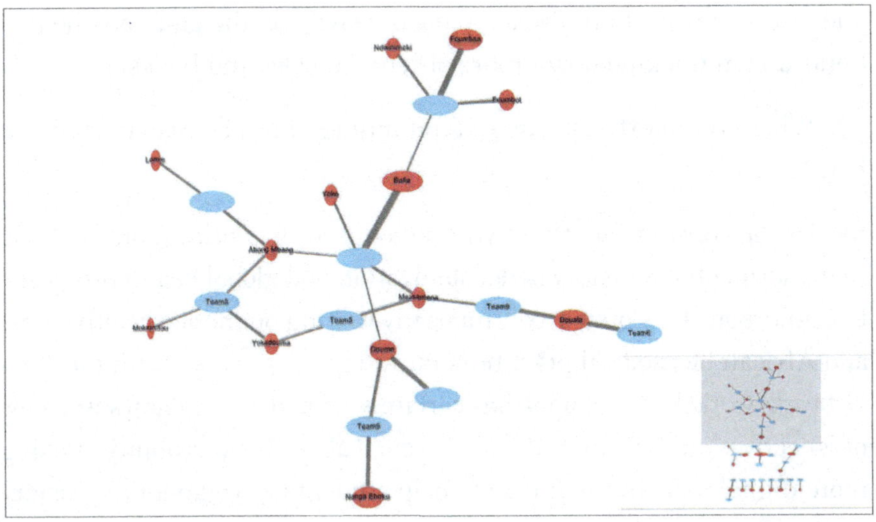

FIGURE 1.3 • Removes all information about the team head and highlights the administrative designation of the team, when available

who study colonial Africa, and certainly colonial medicine, have been discussing this issue for a long time. In thinking through this concern for the purposes of network analysis, I found the work of other scholars writing on digital humanities to be very helpful. In my chapter I discuss the work of Lauren F. Klein; her analysis of how the stories of the enslaved can be reframed away from merely "absences" in the archival record was very useful to me. I began to see that I had choices in how I used my data, choices that could be driven by my interest in understanding the work of Africans themselves as practitioners of biomedicine in the colonial period and beyond.

CN: How do libraries support the kind of research you do?

SR: Libraries are absolutely fundamental to the research I do. I've relied on libraries around the world, particularly medical libraries, to further my research—everywhere from the holdings of the Pasteur Institute in Cameroon to the library of the World Health Organization in Switzerland. The rare holdings of such libraries have been really crucial to me in uncovering complex transnational conversations between African, French and international health officials that I focus on in the part of my research that moves into postcolonial Cameroonian history. At both my doctoral and current institution, I've also relied heavily on the generous help of librarians in tracking down more obscure articles and books.

CN: What's your next step? Are you continuing a line of research discussed here?

SR: In the coming months, I will be focused on working on my book manuscript on the history of decolonization and global health programs in Cameroon. This project continues my writing on mobile health teams and African biomedical practitioners, and my experience with the *Viral Networks* workshop and book has certainly helped me develop some new perspectives on that work. I'm also excited about the possibility of using more digital tools in the future to help students learn about the history of disease and medicine in Africa.

• • •

Read Sarah Runcie's article in Viral Networks: Connecting Digital Humanities and Medical History, *comprising a collection of research papers resulting from the* Viral Networks *workshop, now available from VT Publishing and NLM Digital Collections.*

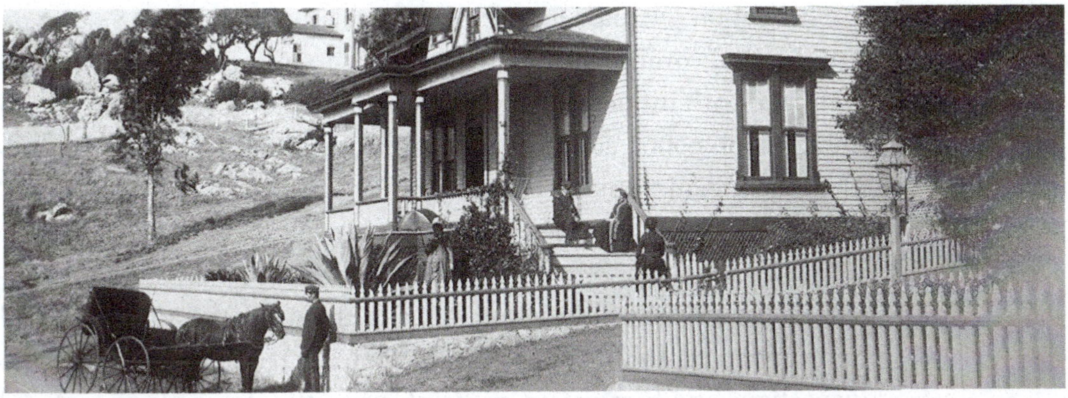

REVEALING DATA: RAIN, EPIDEMICS, AND LIFE ON THE DOCKS IN 1918

https://circulatingnow.nlm.nih.gov/2017/06/01/revealing-data-rain-epidemics-and-life-on-the-docks-in-1918/

June 1, 2017 • Archives & Manuscripts, Revealing Data

ASHLEY BOWEN

United States Public Health Service (USPHS) officers stationed in the San Francisco Bay complained about the rain and deer eating the garden as they carried out the work of inspecting recent arrivals for signs of disease. We know they had a minor deer problem on Angel Island because the Medical Officer in Charge (MOC) made note of it in the station journal, a handwritten log of daily activities. This is but one of the many eccentric, fascinating, and mundane entries in one of the station logs kept by the Marine Health Service that can be found in the Archives and Modern Manuscripts collections at the National Library of Medicine.

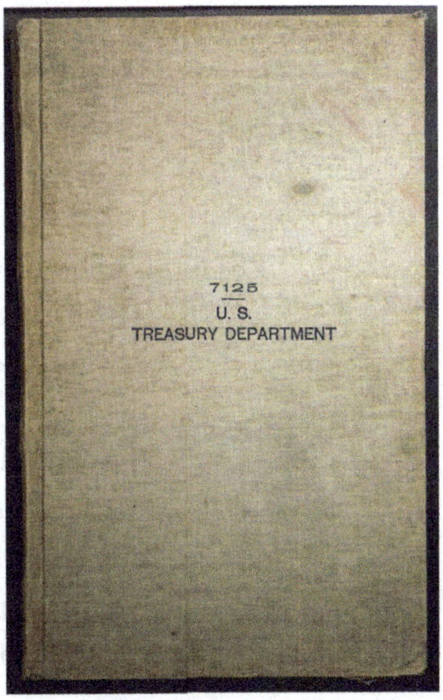

ABOVE Post-hospital Angel Island, CA, ca. 1918 • *National Library of Medicine #101394596*
RIGHT Cover of *San Francisco Quarantine Station Journal*, Angel Island, California, 1903–1943, Volume 4 • *National Library of Medicine #2932180R*

The station journals for the San Francisco Quarantine Station on Angel Island cover forty-three years (1903–1946), spanning two World Wars, the 1918 influenza pandemic, Japanese internment, changes in immigration policy, advances in bacteriology and virology, the development of antibiotics, and so much more. Each day (more or less) the MOC wrote a few lines about the station's activities.

Entries varied slightly by MOC but conform to a fairly standard format, tone, and scope of content. Most of the time, the MOC recorded information on the weather, staff changes or requests for leave, ship inspections and fumigation or disinfection, the status of quarantined patients, building repairs, official visitors to the station, instructions from USPHS leadership, etc. Sometimes, the MOC included newspaper clippings or other pieces of ephemera related to their work. Only the most important events, like the WWI armistice and attack on Pearl Harbor, made it into the log.

The logs offer researchers important data about the workings of a U.S. Public Health Service Immigration Station. Individual entries can be a bit dull (for example, days where the only note was "rain"). They offer up granular, if brief, detail about the work required to keep the station running, individual staff appointments, and specific cases of disease. Taken as a whole, the logs provide a fascinating account of on-the-ground responses to epidemics, policy changes, and life as a USPHS officer (entries mention everything from meritorious service to public intoxication around the holidays).

The notes from MOC W.A. Korn, who managed the Angel Island station through the 1918 influenza pandemic, epitomize the journals' balance of the specific and the general, the local and global.

The 1918 flu pandemic moved through the United States in waves. The first cases broke out at an army camp in Kansas in March 1918 but go unremarked upon in the quarantine station journals. In March 1918, the men working on Angel Island were more concerned about painting the outbuildings and managing the bids for station supplies than the flu. In fact, entries for the entire month of March 1918 take up just a little over two pages. Although it was a more mild infection that spring than it would be in the fall, it is difficult to imagine that Korn and his staff were unaware of the flu in Kansas. If they made any efforts to prepare for a flu

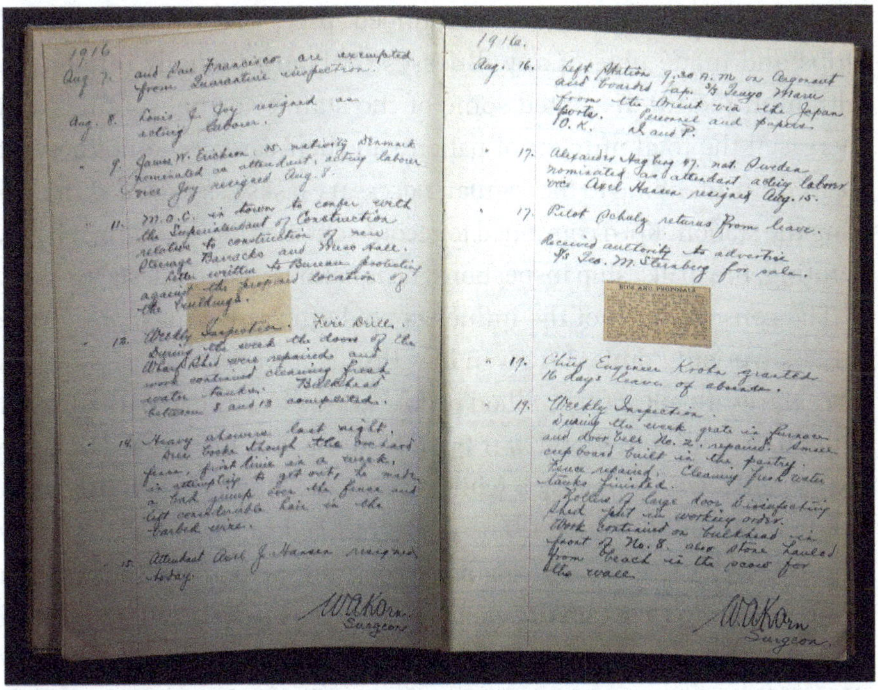

San Francisco Quarantine Station Journal, Angel Island, California, 1903–1943, Volume 4 open to August 7, 1916 • Transcript: 1916 Aug 7. and San Francisco are exempted from Quarantine inspection. • *National Library of Medicine #2932180R*

pandemic, these were not recorded in the station logs. Throughout the spring and summer, the staff reported cases of cerebro-spinal meningitis, small pox ("varioloid"), and an unconfirmed case of yellow fever.

It was the second wave of influenza infection, in the autumn of 1918, that brought the flu to Angel Island. On October 7, 1918 MOC W. A. Korn boarded a ship and discovered "several cases of influenza aboard. Health Officer of San Francisco notified. Otherwise all well." One week later, on October 15, the rate of new influenza cases at the station began to pick up. Thirty-five navy cadets suffering with influenza were transferred to the station for treatment and the Marine Hospital in San Francisco transferred its chronic patients to the Quarantine Station in order to free up space for treating influenza patients. The station also converted one of its dining rooms into an influenza ward. On October 22, one of the assistant surgeons was assigned "special temporary duty during the influenza epidemic" and transferred away from the station. Eventually, over eighty flu patients were on the island.

Nevertheless, life at the station continued apace. The staff still inspected ships and made note of any illnesses on board (usually influenza). Although the flu disrupted some of the staff's normal routines and increased the total number of patients in their care, it did not prevent them from attending to the regular, necessary tasks associated with running the station. Korn continued to record activities like building repairs, painting, fire drills, ship inspections, resignations, and requests for leave.

The consequences of the influenza epidemic rarely make it into the log, a surprising omission given how deadly it was. Modern estimates place the death toll at fifty million people worldwide, dwarfing the sixteen million casualties in World War I! On November 6, Korn noted that one of the clerks was "home sick with influenza." The clerk died nine days later, on November 15, 1918. The report of his death was the only entry Korn made for the day. The log book does not include any information about how Korn or his staff responded to the clerk's death but it is notable that this is the sole influenza death he mentioned. Other people certainly died of the flu on Angel Island; October 1918 was the deadliest month in a deadly epidemic, but those deaths do not make it into the station's log—even as an aggregate number (e.g. "x patients died" or "x buried/cremated/sent to city morgue today"). Korn did not record what, if any, efforts the staff made to mark the passing of a peer.

By early November, the flu recedes from Angel Island and the log book. On the 9th, the last of the naval cadets were discharged and by the 11th a group of ten men from the Naval Training Station at Goat Island (Yerba Buena Island) arrived to participate in experiments to identify the causal agent of influenza. Their arrival and a brief note about the experiment got slightly more attention than the armistice. After November 11th, the log book essentially returns to normal: staff changes, repair work, ship inspections, and a meeting about converting Angel Island into a leprosarium. A few cases of influenza among the staff were mentioned in the following months but not among the passengers or crew arriving in San Francisco.

What makes these station logs fascinating, their ability to juxtapose the mundane and the important, is also their limitation. These short entries hint at much larger stories—about epidemics, serving in the USPHS, immigration, war, crime, climate, and so much more—but by reducing

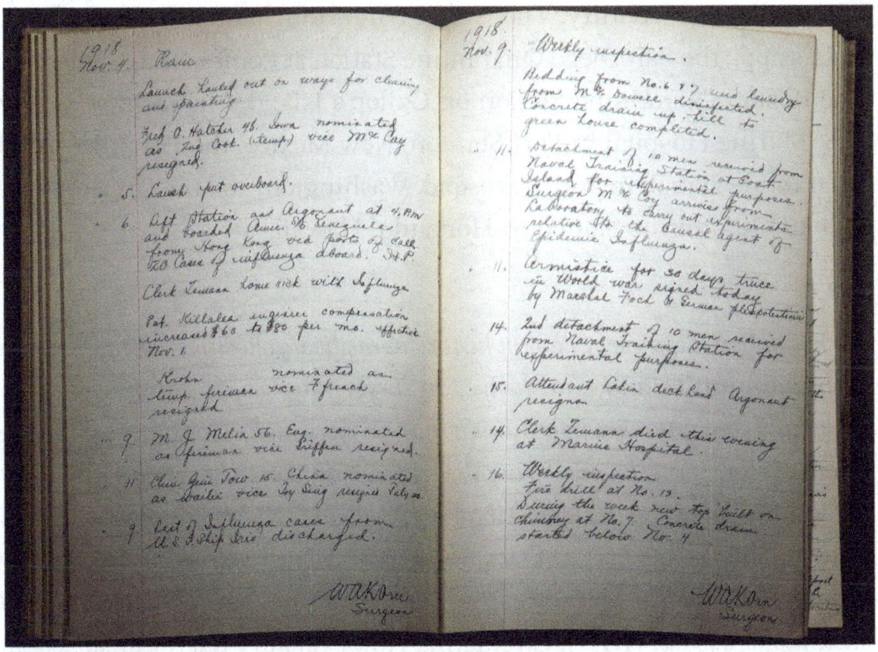

San Francisco Quarantine Station Journal, Angel Island, California, 1903–1943, Volume 4 open to November 4, 1918 • Transcript: 1918 Nov. 4. Rain Launch hauled out on ways for cleaning and painting. . . . • *National Library of Medicine #2932180R*

all of these activities to just a few lines of facts, the log can create a sense of false equivalence between, for example, the arrival of thirty-five sick sailors and repainting the pharmacy.

In addition to this record of forty-three years of daily life at the Angel Island Quarantine Station, the National Library of Medicine has station logs for six additional immigration and quarantine stations that operated

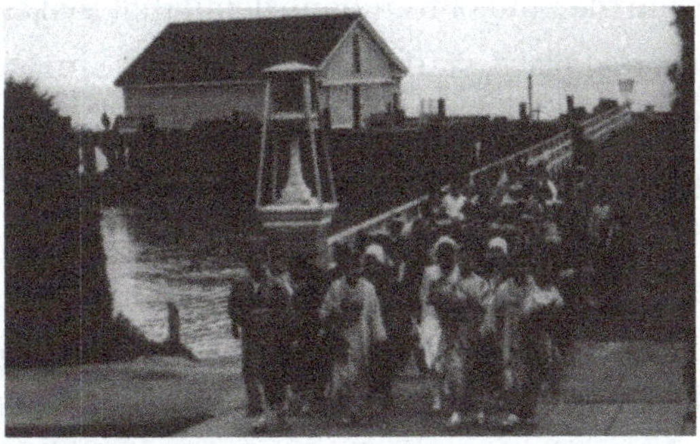

Asian immigrants arriving at the Immigration Station on Angel Island near San Francisco, California, 1931 • *National Library of Medicine #101447221*

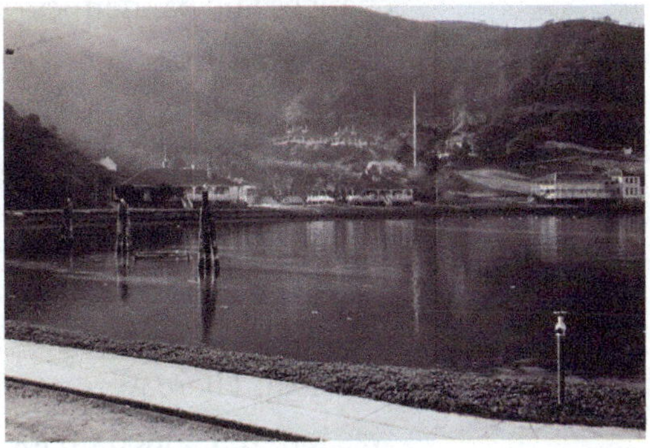

Angel Island Quarantine Station, 1925 • *National Library of Medicine #101416879*

in the twentieth century: The Gulf Quarantine Station on Ship Island, Mississippi; the San Diego Quarantine Station at Point Loma, California; The Boston Quarantine Station on Gallop's Island, Massachusetts; the U.S. Marine Hospital in Fort Stanton, New Mexico; the Port Townsend Quarantine Station in Port Townsend, Washington; and the United States Insular Quarantine Station in Honolulu, Hawaii.

• • •

We hear about data every day. In historical medical collections, data abounds, both quantitative and qualitative. In its format, scope, and biases, data inherently contains more information than its face value. This series, Revealing Data, explores how, by preserving the research data of the past and making it publicly available, the National Library of Medicine (NLM) helps to ensure that generations of researchers can reexamine it, reveal new stories, and make new discoveries. As the NLM becomes the new home of data science at the National Institutes of Health (NIH), Circulating Now *explores what researchers from a variety of disciplines are learning from centuries of preserved data, and how their work can help us think about the future preservation and uses of the data we collect today.*

Reflection

Some sources just beg to be spotlighted. As a historian of medicine with a longstanding interest in making that history accessible, interesting, and relevant to people outside the field, I am always thrilled when I find sources like the San Francisco Quarantine Station Journal. These handwritten logbooks—chronicling everything from the weather to staffing changes and pandemics—provide the kind of mundane detail that makes the quarantine station feel like a real place, staffed by real people. Simply put, this is gold for a historian like me.

I encountered these logbooks while conducting research in support of the NLM exhibition *Outside/Inside: Immigration, Migration, and Health Care in the United States*. I wanted to find a way to do more with these materials. *Circulating Now* provided an excellent platform for achieving this goal. There were so many threads here to pull that selecting just one was tough. I ended up focusing on the 1918 influenza pandemic because it was a discrete topic. The entries were contained by a clear date range, they were dramatic, and they illustrated the value in these kinds of short reflections on a major event made by a professional in the moment. The resulting post previewed the content of the exhibition, raised my own profile as a public historian of medicine, and served as a stand-alone article highlighting a fascinating primary source in the NLM collection, bringing to life the history of the U.S. Public Health Service in ways that are relatable and relevant today. —Ashley Bowen, 2023

CHAPTER 5

FROM WHERE YOU AND I SIT

INTRODUCTION • HEIDI MOREFIELD

Before the COVID-19 pandemic, it was challenging to imagine an academic conference in which you could participate from the comfort of your home, presenting your research from where you sit not only to those who traveled to the site of the meeting but also to anyone around the world, in any field, who chose to participate. Few could have envisioned the virtual conference that has now become commonplace and looks to be a model for the future. In this new space, rather than the standard one or two connections you might make with scholars in the few minutes of downtime between panels, you can be approached by many more people who read your work with interest and have something to ask or contribute. Now imagine an added aspect to this virtual conference: many scholars presenting on and drawing from the same expansive source and knowledge base—what might you learn from one another, and what opportunities and further dialogue might arise? From where I sit as a researcher, I am happy to say that such an expansive source and knowledge base existed before the pandemic, and has continued to flourish during our COVID times, as this book reflects. Since its launch in 2013, *Circulating Now* has provided researchers with a dynamic platform to share what they have discovered in the historical collections of the National Library of Medicine (NLM), encourage public dialogue, and advance knowledge about the past and its relevance to the present and the future.

Circulating Now brings together a network of individuals, wherever they might be located in the world, around a shared and valuable institutional collection. It enables readers to keep apprised of current historical research at the NLM, whether on site or remotely. *Circulating Now* is also a research venue—like a twenty-first-century Republic of Letters—a growing knowledge base of the intellectual depth and breadth of the historical collections of the NLM and the changing research trends in the history of medicine. This aspect of *Circulating Now* is particularly important given the long lead time it takes to have work published in traditional venues. *Circulating Now* offers researchers, and especially younger and early-career scholars, the opportunity to introduce themselves and their work to the broader field in more open and immediate ways. During a time when many scholars are working outside of the academy, *Circulating Now* is even more crucial—making fascinating historical research accessible to a broad range of public and professional audiences.

Like many others, I was fortunate enough to have my own work featured in *Circulating Now*. As an NLM Michael E. DeBakey Fellow in the History of Medicine, I spent a very productive year researching the life and work of DeBakey at the NLM. Writing for the blog was a way of launching a new facet of my research and connecting with scholars working in similar topics—the correspondence I received from fellow academics and medical professionals after publishing my short post led to some very valuable conversations and feedback that informed my further work on the topic. As useful as *Circulating Now* is for historians of medicine, its real strength is in the way it opens up the NLM historical collections—and the history of medicine as a field—for popular interest and engagement. At a moment when our historical research is increasingly relevant to present challenges, bringing the broader public into our conversations is incredibly valuable.

The posts presented in this chapter represent the research findings of a diverse group of stakeholders who find themselves drawn in to the historical collections of the NLM in unique ways, whether as students, interns, subject matter experts, archivists, or historians. Each author focuses on a particular holding, showcasing its importance to medical research and historical understanding of that research.

Through a multi-part interview on *Circulating Now*, psychoanalyst Kerry Kelly Novick discussed her father, Gene Kelly, the renowned actor, dancer, singer, filmmaker, and choreographer, and his role in the film *Combat Fatigue Irritability*, as well as how what is now known as post-traumatic stress disorder was depicted in 1945 and her reflections on training with Anna Freud. Psyche Williams-Forson of the University of Maryland-College Park took to *Circulating Now* to highlight some of the most important revelations from the exhibition she curated at the NLM, titled *Fire and Freedom: Food and Enslavement in Early America*. Writing about the experiences of Black women in the Middle Passage, Williams-Forson centers the importance of food cultures and the contributions enslaved women made to the economics of the New World markets.

Many authors point to the ways that unique holdings in the historical collections of the NLM have led to a new understanding of their field. In her post, "In Search of Sol Spiegelman," Susie Fisher of The Open University of Israel described what is a familiar realization to many who have worked in the NLM historical collections—how far *beyond* the typical narratives of the history of medicine, science, and technology the collections can take you. For Fisher, it was seeing the handwritten note that renowned scientist Salvador Luria had sent to Sol Spiegelman along with a news clipping from *The Boston Globe* that conveyed, very concretely, how important personal relationships are to the making of a scientific field. In her post "'Wrapped in Flesh': Views of the Body in East Asian Medicine," Yi-Li Wu of the University of Westminster looked to the 1808 text of Chinese doctor Qian Xiuchang to show how typical western conceptions that East Asian medicine is focused almost exclusively on the body's energies are not accurate. Rather, Qian's text, with innovative features like drawings of the front and back of the human skeleton and discussion of how to assess broken bones, proves that early East Asian healers were also concerned with bodily structures and anatomy.

The historical collections of the NLM contain an impressive array of visual materials appreciated by researchers of multiple disciplines who value such sources as windows on the human condition. Visual artist and professor at the University of South Carolina, Dawn Hunter, wrote in her post "Drawn To, Drawn From Experience" about her exploration and interpretation of the scientific drawings of the visionary neuroscientist Santiago Ramón y Cajal. His art drew Hunter in as she learned more about his personal history, which inspired her own art series. Medical student Benjamin Forrest drew from first-hand accounts of the Union Army's Ambulance Corps to write a nuanced assessment of how the Ambulance Corps was received by the larger Union Army when it was first established. Generating a far-reaching conversation in the comments, Forrest's contribution "Following the Rear: Travails of the Union Army's Ambulance Corps," testifies to how *Circulating Now* has encouraged public dialogue. Academics, archivists, and even relatives of those involved in the Ambulance Corps effort commented on Forrest's post with questions, their own viewpoints, and related research findings. Forrest not only advanced his own research through this dialogue but also experienced having a public impact with his work as he shared valuable insights into the experiences of some of the readers' cherished ancestors. His contribution represents how *Circulating Now* has served well as an open platform for sharing fine research and facilitating public dialogue to advance the historical research enterprise.

As suggested, the personal connections authors make to their historical subjects is one of the reasons *Circulating Now* is so captivating. For many researchers, archives and historical collections are more than just repositories to be mined—their relationships with the collections cut both ways. Ashley Bowen, editor of the American Historical Association's *Perspectives on History*, described in "Finding Hope: A Woman's Place is in the Lab" how she was inspired to improve collection descriptions through an immense effort to track down an unidentified female lab technician so that she could be properly credited and named. Naming the technician—who we now know was Hope Hopps, an integral member of the Laboratory of Viral Immunology in the 1960s—was Bowen's way of giving back to the archive and making sure that women's contributions to science and NIH history were not forgotten by future generations of researchers.

Others have also improved the accessibility of the collections. Writing in 2014 as a college sophomore and summer intern at the NLM, Shannon Lu recounts in her post "A Peek at Some Pamphlets" the insights she gleaned while cataloguing public health pamphlets in Chinese, Russian, Ukrainian, Bulgarian, Serbian, and Macedonian. Though cataloguing materials in non-Latin alphabets presented a challenge, she found that many of the public health themes present in the pamphlets transcended linguistic and geographic barriers. Emma Carter, writing in 2018 as a college junior and an intern with the Historical Audiovisuals program, took on the project of identifying the copyright status of the most requested films in the collection so that they might be made more available. In doing so, she stumbled upon the film *The Forgotten Frontier*, a popular and pioneering woman-made film from 1931 about Mary Breckinridge and the Frontier Nursing Service of Kentucky. Carter was struck by the film, which offers a rare glimpse of life in 1930s Appalachia, and shared her discovery and excitement with *Circulating Now* readers.

Through these collected posts I hope that, like me, readers will gain deeper appreciation of the wide-ranging value of the collections for a variety of purposes—there is no other resource like it in the United States. And yet, as Kerry Kelly Novick points out at the end of her interview, the NLM remains under-recognized for its historical collections. This is a shame. Historians of medicine know reflexively that these collections are integral to the study of the broader social and cultural history of our world. Current events continue to bring that idea home to a global public and grant it greater urgency. The history of medicine is critical to making sense of our modern world, and the NLM is the primary public institution dedicated to maintaining and furthering this collective cultural inheritance within the United States. As Kelly Novick said: "So . . . roll on history into the present and the future, because history is about how we got here. It created the present and we are now creating the future. So, let's make some history more accessible." *Circulating Now* allows historians and researchers, from where they sit, to connect with each other, share their perspectives on the historical collections of the NLM, and spark conversation and new discoveries.

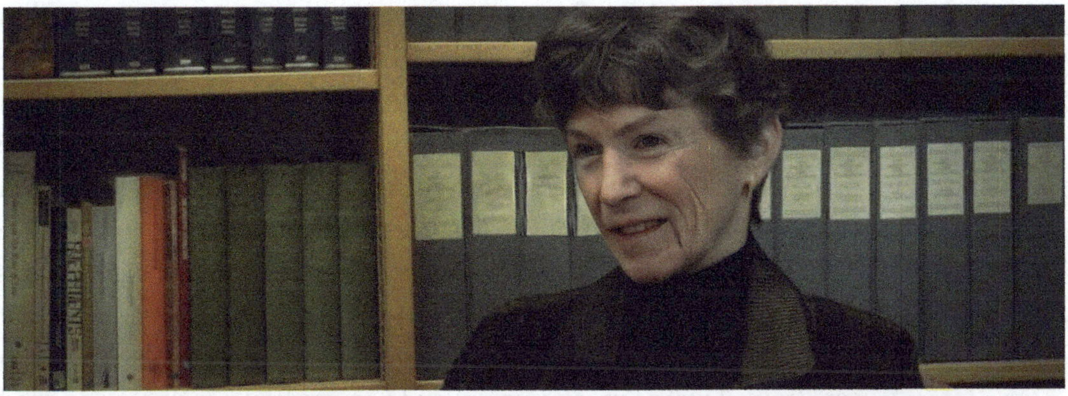

ON COMBAT FATIGUE IRRITABILITY: KERRY KELLY NOVICK PART III

https://circulatingnow.nlm.nih.gov/2014/03/28/on-combat-fatigue-irritability-kerry-kelly-novick-part-iii/

March 28, 2014 • Films & Videos, Revealing Data

KERRY KELLY NOVICK

Last fall Circulating Now *featured a unique film in the National Library of Medicine (NLM)'s vast historical audiovisuals collection, the World War II U.S. Navy training film* Combat Fatigue Irritability. Combat Fatigue Irritability *(1945), was directed by and starred Gene Kelly, who was then a rising Hollywood star. This is the third and final part of a three-part interview with Kerry Kelly Novick, a practicing psychoanalyst and the daughter of Gene Kelly and actress Betsy Blair. This series is an edited transcript of our longer conversation with Mrs. Novick, in which she discusses* Combat Fatigue Irritability, *Gene Kelly, and her own life and career as a psychoanalyst specializing in the treatment of children.*

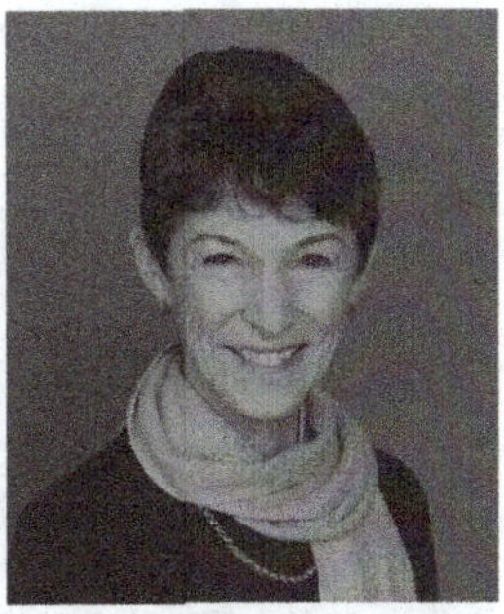

Kerry Kelly Novick, 2014 • *Courtesy Kerry Kelly Novick*

• • •

Circulating Now: Let's turn to your work and career as a psychotherapist. Can you tell us about your training with Anna Freud? What was that like and how did you come to work with her?

Kerry Kelly Novick: Well, I was going to go visit my mother who lived in London, right after college, . . . when I was twenty-one . . . And at that point I was still uncertain about what I wanted to do with my life. I'd always had being a psychoanalyst on my list, but in those days, which was the early '60s, the only way to become a psychoanalyst in this country was if you were a medical doctor. And I had an undergraduate degree in comparative literature. So there was no way that I was going to get psychoanalytic training in this country. But, of course, the tradition was completely different in Europe. In Europe, from the very beginning of psychoanalysis, women were trained just as much as men, and non-medical people were trained just as much as medical people. And so I was kind of casting about in my mind about how I was going to go about getting training. . . . And so at some point in the course of the first few months there, I decided yes, indeed, I did want to be a psychoanalyst. I considered going to medical school but, as they said to me in England, I was a woman, I was a foreigner, and I had an arts background. So medical school was not going to happen. So I started exploring other avenues and I'd always wanted to work with children. So I investigated the three places in London at the time that one could train as a child analyst. . . .

So, I read Anna Freud's book and Melanie Klein's book and Margaret Lowenfeld's book and I visited the three training places and decided that the best fit for me was Anna Freud's approach, her training place, her book, and presented myself. And they looked at me like I was crazy because here was this twenty-one-year-old American comp-lit person and they said well, you're too young and you don't have a psychology degree and you've never worked in the field. So, I went off and got a psychology degree the next year and came back and said, "I have the degree." And they said, but you've never worked and you're still pretty young, because now you're 22. And so I went off and got a job with the Medical Research Council and volunteered in a psychiatric hospital and then came back to them and presented myself and said, "Okay guys, take it or leave it. . . . I've done what you wanted." So they said yes, okay, you will be our experiment in youth. We'll admit you to

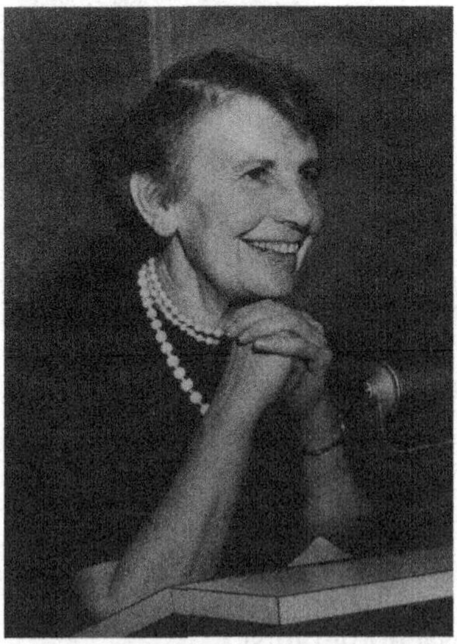

Anna Freud, ca. 1970 • *National Library of Medicine #101415573*

psychoanalytic training. So, I'm kind of an odd bird in the field because I don't have a prior professional identity. I am only a psychoanalyst and most people in my field have an alternative professional identity that they had first as a psychiatrist or a social worker or a psychologist. And so I trained as a child analyst, and at that point Anna Freud was in her seventies, and at the peak of her productivity and . . . her pre-eminence in the field. She was the most important psychoanalyst in the world. . . . There was some survey done at that time of psychiatrists and psychologists. And she was the top ranked person in the field. So it was an extraordinary experience to train there. I was there for four years as a trainee and then on staff at the Hampstead Clinic until we left England in '77. She was the most brilliant person I've ever met; funny, shy, slyly witty once she felt comfortable. Completely fluent at formulating, could take detail and put it together in a way that I've seen no one do ever since. When she would give a talk, a scientific presentation or a talk at a university, . . . or get an honorary degree or whatever, she'd have a yellow pad with four sentences written on it and deliver a publication-ready talk. She was formidable and amazing. Also very clear in her ideas, a combination of decisive in her thinking but extremely open minded. If you were intelligent and you could back up what you said, she'd listen to anything. So, being a rather feisty American young person, I've never been one to not speak my mind. I was brought up in a liberal household where the idea of saying what you think, and your right to speak up, was very fostered. It was a very interesting experience to be in the presence of somebody like Anna Freud.

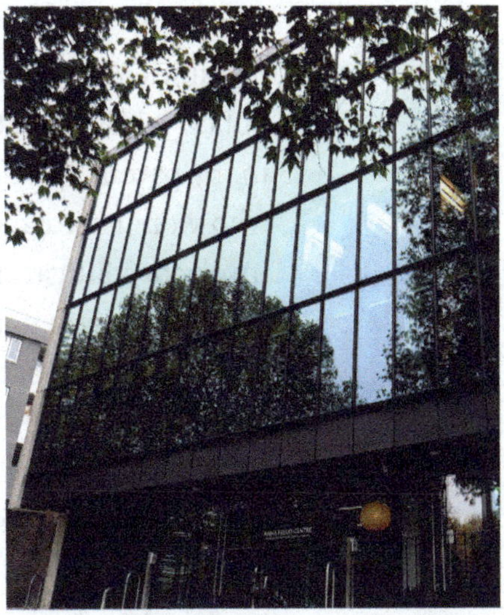
The Anna Freud Centre today • *Courtesy of the Anna Freud Centre*

The other thing that was very interesting about the Hampstead Clinic was that it was a non-profit institution and therefore had independent funding. So it could offer clinical services and various kinds of community services at little or no cost. So the eighty or ninety children or adolescents who were in treatment there at any given time . . . donated what they could to subsidize their treatments, and those of us who were studying there did not pay any tuition. We were also not paid any stipend, but there were various foundation grants that many of the students were able to have. But the clinic ran a well-baby clinic, a blind babies nursery, a nursery school for the community, all kinds of research departments. So, there was a tradition, that came from Vienna, of free clinics run by psychoanalysts in the community and work with disadvantaged groups like the group of concentration camp children that Anna Freud and her colleagues took care of through and after the war. So all of us who trained there also identified with that tradition of what we called altruistic analysis. And so anybody who trained with Anna Freud, all the people who came to this country as child analysts either as émigrés at the end of the war or subsequently because they trained with Anna Freud in London, we've all been active in community efforts. . . . It's a very strong and powerful identificatory influence on all of us and a very identity-forming experience to train with her.

CN: Let's get back to *Combat Fatigue Irritability*. What was the political atmosphere like when it was made?

KKN: My father was always what one would call a Jeffersonian Democrat, very liberal, very open minded, very invested and steeped in American history. And very clear in his own ideas about what was right, you know, ready to die for the Constitution and the Bill of Rights particularly, very upstanding and loyal to his friends, most of whom were much further left than he, including my mother. Certainly during the war everybody was on the Soviet American Friendship Committee, because they were our allies. And my mother was never a member of the Communist Party, but certainly went to a few meetings and we certainly had many friends in my parent's circle who were members of the party and certainly many who were later called fellow travelers. . . . I did grow up in an intensely involved political household . . . and can't remember ever not hearing about what was going on politically at every level, from local politics to state politics to national politics to international politics. So, it was in a sense a very sophisticated political upbringing and it continued to be in the atmosphere all my life. But, certainly during the war and right after the war, things were very lively, and again I can't remember dinner table conversations that weren't all about all that stuff all the time. And because I was an only child in a household of adults who was included in everything, I was listening all the time to everybody debating and talking and thinking about strategies. . . . I can remember the 1948 presidential campaign. That's the first one I have any real memories of, and then I remember working in the next few elections, working very hard for Stevenson . . . All of that was pretty par for the course around our house. My mother was blacklisted and that coincided pretty much with the time that my family moved to Europe for eighteen months in 1952, '53. . . . There was a tax thing where if artists went abroad for eighteen months they could save on their income taxes. So that was the structure of our sojourn abroad, but it did also coincide with my mother's being blacklisted. And then she was kind of reinstated when Hecht Lancaster made *Marty* and they employed blacklisted writers, directors, and actors under their own names. But, certainly the whole circle of friends growing up right after the war and into the '50s, . . . many of our friends went to jail, many of our friends were in the Hollywood Ten. My father went with a group of people from Hollywood to Washington to support the Hollywood Ten at the hearings. The first television we had in our house was bought for the Army-McCarthy hearings and I was kept home from school to watch that on television. So, the political climate was pretty distinct.

CN: Let's talk now about post-traumatic stress disorder (PTSD), and how the treatment of patients is depicted in *Combat Fatigue Irritability*, compared to current treatments of PTSD (which now includes all sorts of traumatic experiences, including criminal assault, sexual assault, accidents, bullying, etc.).

KKN: Yes. I found it fascinating that in the film we see those two treatment methods [abreactive talking therapy and medication], as well as the corpsman's practical methods. And I thought it was very interesting that there is still this same duality in our treatment approaches, and a continuing ambiguity and tension and confusion . . . about how to gauge the relative effectiveness of those different approaches and how to combine them for the maximum effectiveness. And we're in

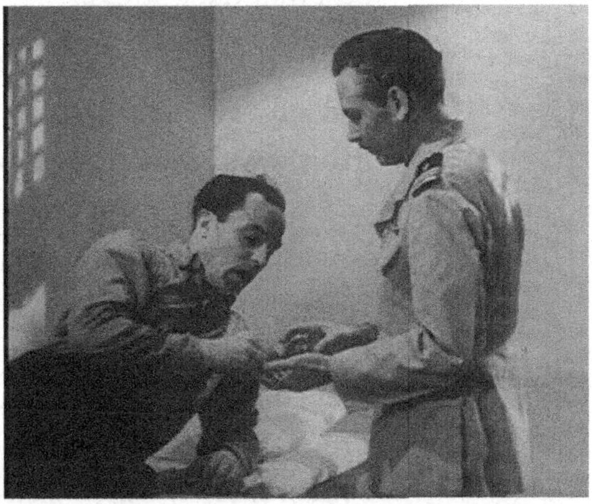

Lauren Gilbert, who plays a military psychiatrist, gives medicine to Gene Kelly playing Seaman Bob Lucas. • *United States Navy, National Library of Medicine #9300763A*

a period of time of ferment in psychology and psychiatry, at the moment where we had a biological psychopharmacologic revolution, starting in the early '80s, and that really swept the board. And now we are getting the pendulum swinging back a little bit, for two reasons. One, because the psychopharmacologies did not fulfill their early promise. They turn out not to help as much as people wished they would. And two, because the data that they were supposedly based on is increasingly found to be suspect at best and fraudulent at worst. So, we're really struggling with "oh wait a minute," we have to go back to more humanistic, more whole person, more psychological methods. . . , and reexamine all the talk therapies and really look at what can we glean from the various traditions and the new methodologies in that realm. So, I think the direction of research and clinical research now is a promising one from my point of view. Because . . . we're beginning to look again at stuff that I'm pretty convinced is relevant, which has to do with relating to people as people and not as conglomerates of chemicals. . . . We just don't know enough to think that we can fine-tune things neurologically, chemically yet. Maybe we will someday, but in the meantime, I want to communicate with people's minds.

CN: Could you say something about the use of history as a resource for us to understand and appreciate where we've come from and how we grapple with issues today concerning the care of service members with post-traumatic stress?

KKN: . . . Harold Bloom said only barbarians are not interested in history and talked about the importance of knowing our history. And there are many ways in which, as a psychoanalyst, I am deeply invested in history, and as a developmentalist I'm deeply invested in history, personal history, because I deal with individuals and individuals within families. But individuals and their families are part of a community. So we are by definition embedded in our cultural and social history as well. What's fascinating about this film is the way it crystallizes so many of those dimensions. . . . I think of it as a Russian doll, that . . . encapsulates all those layers in extraordinarily condensed economical form. . . . This particular film could be very useful in a number of ways. It's a lovely slice of what people looked like and seemed like then. The homefront scenes, when Seaman

Lucas goes home on leave, are charming. The wardrobe, the costumes, the setting of the household, the way the staircase and the doorways are made—the whole thing is wonderful as a bit of cultural history.

In terms of the medical history: the treatment methodology . . . There's a detail that fascinated me. On the blackboard behind the doctor, the psychiatrist, there's written up in chalk a list of symptoms and those are the same symptoms that are the constellation that we talk about now. On the blackboard it said "insomnia, vomiting, tremor" and that's what we deal with now. That's what state-of-the-art current PTSD literature talks about. At a professional conference in New York just this past January 2014, at a discussion of PTSD in veterans, the predominance of insomnia as the first symptom to address, because without addressing sleep disturbances almost nothing else can be dealt with. These things are right there in this movie. So I see this film as a very useful, also because it's short, a very useful discussion starter. A discussion starter about, how does society think about soldiers? How do we think about mental illness? How do we think about masculinity? How do we think about adult development and the changes that experiences bring in our identities? How do we think about relationships and their evolution? Because there is an emblematic picture of a relationship that was frozen in time. They were engaged right out of high school and then he went away to the war and he comes back two years later. Are they the same people? Can they pick up where

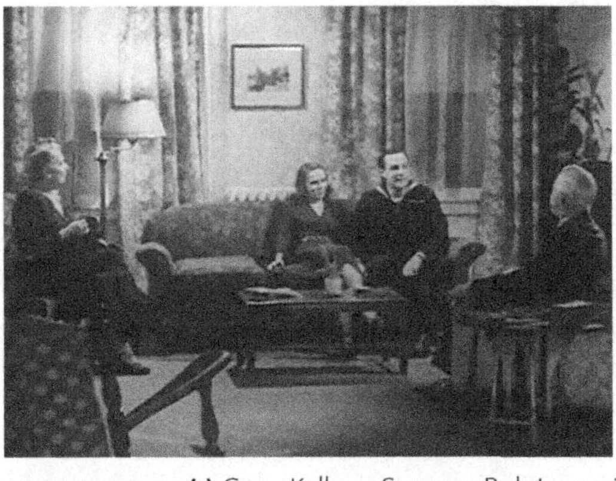

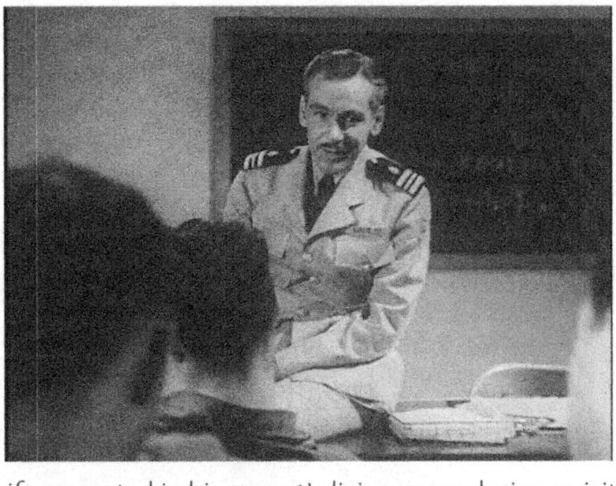

LEFT TO RIGHT (1) Gene Kelly as Seaman Bob Lucas in uniform seated in his parent's living room during a visit home • *United States Navy, National Library of Medicine #9300763A* **(2)** Lauren Gilbert plays a military psychiatrist speaking to a group of patients. • *United States Navy, National Library of Medicine #9300763A*

they left off? No. Their relationship has to evolve, etc. So, I think there are all kinds of groups that could use this film to start very interesting discussions and those could be medical groups, sociocultural historians, film historians, all kinds of people could find this film fascinating. And I am now terribly intrigued by the rest of your collection of films. So, the other thing that seems very important is to publicize what you guys have here, because . . . I'm kind of an informed consumer and certainly an informed citizen. And I didn't know about the National Library of Medicine. I didn't know it existed. Everybody needs to know about this. This is our National Library of Medicine. We own this. So, I want us all to have access to what you have. I think different professional groups need to know, not just doctors, even though it's the National Library of Medicine, but all kinds of professional groups need to know what you have here. So . . . roll on history into the present and the future, because history is about how we got here. It created the present and we are now creating the future. So, let's make some history more accessible.

Watch the Video on YouTube

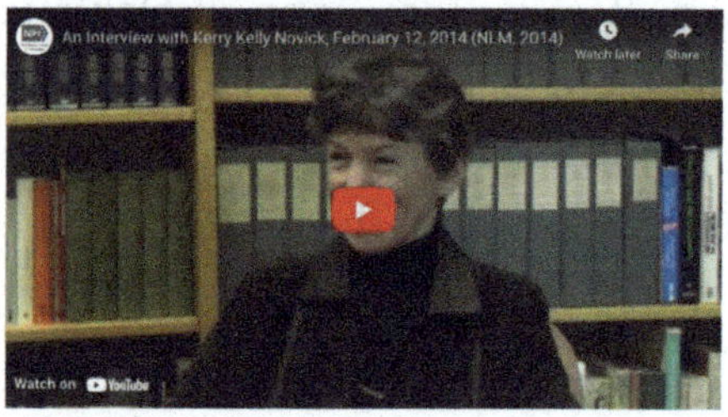

An Interview with Kerry Kelly Novick, February 12, 2014 (NLM, 2014)

• • •

Preceding Mrs. Novick's interview in the NLM's History of Medicine Division, she offered a presentation to the NLM's Board of Regents and Friends of the NLM, entitled "Unique Perspectives on Gene Kelly's 1945 Film Combat Fatigue Irritability."

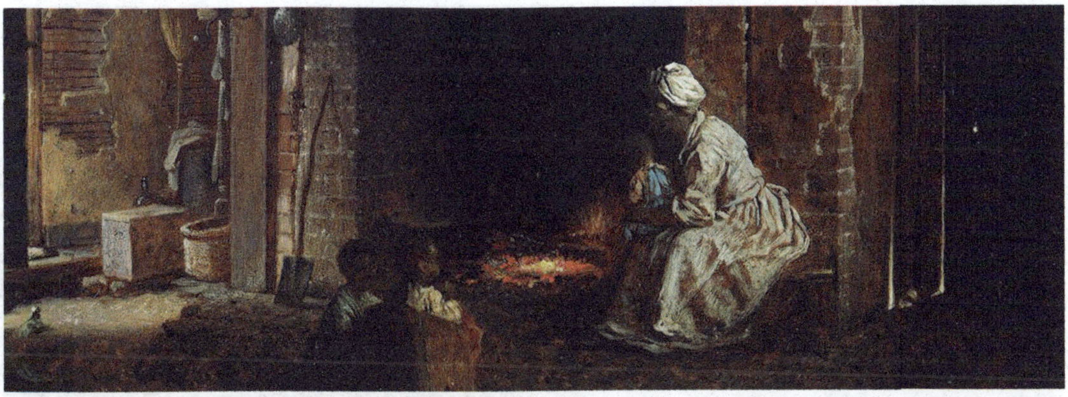

SITTING BY THE FIRESIDE: AFRICAN AMERICAN HISTORY, WOMEN'S HISTORY, AND FOOD

https://circulatingnow.nlm.nih.gov/2017/03/01/sitting-by-the-fireside-african-american-history-womens-history-and-food/

March 1, 2017 • Exhibitions, Guests

PSYCHE WILLIAMS-FORSON

Circulating Now *welcomes guest blogger, Psyche Williams-Forson, PhD. Dr. Williams-Forson is an associate professor and chair, Department of American Studies, University of Maryland-College Park and the guest curator of the National Library of Medicine (NLM)'s exhibition,* Fire and Freedom: Food and Enslavement in Early America.

• • •

Leaving the month of February, when we celebrate Black History Month, and entering March, when we highlight the achievements of women, seems a fitting time to discuss *Fire and Freedom: Food and Enslavement in Early America*. The exhibition recognizes the ways in which meals can tell us how power is exchanged between and among different peoples, races, genders, and classes. Food, as an object or set of objects, reveals a

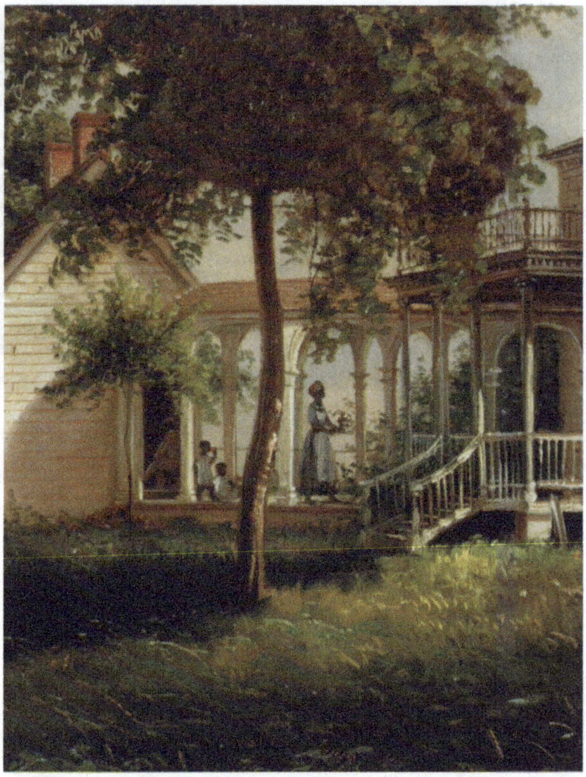

Detail of *East Front of Mount Vernon*, by Joachim Ferdinand Richardt, 1870 • *Courtesy of the Mount Vernon Ladies' Association*

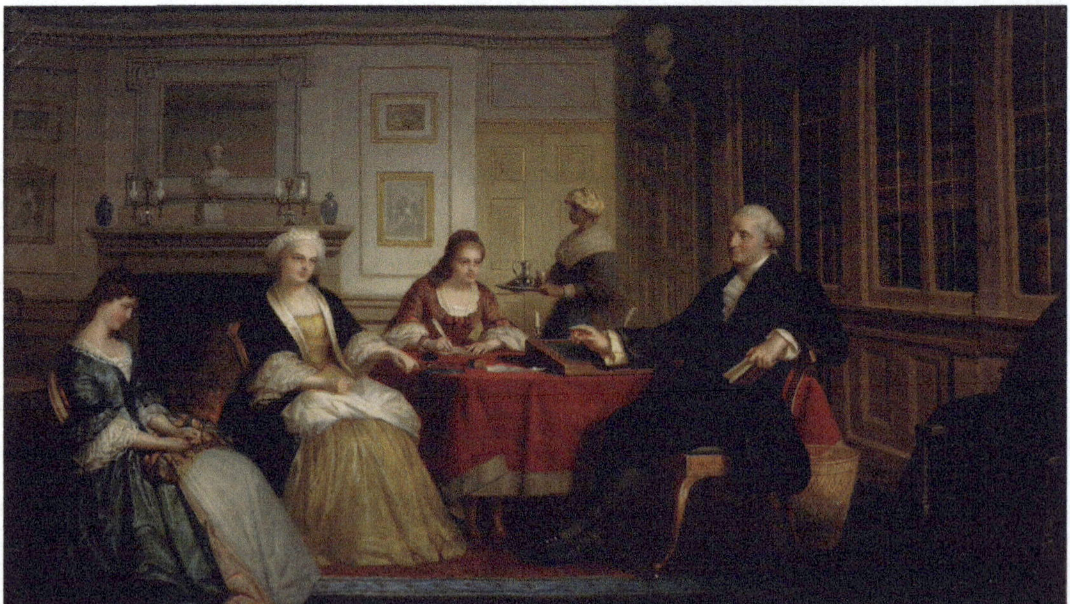

George Washington and Family, by Thomas Prichard Rossiter, ca. 1858–1860 • *Courtesy of the Mount Vernon Ladies' Association*

great deal about who we are, and some of the life experiences that we have and have had.

Only in the last several decades have food and cooking as a cultural process been given serious attention. Prior to this, the discussion was deemed less significant. But food and eating are different sides of the same coin—one may involve the process of acquisition, preparation, and presentation, while the other is the act of consumption—they are both activities basic to human life. And, far from simply resting in the domain of women, food permeates every element of our existence.

Fire and Freedom recognizes the importance of food cultures, as well as the intersections of race and gender in the discussion. Centering this discussion during the era of enslavement—and especially in the colonial period—we learn more about American and African American history, as well as women's history. For example, those interested in the subject of slavery have undoubtedly heard of the Middle Passage—so named as to reflect the part of the horrific journey that brought the slaves from West Africa to the West Indies, often before moving on to other parts of the New World. Established in the early 1500s by slave traders primarily from Spain and Portugal, the Passage bore witness to horrors to come. Enslaved men, women, and children were tightly packed onto a ship to make the three- or sometimes four-week journey. Many slaves did not survive the journey due to starvation, disease, and undoubtedly, brokenheartedness.

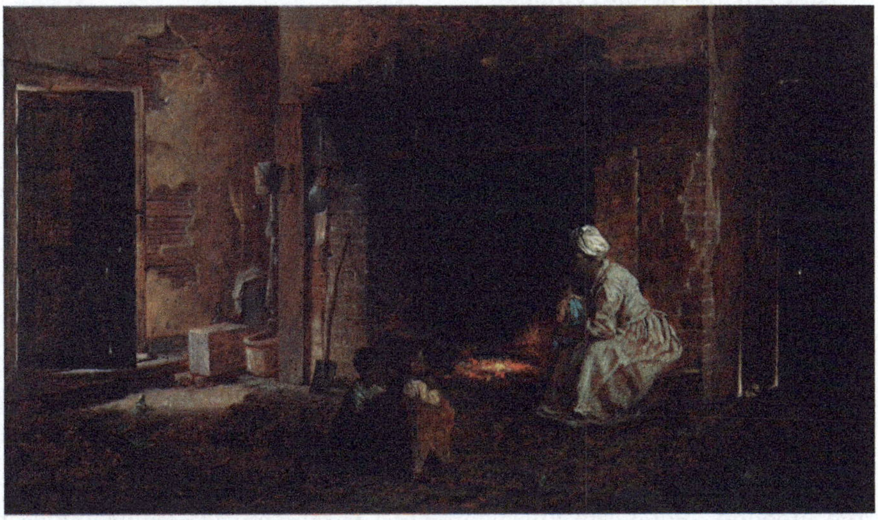

Washington's Kitchen, Mount Vernon, by Eastman Johnson, 1864 • *Courtesy of the Mount Vernon Ladies' Association*

By studying the Middle Passage alone, we not only learn a great deal about trade, early maritime practices, and more, but also we learn about food and foodways—the intersection of food, culture, and economics. Perhaps more importantly, we learn about African American food cultures and roles that women played. As written in the higher education module for *Food and Freedom*:

> Africans came to the Americas not only with intimate memories of traditional culinary practices and cuisines but also with particular regionally based agricultural knowledge. These, and other skills were called upon to benefit New World markets, especially the tending of new kinds of crops. African foods and livestock made their way to the Americas during the Middle Passage when Europeans stocked and restocked slave ships. African women, in particular, prepared foods both during transport and once they arrived using their customary methods as well as borrowing from Native Americans and Europeans. They introduced plants and herbs such as tamarind, hibiscus flowers, and the kola nut to improve tastes and to fight diseases resulting from vitamin deficiency. Africans contributed other foods such as yams, okra, black-eyed peas, plantain, pigeon peas, rice, watermelon, peanuts, sesame seeds, and melegueta or red peppers along with cooking techniques such as slow cooking (stewed) and deep-frying.

As we move to celebrate the enormous contributions of women to American society, we should take a moment to recognize women of all statures—the most notable as well as the lowly. Perhaps understanding the ways in which these women helped others and themselves to survive, the ways that they forged new paths through unbearable odds, and the ways that they helped to build our American food traditions, enables us to be a bit more knowledgeable about and appreciative of the world around us.

• • •

To learn more about colonial era foodways, read an interview with Psyche Williams-Forson and watch her recent lecture at the NLM. Also check out Fire and Freedom: Food and Enslavement in Early America *online and visit the Exhibition Program website to find out when the traveling exhibition is coming to your town.*

Reflection

As I write this reflection on my post "Sitting by the Fireside: African American History, Women's History, and Food," Judge Ketanji Brown Jackson has been confirmed as a justice of the Supreme Court of the United States. Though seemingly unrelated to the Black woman seated hunched over the flaming hearth, it is not. Judge Jackson endured tortuous confirmation hearings and "weeks and weeks of racist, misogynistic and stomach-churning attacks," according to Derrick Johnson, president of the National Association for the Advancement of Colored People (NAACP), despite having stellar credentials and more judicial experience than any other justice when they were nominated. I understand this experience, more than I should. It indelibly informs how in creating the NLM exhibition *Fire and Freedom: Food and Enslavement in Early America*, I was able to speak to the ways in which Black people have always searched for and lived in the struggle for physical, social, emotional, and psychological freedom despite the—real and perceived—boundaries of oppression that surround us. Whether it be the chains of slavery that sought to deny us our culinary traditions, innovations, and resilience; or the era of Jim Crow that denied us basic liberties like sitting at a lunch counter; or even contemporary moments where we can be arrested for waiting on friends in a coffee shop—we have always fought and continue to fight for our freedoms, even with food. After all, we live in the land of "liberty and justice for all," and foods tell stories, so I was honored to be able to shed a bit of light on the food and freedom experiences of African Americans in the Chesapeake. —Psyche Williams-Forson, 2023

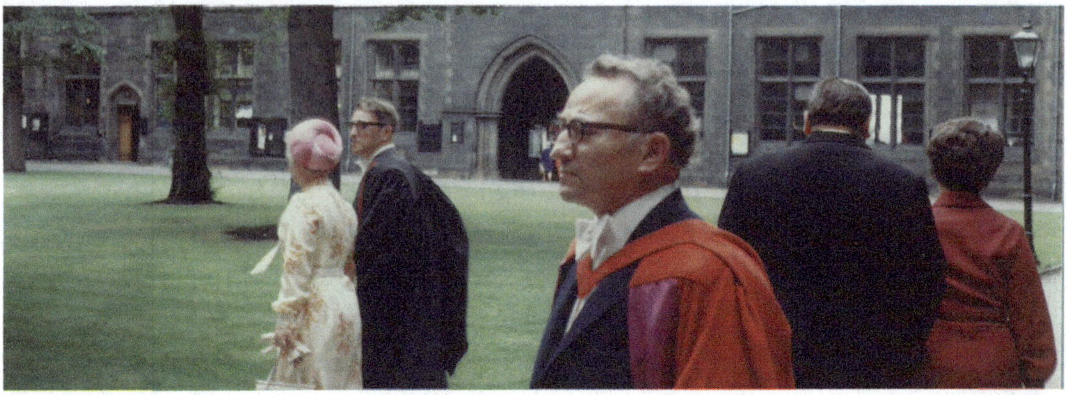

IN SEARCH OF SOL SPIEGELMAN

https://circulatingnow.nlm.nih.gov/2015/10/27/in-search-of-sol-spiegelman/

October 27, 2015 • Archives & Manuscripts, Guests

SUSIE FISHER

Circulating Now *welcomes guest blogger Susie Fisher who brings us this post highlighting her work with the National Library of Medicine (NLM)'s archival collections for American Archives Month. Dr. Fisher is an academic teaching faculty-member for the MA program in Biological Thought at The Open University of Israel. Her article "Not just 'a clever way to detect whether DNA really made RNA': The invention of DNA-RNA hybridization and its outcome" on Sol Spiegelman, based on research at the NLM, was recently published in* Studies in History and Philosophy of Biological and Biomedical Sciences.

• • •

Fly 9,000 miles, really? Just to examine a historical collection at the NLM? Well, the editor seemed quite insistent and The Open University of Israel forthcoming. So I arrived in Bethesda on a sunny but freezing winter day in January to have a look at Sol Spiegelman's papers. Unlike the weather, the reception at the Library was warm and welcoming and the personnel were very helpful and efficient. My particular interest was Sol Spiegelman and Ben Hall's invention of DNA-RNA hybridization. This technique had, during the 1960s, a powerful impact on the theory and discourse of molecular biology. Since the mid-1970s, it has become a core component of many DNA technologies that have revolutionized the study of biology.

Although I had found online at *Profiles in Science* several original documents of Spiegelman, the real measure of his scientific enterprise and recognition was revealed to me in nintey-five boxes full of Spiegelman "material." I was surprised to see how much his work was appreciated both by the scientific community and the public. This is far from what one can gather from reading traditional histories of molecular biology. For example, the renowned scientist Salvador Luria, in an interview published in *The Boston Globe* pointed out Spiegelman's contribution to

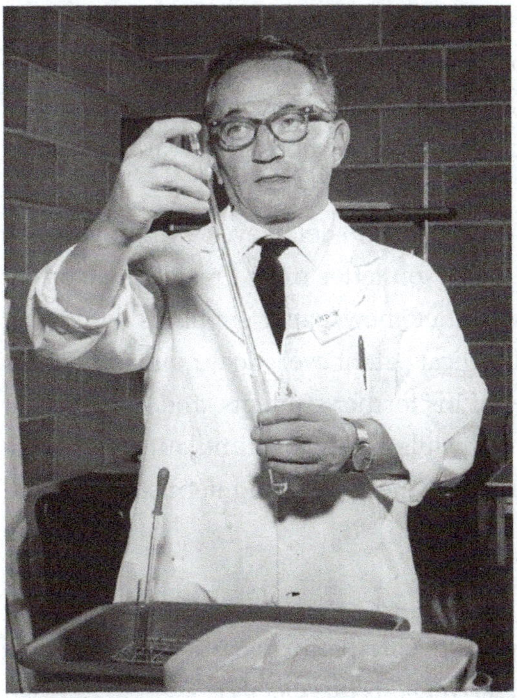

Sol Spiegelman in lab with pipette, ca. 1965 • *Courtesy of the University of Illinois at Urbana-Champaign Archives, Sol Spiegelman Papers,* Profiles in Science, *National Library of Medicine MS C 561*

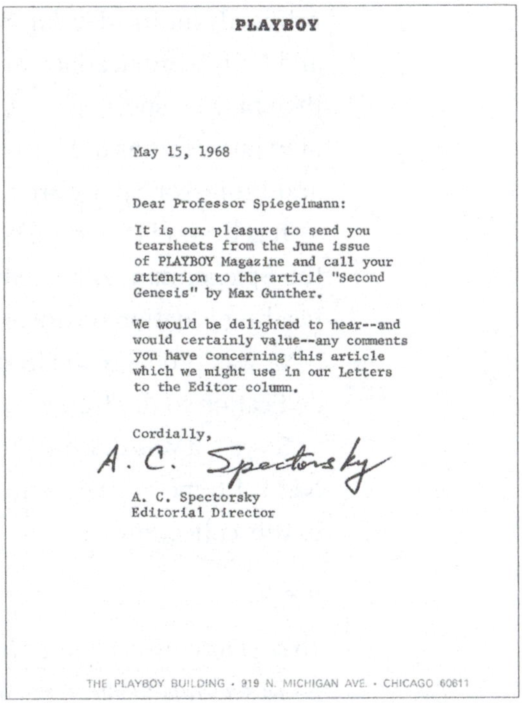

PLAYBOY

May 15, 1968

Dear Professor Spiegelmann:

It is our pleasure to send you tearsheets from the June issue of PLAYBOY Magazine and call your attention to the article "Second Genesis" by Max Gunther.

We would be delighted to hear--and would certainly value--any comments you have concerning this article which we might use in our Letters to the Editor column.

Cordially,

A. C. Spectorsky

A. C. Spectorsky
Editorial Director

THE PLAYBOY BUILDING • 919 N. MICHIGAN AVE. • CHICAGO 60611

Letter from *Playboy* to Spiegelman, May 15, 1968 • *Sol Spiegelman Papers, National Library of Medicine MS C 561*

the new field, but even more interesting, on the clipping itself, he wrote: "A small effort to set the record straight! And happy New Year! Salva."

Playboy Magazine surprised me with an article that described the new field of molecular genetics specifying Spiegelman's contributions to it. The cover page of the article is a prescient vision of the potential of the new genetics. It suggests that molecular genetics could be used to revolutionize biology and improve humankind (eugenics). Another major accomplishment of Spiegelman and his team, during the 1960s, was the isolation of a viral enzyme that they used to make, in-vitro, copies of the virus's RNA. The finding generated much excitement and was described by one newspaper as creating "life in a test tube."

A fellow historian of biology once told me that Spiegelman was disappointed not to be awarded a Nobel Prize. I noted this in an article that I submitted for publication. However, one of the peer reviewers thought that my claim needed better support. Luckily I came across a note by Spiegelman in which he indeed contemplated the possibility: "If the Nobel committee for Chemistry considers that this award should be made primarily for the development of the RNA:DNA molecular hybridization and for the implications to biology of these macromolecular interactions, then may I respectfully suggest that the committee consider the possibility of making this award jointly to Professor Paul Doty of Harvard University and Professor Spiegelman of Columbia University."

It is beyond the scope of this brief note to detail everything I found in the Spiegelman collection: a thank-you letter from President Nixon for heading a national cancer committee; newspaper clippings describing what was probably the first biological patent ever; documentation of his dedication to the future career of his former students; and much more.

So yes, it was definitely a worthwhile and most stimulating trip to the NLM. I hope to make further use of the fascinating items that I found in this collection.

• • •

To celebrate American Archives Month Circulating Now *is highlighting the NLM's archival collections with several posts this October.*

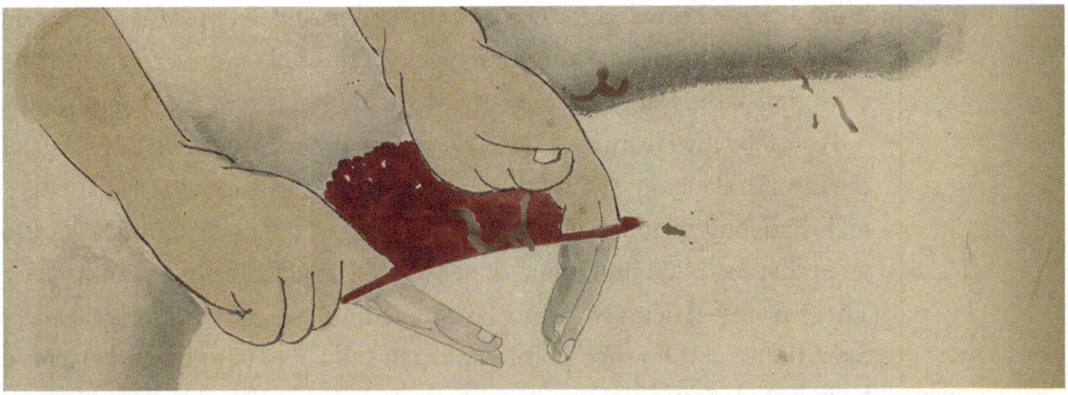

"WRAPPED IN FLESH": VIEWS OF THE BODY IN EAST ASIAN MEDICINE

https://circulatingnow.nlm.nih.gov/2015/12/03/wrapped-in-flesh-views-of-the-body-in-east-asian-medicine/

December 3, 2015 • Rare Books & Journals, Guests

YI-LI WU

Circulating Now *welcomes guest blogger Yi-Li Wu. Dr. Wu is a Center Associate of the Lieberthal-Rogel Center for Chinese Studies at the University of Michigan, and a Research Fellow of EASTmedicine, University of Westminster and an organizer of the recent workshop* Comparative perspectives on body materiality and structure in the history of Sinitic and East Asian medicines. *Today she explores some of the topics discussed at the workshop.*

•••

How do you assess the state of a broken bone when you can't directly see it? Writing in 1808, Chinese doctor Qian Xiuchang discussed a problem shared by healers worldwide prior to the X-ray age: "When someone has a dislocated or fractured bone, the bone and joint are wrapped in flesh. Looking at it from the exterior, it is hard to get a clear understanding, and there is the danger of making an error." To improve the state of bonesetting knowledge, Qian compiled *Supplemented Essentials on Medicine for Injuries* (*Shangke buyao*). That book can be found in the collection of the National Library of Medicine and is now accessible online.

An innovative feature of Qian's text is that it includes two drawings of the human skeleton, shown from the front and the back. Chinese medical texts had long included written descriptions of the body's "bones" (*gu*), a term that included individual bones as well as palpable bony landmarks. These were particularly important in acupuncture, where practitioners used them as reference points to locate the spots where needles could be inserted. Some acupuncture diagrams also outlined the positions of major bones. However, prior to the nineteenth century, Chinese texts on therapeutic medicine did not contain diagrams of the full skeleton. In 1742, when the Imperial Medical Academy compiled a textbook on bonesetting, the illustrations only indicated the position of bones by labels on the outside of human figures. In 1770, however, the Qing imperial

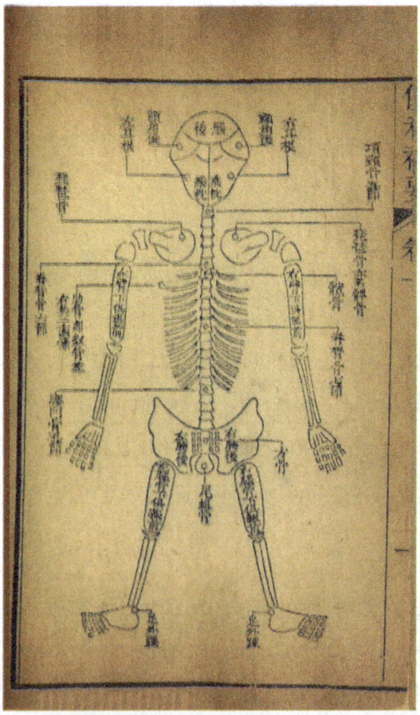

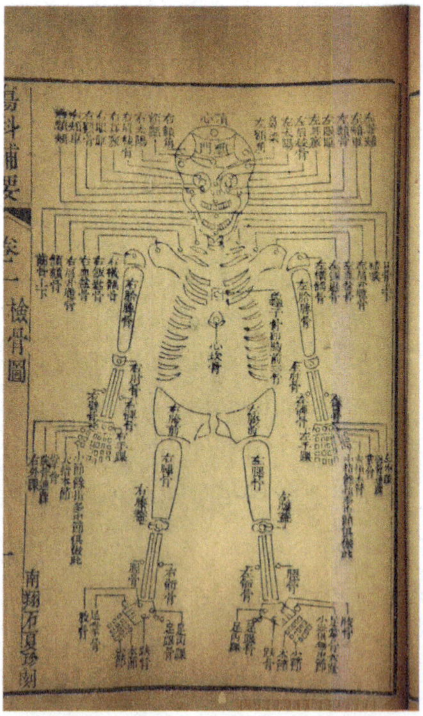

LEFT TO RIGHT (1) Skeleton Diagram, Back View, in Qian Xiuchang, *Supplemented Essentials of Medicine for Injuries*, 1818, first printed 1808. • *National Library of Medicine #46810390R* **(2)** Skeleton Diagram, Front View, in Qian Xiuchang, *Supplemented Essentials of Medicine for Injuries*, 1818, first printed 1808. • *National Library of Medicine #46810390R*

government promulgated a set of official inquest forms in order to standardize forensic investigations on skeletal remains. It was these forensic diagrams of the skeleton that Qian Xiuchang borrowed and reproduced in his work on treating injuries, so that readers could more easily learn the forms of bones hidden beneath the skin.

Qian Xiuchang, a native of Shanghai, had received some degree of classical education and he had presumably once aspired to success in the civil service examinations that defined members of the Chinese sociopolitical elite. He became interested in injury medicine after he broke his leg. He apprenticed with the doctor who cured him and eventually became successful enough to attract disciples of his own. Seven of them helped to collate his *Supplemented Essentials*, which discussed a wide range of traumatic injuries caused by weapons, blows, and falls. It also featured a laudatory preface from Su Chang'a, a former Shanghai magistrate who became a supporter after Qian saved the life of a prisoner who had attempted suicide.

It was an era when the Chinese were critically re-evaluating received teachings, including those on medicine. At the time that Qian's text was printed, another doctor, Hu Tinguang, was completing his own manuscript on injury medicine and also incorporated forensic diagrams of the skeleton. Both books sought to address the shortcomings of the imperial bonesetting manual. Besides using forensic medicine—and diagrams of the human skeleton—to improve their readers' knowledge of the bones, they also incorporated forensic teachings on "mortal points," namely spots on the body where injuries were particularly dangerous.

Qian's *Supplemented Essentials* thus leads us to consider an understudied aspect of East Asian medical history: how doctors investigated and understood the body's material structures and components. The present-day view is that "traditional Chinese medicine" is primarily interested in the body's energies and vital functions and not in anatomy or body structures. Historically, however, that was not precisely the case. East Asian healers argued about how to define the parts of the body and their relation to health, injury, and disease, and like Qian Xiuchang, pursued different methods for improving their knowledge of the body: textual study and introspection, the dissection and observation of corpses, careful observation of healthy and diseased people.

These issues took center stage at an extraordinary workshop. Held October 2–4, 2015 at the University of Michigan, *Comparative perspectives on body materiality and structure in the history of Sinitic and East Asian medicines* brought together an international group of scholars (including historian Michael Sappol of the National Library of Medicine) to discuss medical portrayals and practices of the body, from the first century A.D. to the nineteenth, in China, Japan, Korea, Vietnam, the Mongol Empire, and Tibet.

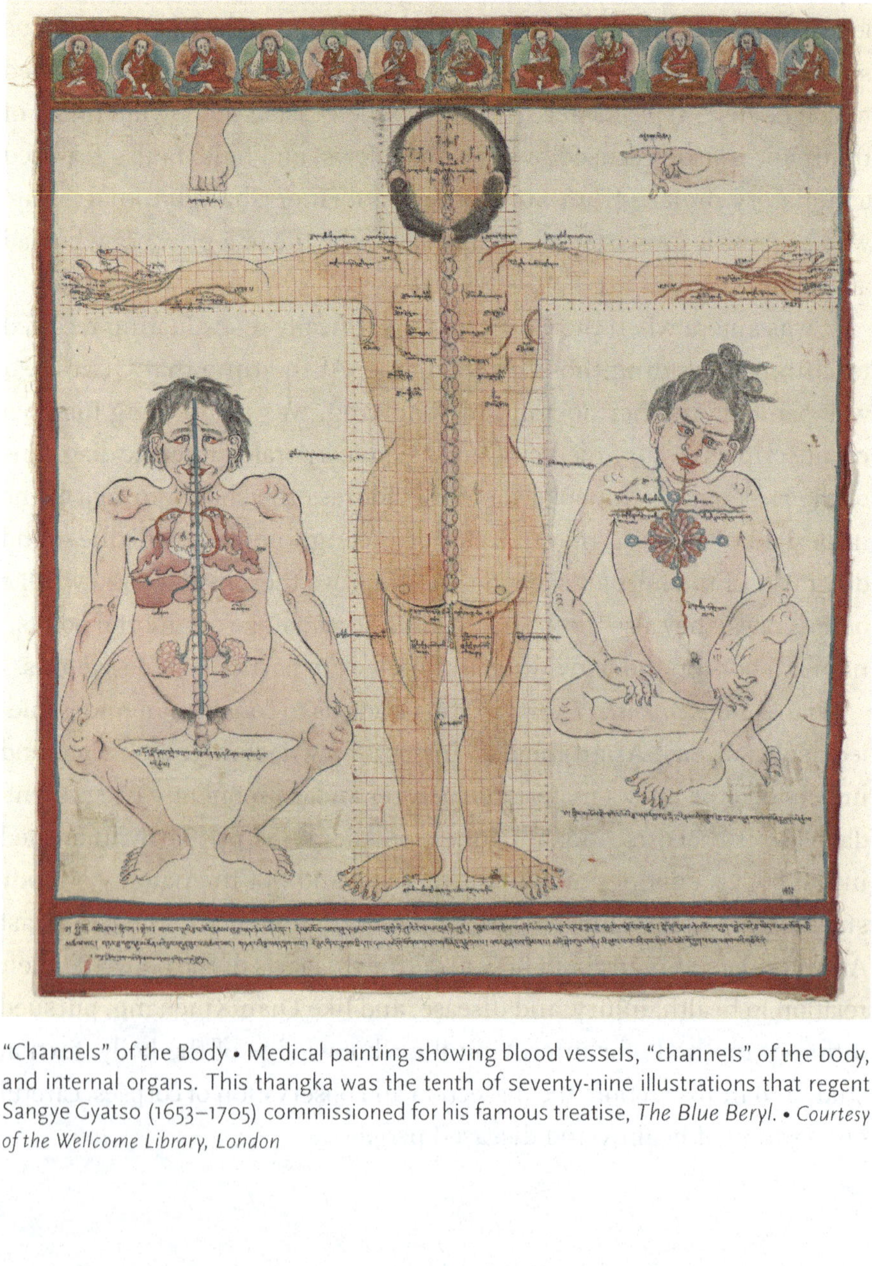

"Channels" of the Body • Medical painting showing blood vessels, "channels" of the body, and internal organs. This thangka was the tenth of seventy-nine illustrations that regent Sangye Gyatso (1653–1705) commissioned for his famous treatise, *The Blue Beryl*. • *Courtesy of the Wellcome Library, London*

The workshop explored a number of questions. How did different representations of the body co-exist with each other within a given cultural context? The anatomical images and descriptions in Tibetan medical treatises, for example, included those based on examination of corpses as well as those elaborating humoral and vitalistic beliefs and those metaphorically comparing the body's components to a palace or to a kingdom's rulers and ministers. Different body views were linked to different explanations for how and why illness afflicted the body, and to different therapeutic methods.

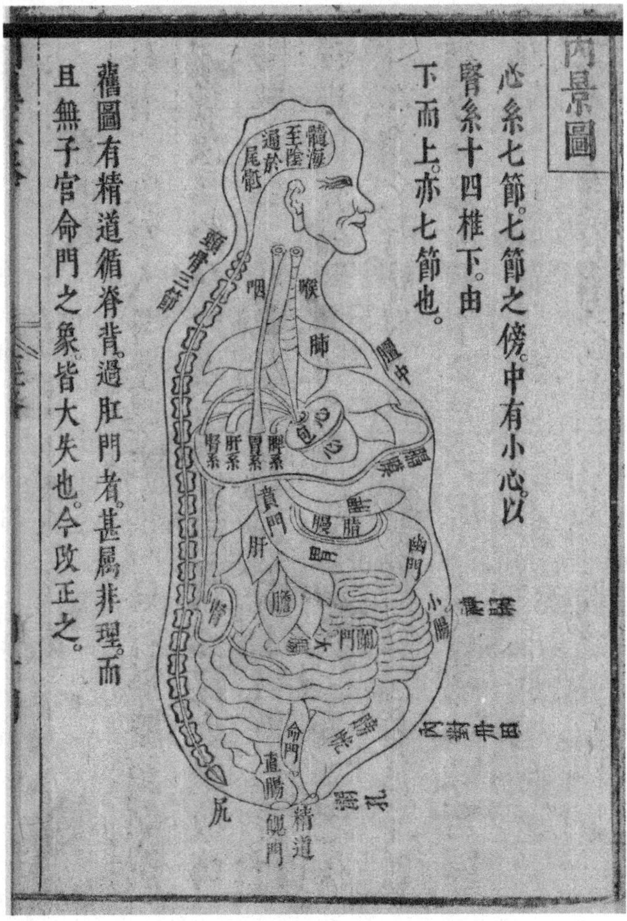

"Internal Landscape," by Zhang Jiebin, Illustrated Wing to the "Classic, Arranged by Category," *Leijing tu yi*, 1624 • Zhang revised older images by adding a new organ between the rectum and bladder, claiming that this was the true location of the so-called "vital gate." • *Courtesy of the Chinese Collection, Harvard-Yenching Library, copyright President and Fellows of Harvard College*

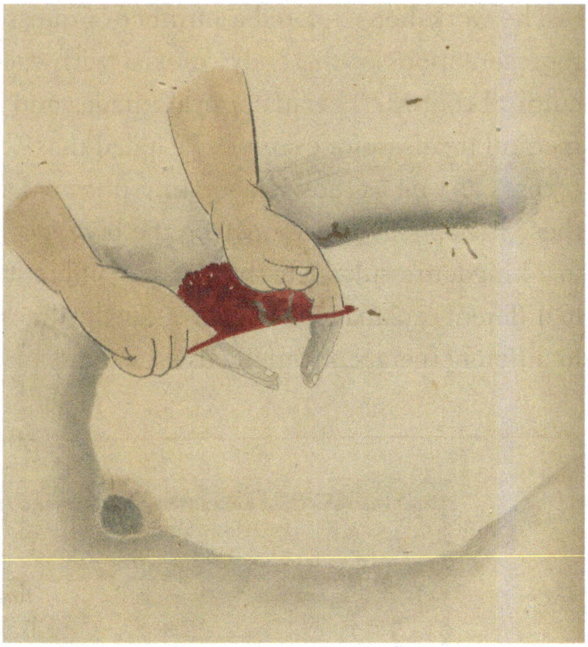

Breast Cancer Surgery, Hanaoka Seishū (1760–1835), in *An Illustrated Book on External Treatments for Unusual Diseases (Kishitsu geryō zukan)* • *National Library of Medicine* #101147736

Competing images of the internal organs circulated in China, Japan, Korea, and Vietnam, and were the subject of debates about how internal structures were connected to each other and to imagined centers of primordial vitality.

The conference also explored the status and value assigned to medical illustration compared to textual descriptions of the body, and how visual conventions from various realms of medicine influenced each other. In early nineteenth-century Japan, for example, both the bonesetting expert Kako Ryōgen (1810) and the surgeon Hanaoka Seishū (1760–1835) employed images in which the body's flesh was transparent or invisible. Finally, the conference highlighted the historical importance of surgery, bonesetting, and other manual therapies that required healers to physically manipulate the body's components.

The rich diversity of presentations, the wealth of ideas and material, and the lively discussions that ensued, showed the creative vigor of contemporary scholarship on East Asian medicine, enormously facilitated by the increasing number of rare books and manuscripts that have been digitized by the National Library of Medicine and other libraries and made accessible online for researchers throughout the world.

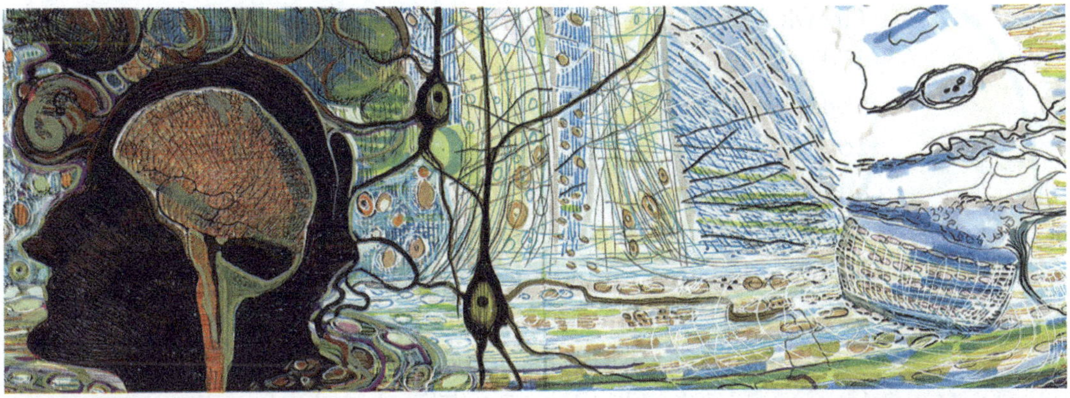

DRAWN TO, DRAWN FROM EXPERIENCE

https://circulatingnow.nlm.nih.gov/2017/11/14/drawn-to-drawn-from-experience/

November 14, 2017 • Rare Books & Journals, Guests

DAWN HUNTER

Circulating Now *welcomes guest blogger* *Dawn Hunter, Associate Professor, School of Visual Art and Design, University of South Carolina and Fulbright España Senior Research Fellow at the Instituto Cajal in Madrid, Spain. Her new body of work is a suite of biographical drawings and paintings about Santiago Ramón y Cajal, the father of modern neuroscience. Her series is comprised of creative works and formal investigations of Cajal's scientific drawings that are currently on display at the John Porter Neuroscience Research Center at the National Institute of Health, Bethesda, Maryland.*

• • •

> "Every great drawing—even if it is of a hand or the back of a torso, forms perceived thousands of times before—is like the map of a newly discovered island. Only it is far easier to read a drawing than a map; in front of a drawing it is the five senses that make a surveyor."
>
> —John Berger, from *A Painter of Our Time*

The wholly integrated experience of phenomena is powerful. The union of the mind's curiosity, the heart's passion, and the body's senses sing a chorus that reminds us of the wonder of our own existence. The U.S. 2017 solar eclipse was that experience for many. However, it was also predictable. Sitting on the front steps of my home in South Carolina, steeped in the avalanche of media coverage, I experienced the path of totality only with my mind; my brain perfectly primed with expectations. The forecast sound bites focused the quality of celestial delivery, and by doing so reduced the universe to a branded experience. It may sound like I am complaining, but I am not. The obstacle of mediated experience served as a reminder to value those encounters when I experience the extraordinary, nonaligned, for myself. While ignorance is not bliss, on rare occasions, it can be a blessing—allowing new, unexpected experience of phenomena to rival the first time one bit into a luscious strawberry or walked across hot sand. Encountering Santiago Ramón y Cajal's scientific drawings of the nervous system for the first time was one such extraordinary experience for me.

I am an artist, and I draw every day. It is how I know and understand the world. One day back in 2012, I was looking up neuroscience terminology to supplement an article I was reading on the claustrum, I stumbled across Cajal's scientific drawings. In the midst of trawling visuals on the web, I was swept away within "gesturely expressive" cellular images drawn in implied space. I was dwarfed and transported into Cajal's microscopic world. Other neuroscience drawings were in the image cache, like those of Camillo Golgi. However, I was not as taken with them, because Golgi's

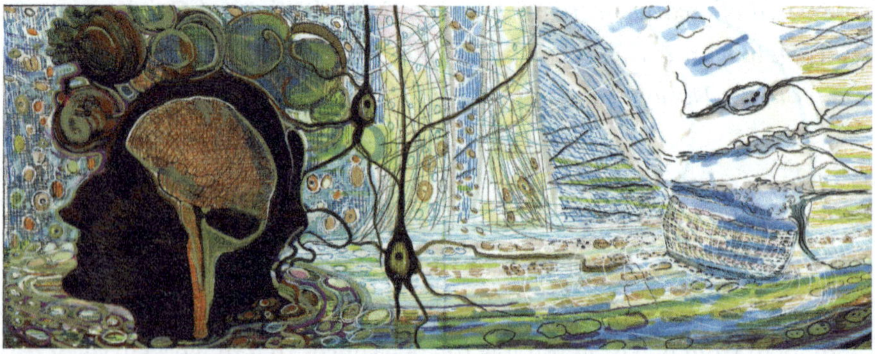

Surreal portrait of Cajal, 2015 • From my handmade sketchbook, pen, marker and ink on paper, 5.5" x 13" • *Courtesy Dawn Hunter*

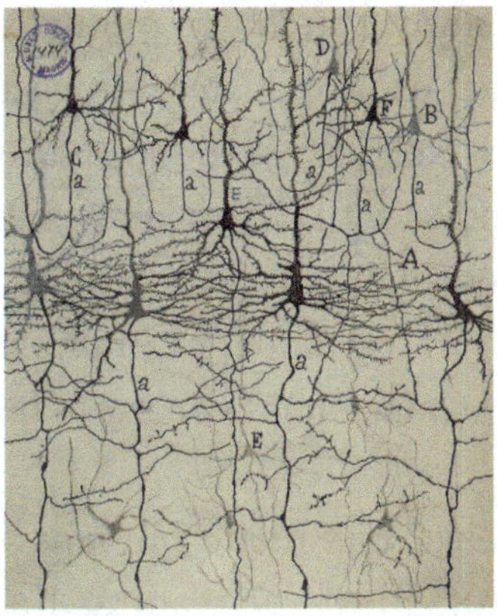

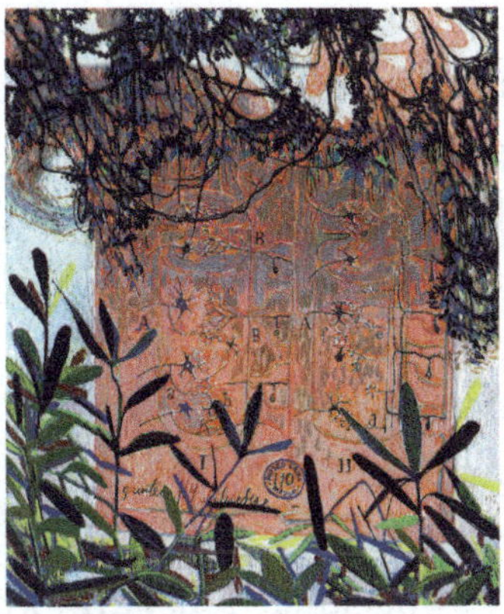

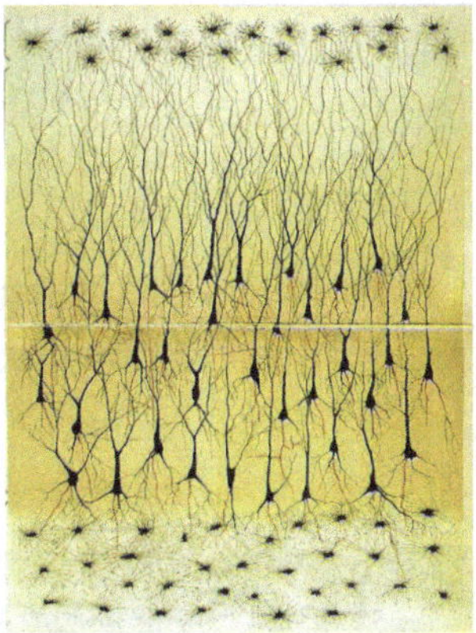

LEFT TO RIGHT **(1)** Cajal's Drawing of Pyramidal Neurons, n.d. • *Courtesy of the Legado Cajal at the Insituto Cajal* **(2)** Cajal and Golgi, 2015 • Cajal and Golgi juxtaposed against Cajal's drawing of their opposing theses, acrylic and ink on paper, 11" x 14" • *Courtesy Dawn Hunter* **(3)** Golgi's Drawing of Pyramidal Neurons, 1885 • *Courtesy of Museo Golgi, University of Pavia*

illustrations were surrounded by a border that created closure and containment and possessed a topographical mannerism. Based on those visual qualities, I felt Golgi's drawings were "designed," and that construction revealed a particular point of view regarding the role of drawing in his work: that drawing was a vehicle to guide, transcribe, and organize nature in a manner that demonstrated a theory. Instead of creating drawing from a designer's perspective, Cajal's work in comparison is drawn with a type of perceptual observation, one in which the inherent design of nature is discovered through sighting. Drawing was a tool to observe, discern and recount microanatomy structure. Cajal's drawings are filled with actual lines and drawn with implied space. I believe they demonstrate a philosophy that he was at the service of nature—recording and reporting the truthfulness of sight's journey.

Intrigued and invigorated, I felt an urgent need to learn more. I pursued my interest in Cajal without any foreknowledge of his monumental identity within modern neuroscience. I quickly learned the basics: Santiago Ramón y Cajal (May 1, 1852–October 17, 1934) was a Spanish histologist and the first person to demonstrate that the nervous system was made up of individual units (neurons) that were independent of one another but linked together at points of functional contact called synapses. Cajal was a 1906 Nobel Laureate in Physiology or Medicine awarded jointly to another neuroscientist, Camillo Golgi, "in recognition of their work on the structure of the nervous system;" however, their research was mutually exclusive and embraced opposing theses. Cajal used and later refined a silver staining technique developed initially by Golgi to see the structure of neurons. He illustrated the results of his studies with elegant drawings of the neurons that he proposed worked independently or collectively, each individual unit participating simultaneously in individual or multiple neuron functions. Santiago Ramón y Cajal is considered by many to be the father of modern neuroscience.

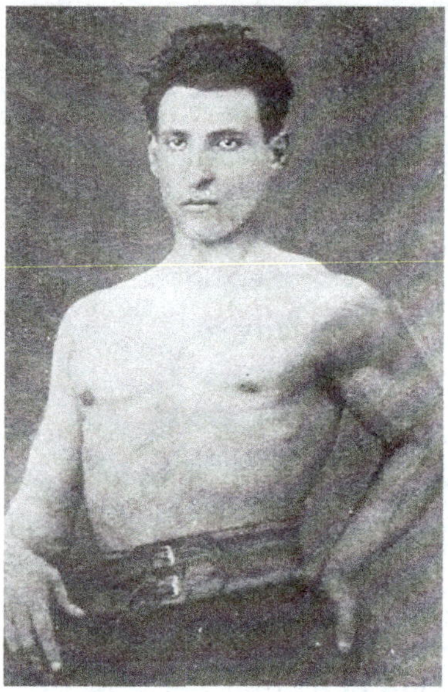

Ramón y Cajal, 1871, in *Recuerdos de Mi Vida*, 1923. • *National Library of Medicine #56120450R*

From the beginning, Cajal has made me laugh because I began "knowing him" by reading his science fiction writing, *Vacation Stories*, published under the pseudonym, Dr. Bacteria. Anyone with that pseudonym has a great sense of humor, right? It framed my perception of the *Vacation Stories* as sublimation for personal and professional frustrations while being intentionally campy. Cajal's psychological complexity revealed itself when I read his memoir *Recollections of My Life*. As I perceive it, the autobiography was written with unguarded honesty, and the breadth of content he shared about himself and his research captivated me. I was particularly struck at times with his humor. Like the devotion of three highly descriptive paragraphs letting the reader know that not only was he very physically fit and muscular in his bodybuilding "selfie" photo published in the book shot at age nineteen, but that in real life he was bigger and more defined than the photo captures. His autobiography also touched my heart, especially when he shared the hardships of his boarding school days and the level to which his particular learning style was misunderstood. Cajal, an experience-based learner, was unable to conform to the educational standards and had great difficulty learning from the method that required memorization and repetition of large amounts of information. He was rebellious, and his teachers were intolerant and unleashed extreme and harsh punishments that were physical and psychological assaults.

Childhood hardships did not diminish Cajal's innate pioneering spirit, a temperament that may have been spurred by a formative experience at the age of eight. On July 18, 1860, Cajal witnessed the totality of a solar eclipse and the excitement surrounding Warren de la Rue's arrival in Spain to record the moment of totality for the first time in history with photography. The occasion inspired a lifelong appreciation of astronomy in Cajal. Many have speculated over the years that this was the seminal event that planted the seeds of his scientific rigor. The eclipse totality dwarfed Cajal in the universe and provided a new context for his existence. Judging from the intensity, directness, and wonder of his drawings, it was a context he never left.

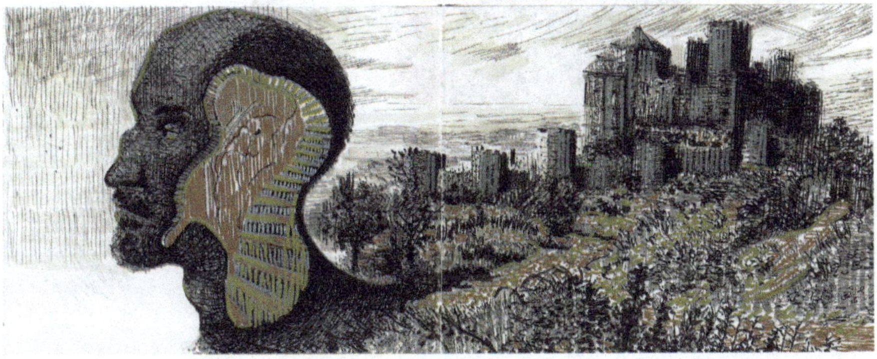

Cajal on May Day, 2015 • From my handmade sketchbook, pen and ink on paper, 5.5" x 13" • *Courtesy Dawn Hunter*

By proxy, with those seeds firmly sown in me, my fascination has grown into a comprehensive visual art project about him titled *Aesthetic Instincts: the Intersection of Art and Science in the Life of Santiago Ramón y Cajal.* I have developed theses about him and inform my project with primary source material. As a Fulbright España Senior Research Fellow at the Instituto Cajal in Madrid, Spain, I am currently researching the archives of the Legacy of Cajal. After I read his autobiography, *Recollections of My Life*, a part of me that felt like some key aspects of Cajal (his humor, and how he imagined himself—particularly in his youth) were absent from the mainstream discourse patterns about him. I view my drawings and paintings as educational tools that address art, history, and neuroscience and that splice and fuse his animated neurons, with representations of biographical elements, fictional narratives, and surrealism. My artwork highlights his personality traits and his private value system essential to his unique scientific insight that led to his great discovery: that the

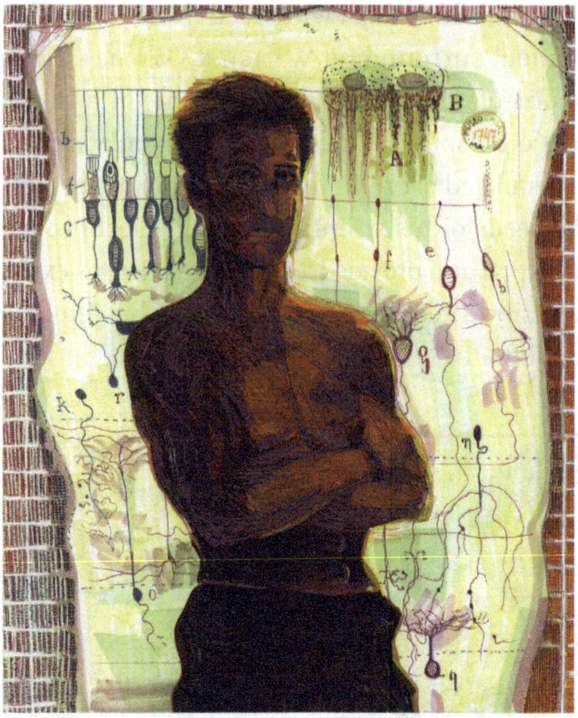

Cajal as Bodybuilder juxtaposed against a retina drawing, 2016 • Pen, marker and ink on paper, 11" x 14" • *Courtesy Dawn Hunter*

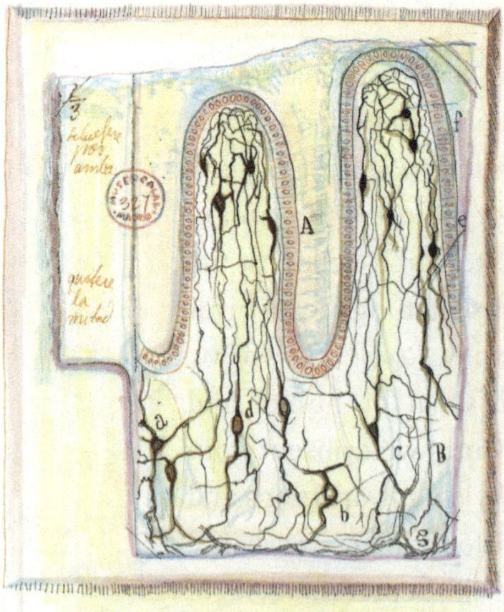

Dawn Hunter's study of Cajal's Intestinal Villi & Interstitial Cells, 2017 • This drawing of Cajal's is currently on display at the John Porter Neuroscience Center of the NIH, 11" x 14". • *Courtesy Dawn Hunter*

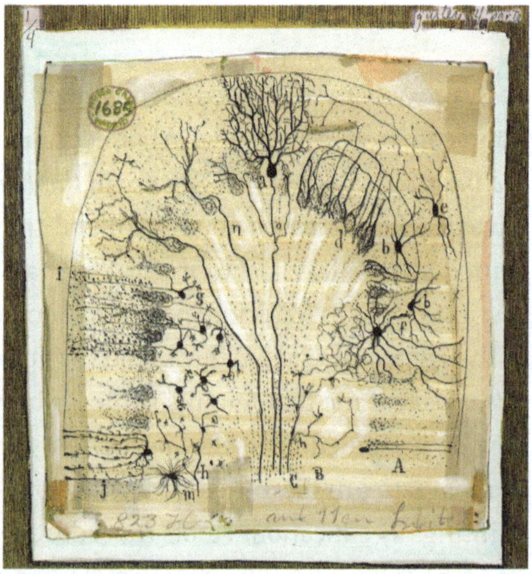

Dawn Hunter's study of Cajal's cerebellum drawing, 2016 • This drawing of Cajal's was part of the first exhibit of Cajal's work at the John Porter Neuroscience Center of the NIH, pen, ink and marker on paper, 11" x 14". • *Courtesy Dawn Hunter*

nervous system is comprised of individual, independent biological units, i.e. neurons.

Because of his complexity as a person and scientist, getting to know Cajal requires investment. Those who take the time are often, like me, completely enthralled, enchanted, and transformed by the phenomenological journey.

Reflection

My life changed when I met Jeff Diamond, Senior Researcher at the National Institute for Neurological Disorders. The world of Santiago Ramón y Cajal opened up for me in ways that I could have never imagined. Jeff invited me to exhibit my biographical artwork about Cajal alongside his (Cajal's) original scientific drawings on display at the John Porter Neuroscience Center at the National Institutes of Health (NIH). I make regular trips to the NIH to research the exhibited Cajal drawings. My process evolved into conducting research in the rare books collection at the National Library of Medicine (NLM), where I met Stephen J. Greenberg. He helped me locate rare editions of Cajal's histology textbooks. Through my many visits to the NLM, I developed my proposal for my Fulbright España Senior Research Fellowship, which I was awarded in 2017. That enabled me to research the archives housed in the Legado Cajal at the Instituto Cajal, Madrid. During my Fulbright, I was invited by Elizabeth A. Mullen to contribute to *Circulating Now,* and I wrote: "Drawn to, Drawn from Experience." It seemed like a full circle experience; however, it was an expansion—the circle and meaningful research connections continue to evolve from that writing. My foray into SciArt, scientifically influenced art, was unexpected. I meet people I would not encounter otherwise through my NLM writings and art exhibits about Cajal. The significant connections resonate with those within the international neuroscience community and Spain. There is always a new adventure waiting and new collaborative opportunities on the horizon. —Dawn Hunter, 2023

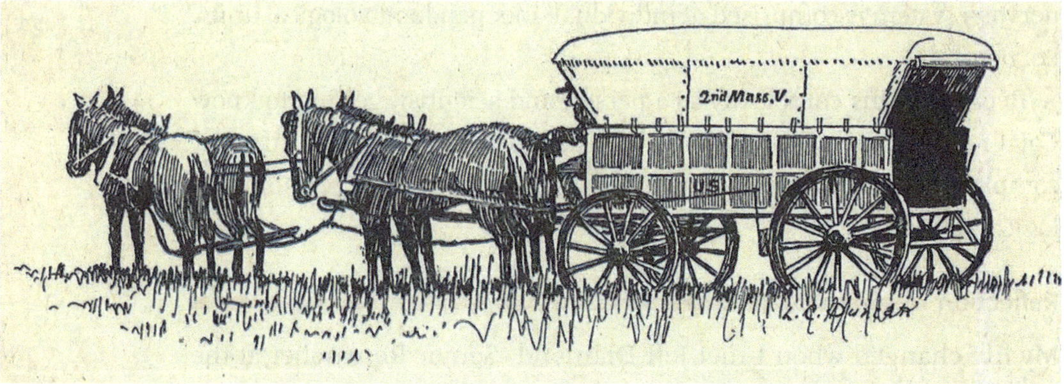

FOLLOWING THE REAR: TRAVAILS OF THE UNION ARMY'S AMBULANCE CORPS

https://circulatingnow.nlm.nih.gov/2019/08/02/following-the-rear-travails-of-the-union-armys-ambulance-corps/

August 2, 2019 • Archives & Manuscripts, Rare Books & Journals, Guests

BENJAMIN FORREST

Circulating Now *welcomes guest blogger Benjamin Forrest, a fourth year medical student at the University of Birmingham, United Kingdom. He has just completed an intercalated degree programme in the history of medicine, which saw him travel to archives and libraries in the United States. Today, he explores the Union Army's Ambulance Corps during the Civil War drawing on first-hand accounts in National Library of Medicine (NLM) manuscript collections.*

• • •

Early in the American Civil War, no organized system of battlefield evacuation existed. Regimental bandsmen were ordered to transport the wounded; the outcome was a muddled system where wounded men could suffer

TOP A detail of American Civil War Ambulance • An 1861 ambulance in *The Medical Department of the United States Army in the Civil War* by Louis C. Duncan, Carlisle Barracks, PA, Medical Field Service School, 1931. • *National Library of Medicine #14120240R*

on the battlefield for over a week. The horror of the unnecessary suffering of injured soldiers compelled officers to improve frontline medical provisions.

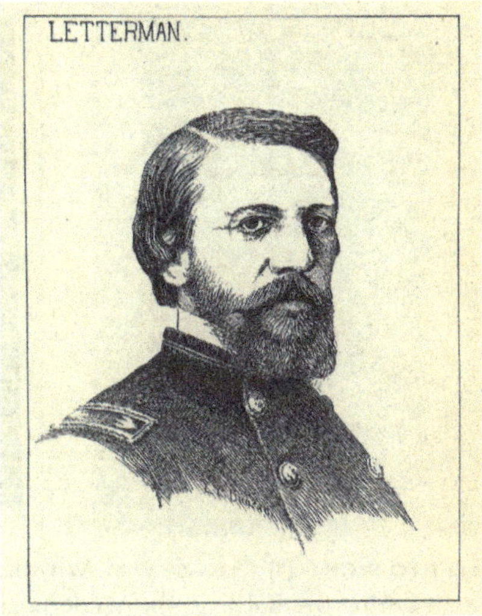

Jonathan Letterman • Engraved portrait in *The Medical Department of the United States Army in the Civil War* by Louis C. Duncan, Carlisle Barracks, PA, Medical Field Service School, 1931. • *National Library of Medicine #14120240R*

On August 2, 1862, under the instruction of Jonathan Letterman, the Medical Director of the Army of the Potomac, General George B. McClellan issued General Orders 147 and created the United States Army's first full-time, dedicated Ambulance Corps. These orders determined the structure, training, and role of the service; and crucially, they were a blueprint for the creation of subsequent Ambulance Corps later in the war. This instigated a major improvement in battlefield medicine. However, the new service challenged contemporary ideas concerning wartime humanitarianism, suffering, and military authority. So, the corps was often met with hostility and neglect from the rest of the army.

In the Army of the Potomac, the Ambulance Corps soon demonstrated its worth. At the Battle of Antietam on September 17, 1862, all the Union wounded were evacuated from the battlefield within twenty-four hours.

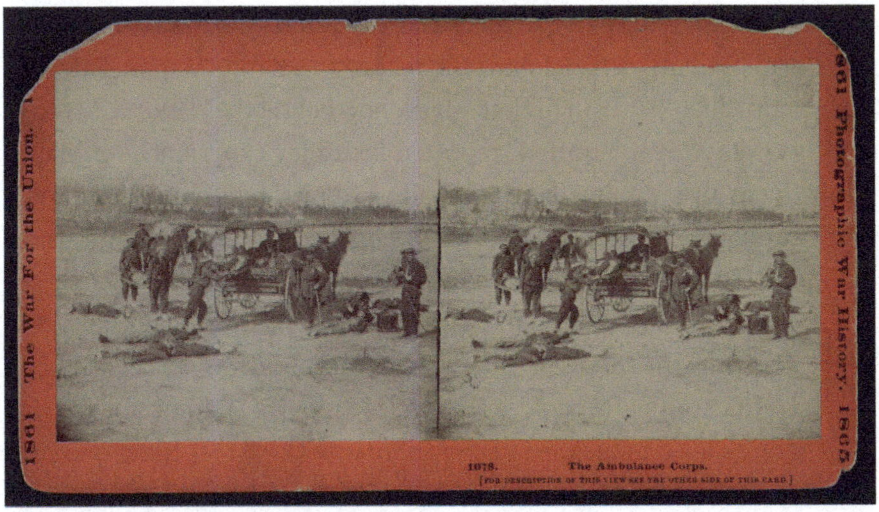

Stereograph Card "The Ambulance Corps," ca. 1865 • Although the Ambulance Corps was dedicated and full-time, training was limited. The staged photograph above shows ambulance-men practicing loading ambulances. However, this was a rare occurrence. • *Library of Congress #2011660482*

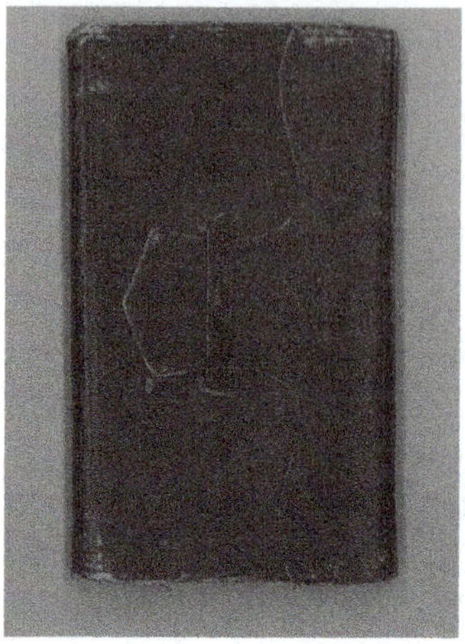

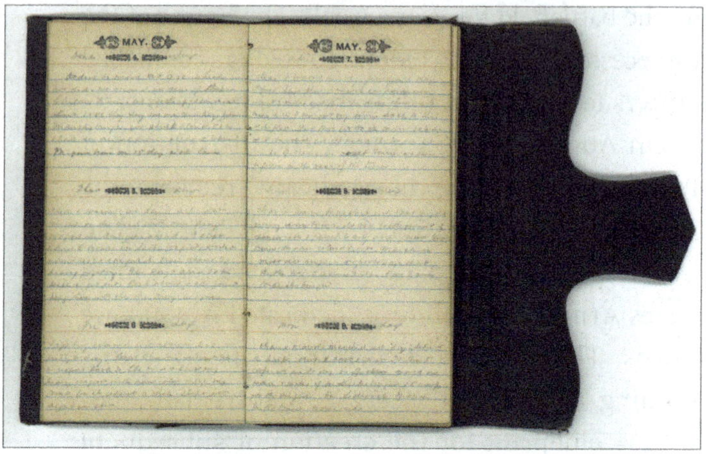

LEFT TO RIGHT (1) Diary of W.H. Whyte, 1864 • On May 7, Whyte's ambulances are at the back of the wagon train during the Battle of the Wilderness. • *National Library of Medicine #100938705* **(2)** Diary of W.H. Whyte, 1864 • Drilling of new recruits is mentioned on Thursday April 14 and Friday April 15 1864. • *National Library of Medicine #100938705*

Nevertheless, despite its success, the service received hostility from the military.

First, the service was opposed due to the supposition that it restricted the military's authority and activity, as officers surrendered power to medics. This point of contention resulted in a physical relegation of the Ambulance Corps. In his diary of 1864, now in the manuscript collections of the National Library of Medicine, Lieutenant W.H. Whyte repeatedly notes that, during the Battle of the Wilderness on May 5–7, his ambulances were neglected and left to follow the rear of the army's wagon train.

Captain Elliot Pierce, in his letter-book now held at the National Archives and Records Administration, reported a similar experience on May 3, 1863; the army's wagons blocked roads and prevented his ambulances from supplying medical assistance to engaged troops. However, most strikingly, Pierce believed that many military officers did not even know the Ambulance Corps existed. Early Civil War medical historian Louis Duncan claims the service is "never mentioned in the report of a general officer"—meaning one could read all these reports and never learn that the Union Army even possessed an Ambulance Corps. So, the service was not only actively opposed by officers who knew of its existence, but was also neglected entirely by others who had no knowledge of it altogether.

Second, besides being held in contempt for its infringement upon military authority, the Ambulance Corps was shunned due to the belief that it was ineffective and staffed by slackers. Thomas McParlin,

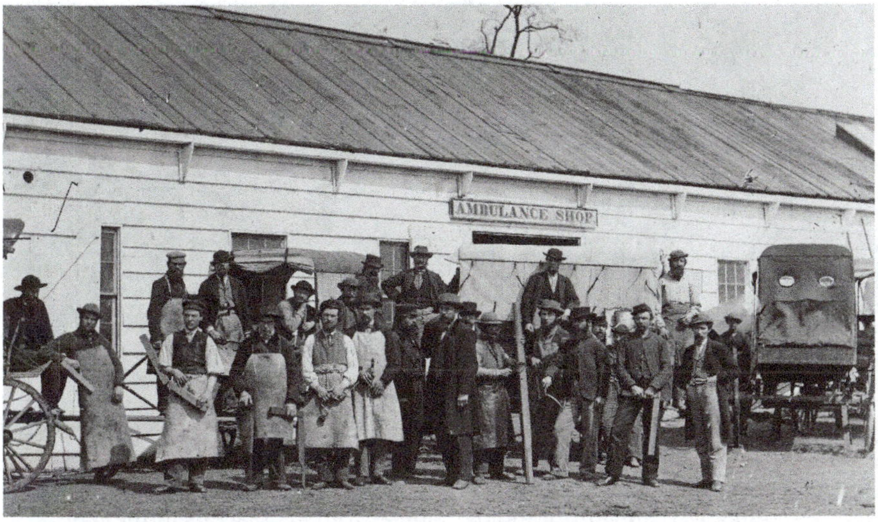

Ambulance Shop • Workmen in front of the Ambulance Shop in Washington, DC, ca. 1865 • *Library of Congress #2018667013*

Letterman's successor as Medical Director of the Army of the Potomac, said the Ambulance Corps did not always follow advancing troops into battle as they should have. However, because of the military's neglect, as described by Whyte and Pierce, ambulance-men often struggled to perform their role effectively. Furthermore, an event from stretcher-bearer Private Heyward Emmell's diary (held by the Madison Historical Society in New Jersey, a transcribed copy is available at the NLM) demonstrates that ad hoc skirmishing meant ambulance-men could not be aware of all ensuing clashes. On October 15, 1863, Emmell records that he and his fellow stretcher-bearers were cooking dinner when a mêlée began nearby. Nevertheless, they rushed into action, even attempting a dangerous shortcut that drew Confederate gunfire, and joined the engaged soldiers. Emmell's account shows that ambulance-men were often unfairly labelled slackers; instead, they were willing to put themselves in danger to perform their role.

The Union Ambulance Corps' efficacy saved countless soldiers the agony of days languishing on the battlefield. In the words of Louis Duncan, "[it was] the best care of the wounded the world had ever seen." And yet it was not appreciated by the American military fully during the war. Nevertheless, the system set a new precedent for humanitarianism on the battlefield and has formed the backbone of American military medicine during every conflict since.

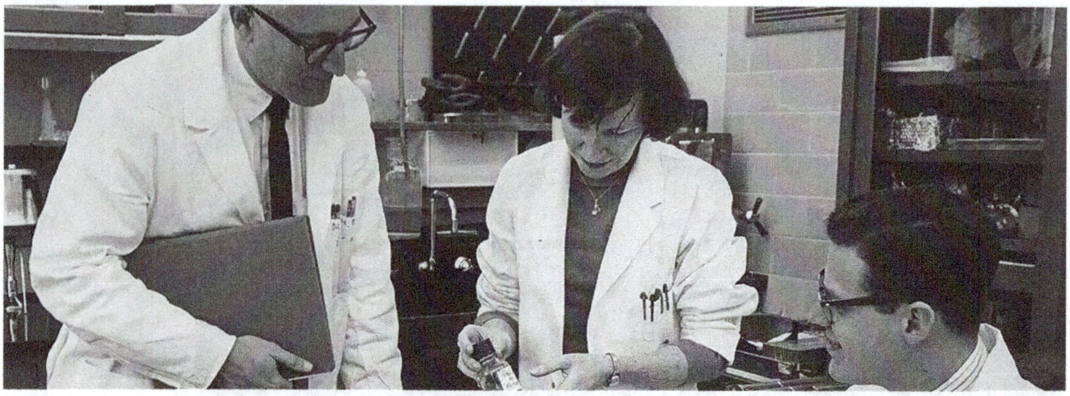

FINDING HOPE: A WOMAN'S PLACE IS IN THE LAB

https://circulatingnow.nlm.nih.gov/2018/09/06/finding-hope-a-womans-place-is-in-the-lab/

September 6, 2018 • Prints & Photographs

ASHLEY BOWEN

While doing some research ahead of the fiftieth anniversary of the rubella vaccine in June 2019, I came across an image of the team that developed the vaccine and an improved blood test. The photograph, taken by National Institutes of Health (NIH) photographer Jerry Hecht, shows Drs. Harry M. Meyer, Jr. (1928–2001) and Paul Parkman (b. 1932) conferring with a female scientist holding a bottle of rubella antigen. When the photograph came into the National Library of Medicine's collections several decades ago, the information associated with it read:

> Drs. Harry M. Meyer, Jr. (light hair), Paul D. Parkman (dark hair), and a female lab technician of the Laboratory of Viral Immunology, Division of Biologics Standard [sic] working with rubella antigen in laboratory setting.

TOP A Detail of Hope Hopps • Drs. Harry M. Meyer, Jr. (left), Paul D. Parkman (right), and Hope Hopps (center) of the Laboratory of Viral Immunology, Division of Biologics Standards working with rubella antigen in laboratory • *National Library of Medicine #101541114*

Just before I came across this photograph, I had been reading about the efforts of other historians and researchers to identify the women present but unidentified in the history of science and medicine. When I looked at this image and read the existing documentation, I wondered if there was more to her role in the rubella research team than is implied by the phrase "lab technician." After all, she is holding a bottle of antigen and centered in two photographs with the men who developed the rubella vaccine. Quite frankly, I couldn't let it go that two male researchers were identified by name while this woman was not.

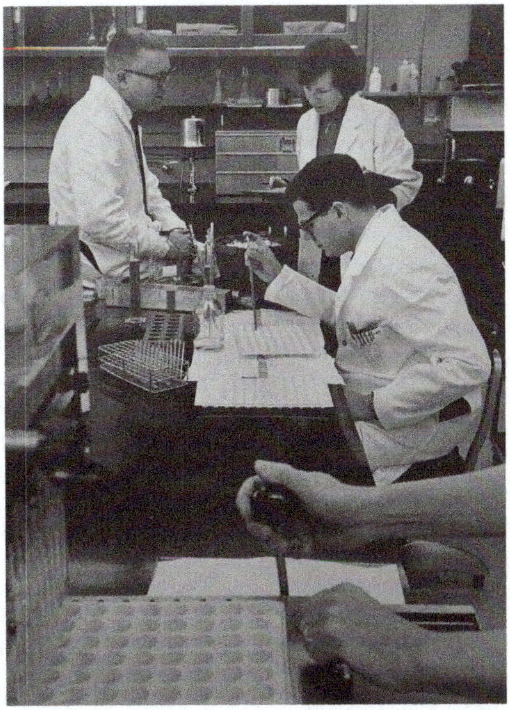

Female Lab Technician • Drs. Harry M. Meyer, Jr. (light hair), Paul D. Parkman (dark hair), and a female lab technician of the Laboratory of Viral Immunology, Division of Biologics Standard [sic] working with rubella antigen in laboratory setting • *National Library of Medicine #101729450*

I wanted (needed) to know who this woman was.

It took over a month but, thanks to some archival sleuthing here at the National Library of Medicine, help from private citizens (including the adult children of former Division of Biologic Standards [DBS] laboratory staff), the generous assistance of professional organizations like Graduate Women in Science, conversations with librarians and historians at various museums, universities, and federal agencies—not to mention a fair bit of luck—we have been able to identify this female lab technician as Hope Hopps (1926–1988).

Hopps was much more than a lab technician. She earned a master's degree in microbiology from the University of Maryland in 1950, an era when few women pursued advanced degrees in the sciences. After working as a bacteriologist for a few years, Hopps joined the staff at the NIH first in the National Institute of Allergy and Infectious Diseases and then in the Division of Biologics Standards' Laboratory of Viral Immunology.

As a staff member in the Laboratory of Viral Immunology in the 1960s, Hopps worked with Drs. Parkman and Meyer on several research projects, is listed as an author on several articles they published in outlets like the *New England Journal of Medicine* and *Pediatrics*, and held a patent with them for the rubella blood test. In a 2005 oral history, Dr. Parkman remembered Hopps as:

> ". . . our—it's an unacceptable term now I suppose—but she was our 'Girl Friday.' She could make any kind of cell culture grow, for example, she developed the BSC-1 cell line, which stands for biological standards culture one. It is still used for things."

When DBS moved to the FDA in 1972, Hopps relocated with it and assumed the role of assistant to the director of biologics. She also served as the acting associate director for program development and operations. After retiring from government service, Hopps continued to work as a consultant and guest worker in the FDA's Center for Drugs and Biologics.

Her achievements in government are matched by her contributions to science. Over the course of her career, Hopps authored or co-authored eighty-nine articles in medical journals and books, was awarded two different patents, served as the national president of Graduate Women in Science, and developed the BSC-1 cell line.

To me, researching this woman's name was an opportunity to surface the role of women in both the laboratory and the historical record. It was an opportunity to ask questions, look deeper, and to reevaluate historical value judgments about who is important, who substantively contributed to the rubella research project, and who is worth knowing about. Things are changing, certainly, but the stereotype that "science is male" remains strong.

Based on this research, Ginny A. Roth, the Program Manager for the Prints and Photographs Program, has updated the catalog record for the photograph. I am thrilled that we could identify her and expand the record to account for her contributions to the research team and help ensure that Hopps' contributions to the development of the rubella vaccine and blood test are remembered in the future.

This "Girl Friday" had a graduate degree, two patents, and a name. That name was Hope Hopps.

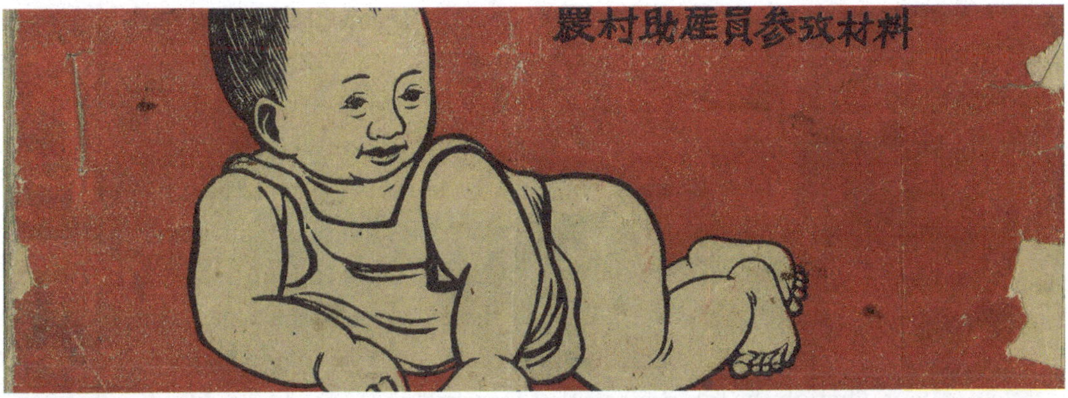

A PEEK AT SOME PAMPHLETS

https://circulatingnow.nlm.nih.gov/2014/01/22/a-peek-at-some-pamphlets/

January 22, 2014 • Rare Books & Journals

SHANNON LU

Every year, with half the school year behind them, high school and college students begin to fret about summer plans, jobs, and internships. I am currently a sophomore at Wellesley College in Massachusetts, pursuing a double major in economics and computer science and a minor in Russian, and I was fortunate enough to have the opportunity to be a Pathways Intern at the National Library of Medicine (NLM) last summer. I spent my time in the Rare Books and Early Manuscripts Section of the History of Medicine Division, where I worked with the Library's vast collection of Chinese and Cyrillic pamphlets, which date from the nineteenth to the twenty-first century. The most important part of my work was to enhance the catalog records, such as this one, of these unique publications to make them more available to researchers and scholars who might otherwise have trouble finding these materials, even in the libraries of the countries of origin.

The National Library of Medicine has a vast collection of English publications about medicine, medical history, and health from the Western Hemisphere. What may come as a surprise to some people, however, is that the NLM also has a large collection of publications in many different languages and from countries in Africa, Eastern Europe, and Asia. During my summer at the NLM, I have flipped through the pages of almost 2,000 different pamphlets, books, serials, and even handwritten manuscripts. Though the two projects that I worked on focused on publications written in Chinese, Russian, Ukrainian, Bulgarian, Serbian, and Macedonian, I also came across languages such as Japanese, Polish, Uyghur, Czech, German, Swahili, Mongolian, French, Romanian, Portuguese, Tibetan, Italian, Spanish, and Latvian.

As I worked though my cataloging tasks, I found many materials that dealt with basic topics of health and medicine. Especially in the Chinese texts that I worked with from the 1940s and 1950s, I frequently saw publications on hygiene, nutrition, sanitation, and first aid. Many of the small books and pamphlets had few words and many pictures. This is likely because the target audiences of these publications were children and mostly illiterate farmers and laborers in villages and rural parts of China. The topics varied from not spitting in public places to eating fruits and vegetables to boiling water and washing hands before eating so as to avoid cholera. In later publications from the 1960s to 1990s, the topics shifted to more advanced healthcare for malaria, parasites, infectious diseases, and, not surprisingly, a number of books on family planning and birth control. The most recent Chinese publications that I found were from 2002 and 2003, reporting on and researching the Severe Acute Respiratory Syndrome (SARS).

While most of the Chinese texts seemed to be aimed at promoting public health, the Cyrillic texts tended to be far more specialized and advanced in terms of research and technology. This may be due to the fact that many publications were from the 1950s during the Soviet Union's immense innovation in science and technology. My favorite Cyrillic publication was one that discussed Ivan Pavlov's experiments, especially those in psychology and of course, Pavlov's dogs. I also came across a wide variety

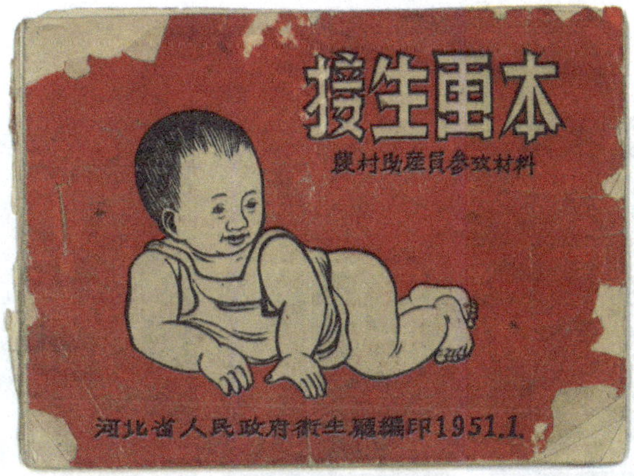

Jie sheng hua ben: nong cun zhu chan yuan can kao cai liao, 1951 • Chinese Pamphlet, Hebei Sheng ren min zheng fu wei sheng ting bian yin, 接生画本: 農村助產員参攷材料 / / 河北省人民政府衛生廳编印 • *National Library of Medicine #101596172*

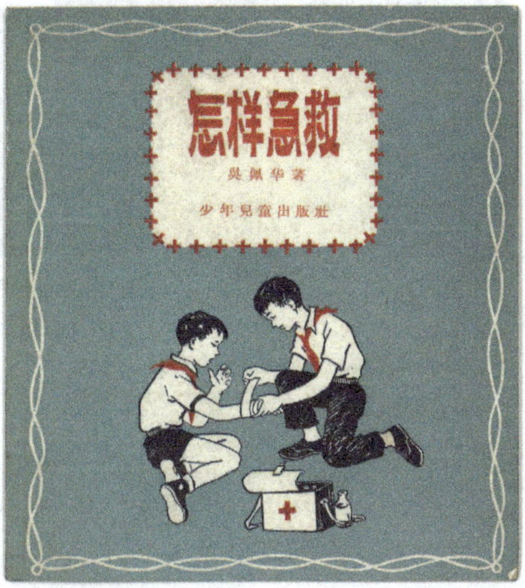

Nong cun bao yu yuan shou ce, 1958 • Chinese Pamphlet, [Shanghai Shi wei sheng ju bian ; Xiong na hui], 农村保育員手册 / [上海市卫生局编; 熊纳繪] • *National Library of Medicine #101592507*

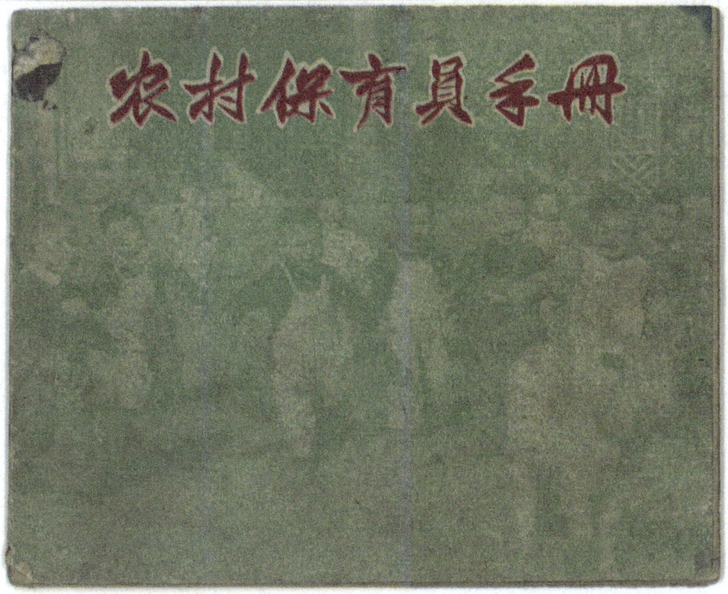

Zen yang ji jiu, 1957 • Chinese Pamphlet, Wu Peihua zhu, 怎样急救 / 吳佩华著 • *National Library of Medicine #101596164*

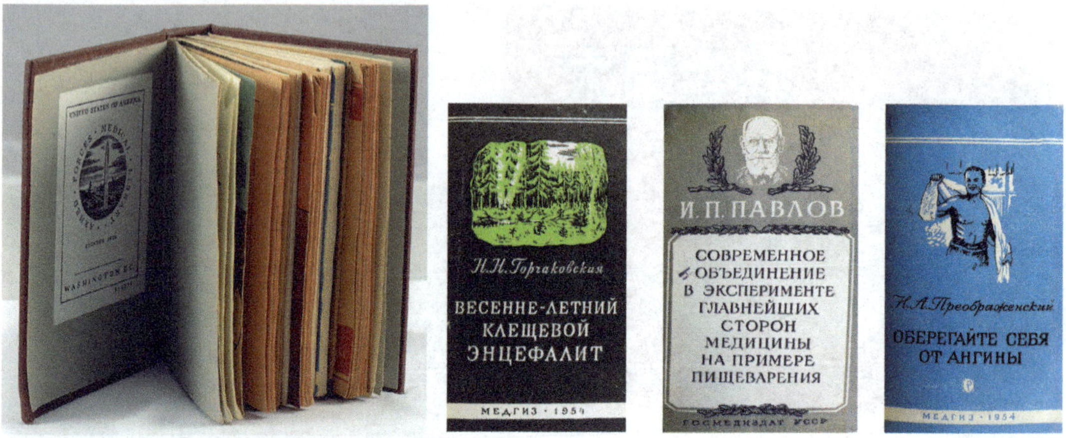

Pamphlets in Russian on tuberculosis, encephalitis, digestion, and angina bound together, ca. 1953–1955 • *National Library of Medicine #26061980R*

of other subjects including alcoholism, oral hygiene, child care, blood transfusions, neurotic diseases, radiation, mental disorders, and even plastic surgery, but the topic I found most frequently was tuberculosis. The juxtaposition of publications on high level scientific research, such as exposure to radiation, against the numerous books on tuberculosis, its prevention, its symptoms, and its manifestation in children was hugely indicative of life in the Soviet Union during the Cold War.

I've only scratched the surface of these subjects simply by browsing through the pages this past summer, but the NLM's staff work daily to preserve and make accessible these and other invaluable collections.

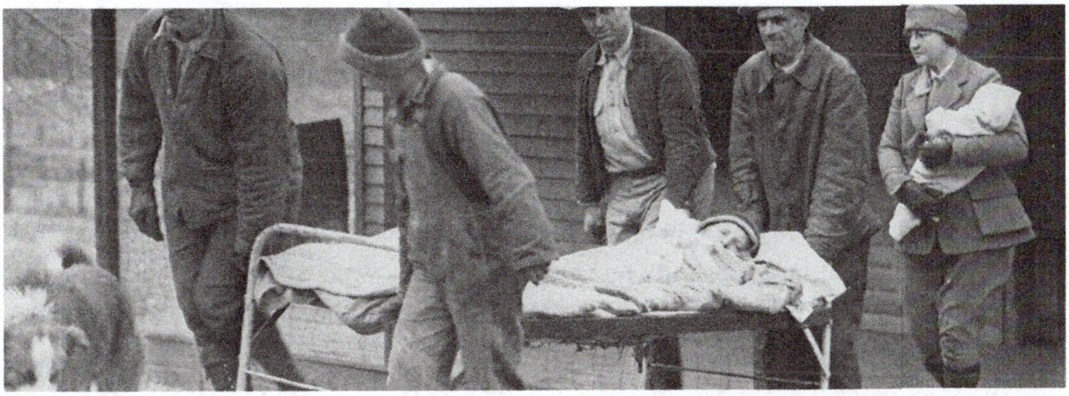

THE FORGOTTEN FRONTIER: NURSING DONE IN WILD PLACES

https://circulatingnow.nlm.nih.gov/2018/09/20/the-forgotten-frontier-nursing-done-in-wild-places/

September 20, 2018 • Films & Videos

EMMA CARTER

"Where do babies come from?" Children have been asking this question for as long as humankind has populated the Earth, and parents have offered many answers: I found her in a cabbage patch, God sent him, the stork dropped by. For many decades, the most likely answer given by mothers and fathers in the Appalachian hills of Leslie County, Kentucky was . . . the ladies from the Frontier Nursing Service (FNS). The proof is in the picture, a swaddled newborn tucked in a saddlebag.

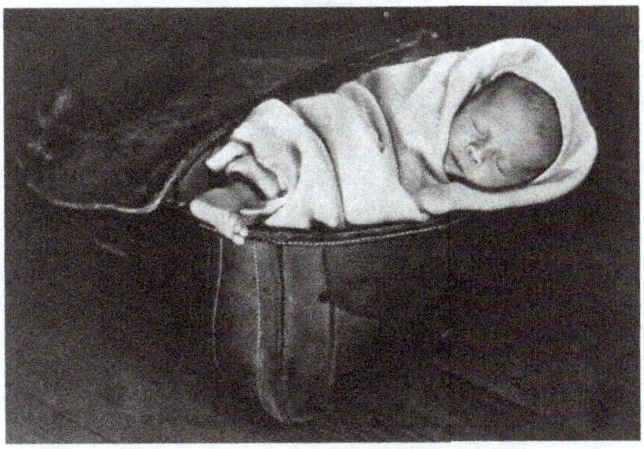

Saddlebag Baby, 1937, in *Wide Neighborhoods: A Story of the Frontier Nursing Service*, by Mary Breckinridge. Lexington KY: The University Press of Kentucky, 1981. Original edition 1952. • *Photo by Marvin Breckinridge, National Library of Medicine #8211678*

The FNS was more than just a cute reply to inquisitive children. Launched in 1925 in Leslie County, the service delivered thousands of babies over many decades in remote hill country where people were poor and doctors were scarce. By the 1980s, the number of births in Leslie County had dropped significantly, but show that 95 percent of the 20,000 births since the 1920s had taken place without a doctor in attendance, with an infant mortality rate consistently below state and national averages.

Fourteen years after FNS began its work, its founder, Mary Breckinridge, started the Frontier Graduate School of Midwifery, sending its graduates all over the country to assist underserved communities. The graduate school evolved into Frontier Nursing University, still operating in Kentucky today.

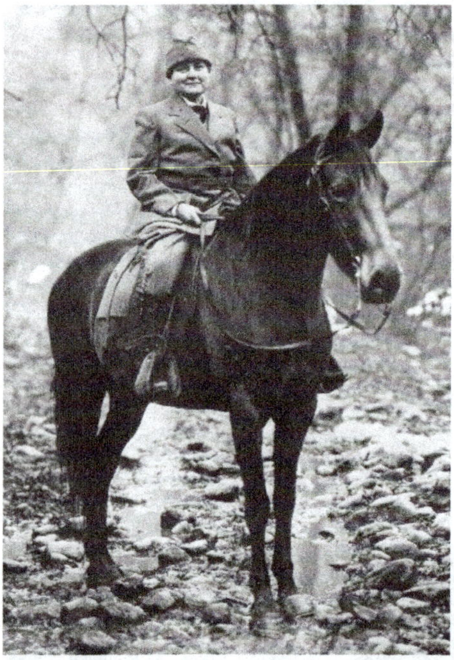

Mary Breckinridge, 1937, in *Wide Neighborhoods: A Story of the Frontier Nursing Service*, by Mary Breckinridge. Lexington KY: The University Press of Kentucky, 1981. Original edition 1952. • *Photo by Marvin Breckinridge, National Library of Medicine #8211678*

Mary was born in 1881, in Memphis, Tennessee, to a wealthy family of statesmen—including members of Congress, ambassadors, and a U.S. vice president, her grandfather John C. Breckinridge. She also suffered great loss, including the deaths of a husband and two children. These experiences, combined with an interest in infant care and a thirst for adventure, led her to service in France post-World War I, then midwifery training in England, and eventually back to Appalachia to serve the communities there. She gave back as much as she was given.

In 1923, Mary undertook, on horseback, an information-gathering trip to assess the availability and skills of midwives in three Kentucky counties (Leslie, Knott, and Owsley), and to determine what they and the childbearing women they served most needed. The National Library of Medicine holds Mrs. Breckinridge's original manuscript, *Midwifery in the Kentucky Mountains: An Investigation*, and it makes for remarkable reading. Included in the manuscript is a data table listing the age, birthplace, literacy status, number of years in practice, cleanliness, and number of children reared for each practicing midwife in the region to whom Mary was able to speak.

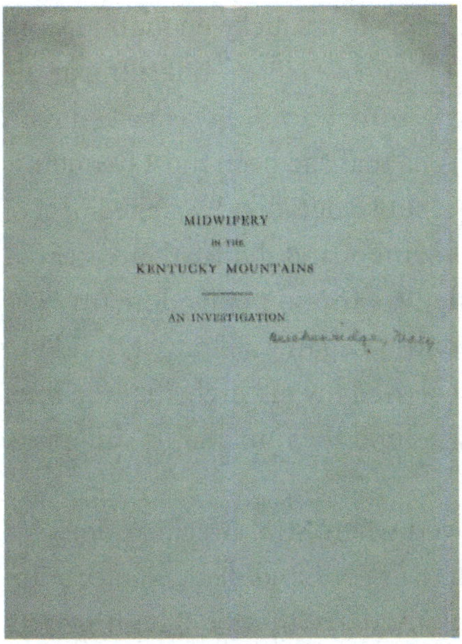

MIDWIFERY
IN THE
KENTUCKY MOUNTAINS

AN INVESTIGATION

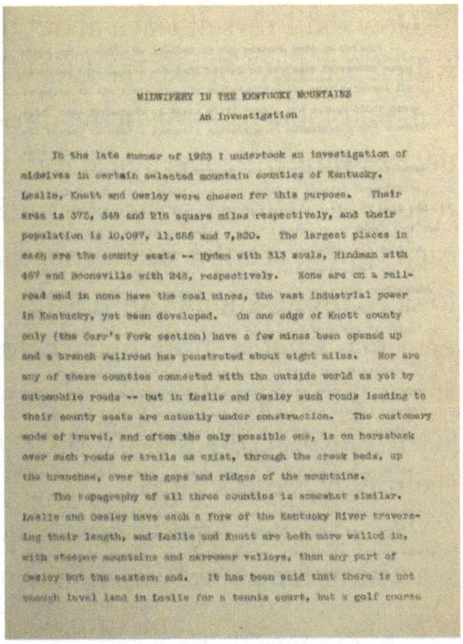

MIDWIFERY IN THE KENTUCKY MOUNTAINS
An Investigation

In the late summer of 1923 I undertook an investigation of midwives in certain selected mountain counties of Kentucky. Leslie, Knott and Owsley were chosen for this purpose. Their area is 375, 349 and 216 square miles respectively, and their population is 10,097, 11,668 and 7,820. The largest places in each are the county seats -- Hyden with 313 souls, Hindman with 467 and Booneville with 248, respectively. None are on a railroad and in none have the coal mines, the vast industrial power in Kentucky, yet been developed. On one edge of Knott county only (the Carr's Fork section) have a few mines been opened up and a branch railroad has penetrated about eight miles. Nor are any of these counties connected with the outside world as yet by automobile roads -- but in Leslie and Owsley such roads leading to their county seats are actually under construction. The customary mode of travel, and often the only possible one, is on horseback over such roads or trails as exist, through the creek beds, up the branches, over the gaps and ridges of the mountains.

The topography of all three counties is somewhat similar. Leslie and Owsley have each a fork of the Kentucky River traversing their length, and Leslie and Knott are both more walled in, with steeper mountains and narrower valleys, than any part of Owsley but the eastern end. It has been said that there is not enough level land in Leslie for a tennis court, but a golf course

LEFT TO RIGHT (1) "Midwifery in the Kentucky Mountains: An Investigation," ca. 1923 • *National Library of Medicine #101175890* **(2)** "Midwifery in the Kentucky Mountains: An Investigation" • "In the late summer of 1923, I undertook an investigation of midwives in certain selected mountain counties of Kentucky." • *National Library of Medicine #101175890*

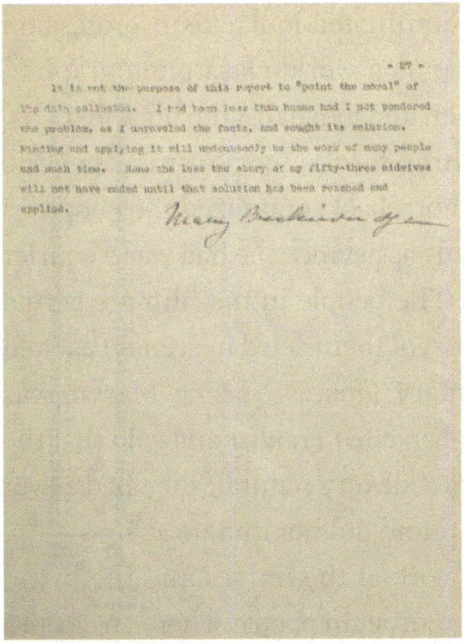

- 27 -

It is not the purpose of this report to "point the moral" of the data collected. I had been less than human had I not pondered the problem, as I unraveled the facts, and sought its solution. Finding and applying it will undoubtedly be the work of many people and much time. None the less the story of my fifty-three midwives will not have ended until that solution has been reached and applied.

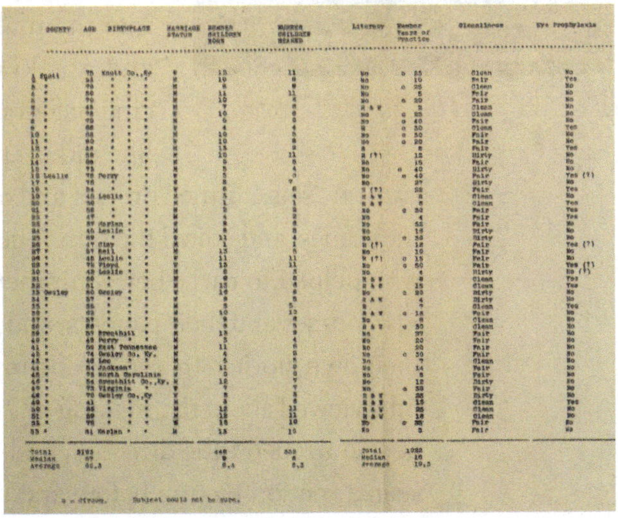

COUNTY	AGE	BIRTHPLACE	MARRIAGE STATUS	NUMBER CHILDREN BORN	NUMBER CHILDREN REARED	Literacy	Number Years of Practice	Cleanliness	Eye Prophylaxis
Total	3193			448	338	Total	1032		
Median	57			9	6	Median	16		
Average	60.3			8.4	6.3	Average	19.5		

Subject could not be sure.

LEFT TO RIGHT (1) "Midwifery in the Kentucky Mountains: An Investigation," page 27, ca. 1923 • "It is not the purpose of this report to 'point the moral' of the data collected. I had been less than human if I had not pondered the problem, as I unraveled the facts, and sought its solution . . . " • *National Library of Medicine #101175890* **(2)** Data on Mothers, in "Midwifery in the Kentucky Mountains: An Investigation," ca. 1923 • *National Library of Medicine #101175890*

How did I myself learn about the FNS? I was lucky enough to work with a primary source, the film *The Forgotten Frontier*. Interning at the National Library of Medicine during summer 2018, I was tasked with determining the copyright status of films that had been most frequently requested by library patrons over the last two decades. I watched part of each film to see if it had a copyright symbol and did further research to determine whether or not the title was in the public domain. *The Forgotten Frontier* made my list, and once I began watching it, I did not stop until I'd seen the entire picture. I started my research after the final scene rolled, trying to learn the story behind the film and its galloping, seemingly fearless nurses.

The Forgotten Frontier was conceived when Mrs. Breckinridge was searching for a new way to promote the FNS and decided a motion picture was the modern answer. The film was written, produced, and directed by Mary "Marvin" Breckinridge, Mrs. Breckinridge's young cousin who was studying cinematography at the time. Marvin adopted a traditionally male name to ease into the male-dominated journalism profession and was known as a world-class photographer, cinematographer, and journalist during the 1930s. She did everything for the movie—managed the natural "sets," filmed on foot and on horseback, organized the people in the scenes, and edited the film. The only assistance she had was a courier who helped to carry her equipment. The people in the film are actual FNS nurses and their patients, and most of them acted in scenes that told their own stories. In a 1984 documentary, *Frontier Nursing*, Marvin was interviewed about the making of *The Forgotten Frontier* and said that the people needed little direction and were all very natural; they had never seen a motion picture before and therefore did not imitate actors.

Watch the Video on YouTube

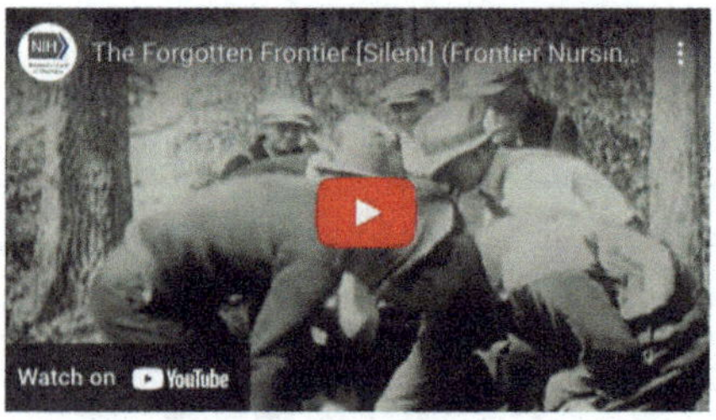

The Forgotten Frontier [Silent] (Frontier Nursing Service, Inc., 1931)

The Forgotten Frontier shows the work of the nurses and the living conditions and needs of the Kentucky mountain people. There are scenes of a nurse racing to a mother in labor and of men and a nurse carrying an injured man for 16 miles on a makeshift stretcher fashioned from wood that was chopped on the scene and lined with men's jackets. All of the scenes in the movie are true stories, and my favorite is the inoculation

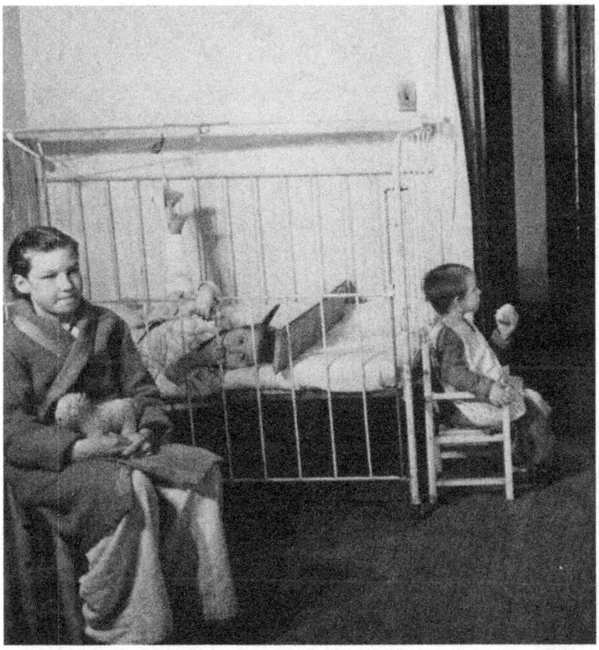

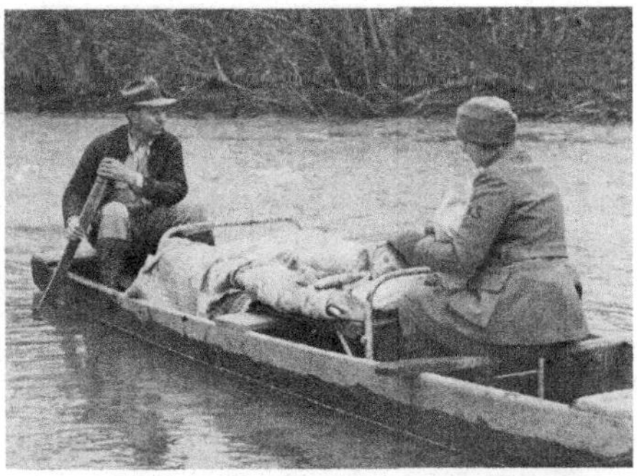

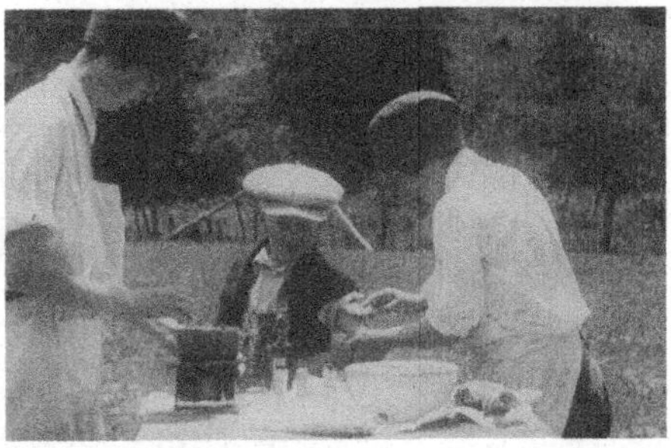

ABOVE Young patients, in *Wide Neighborhoods: A Story of the Frontier Nursing Service*, by Mary Breckinridge. Lexington KY: The University Press of Kentucky, 1981. Original edition 1952. • *Photo by Marvin Breckinridge, National Library of Medicine #8211678*
TOP RIGHT Rural transportation, in *Wide Neighborhoods: A Story of the Frontier Nursing Service*, by Mary Breckinridge. Lexington KY: The University Press of Kentucky, 1981. Original edition 1952. • *Photo by Marvin Breckinridge, National Library of Medicine #8211678*
BOTTOM RIGHT Getting Vaccinated • Still from *The Forgotten Frontier*, 1931 • *National Library of Medicine #8600028A*

of the schoolchildren. Two nurses arrive at the schoolhouse to give the children vaccinations against diseases common in Leslie County. All the children are gathered outside, ready for the nurses to do their work, when a teacher appears. As bold as brass, she says to her students, "You don't want to be inoculated, do you, children? IT HURTS!" The camera cuts to the children, who have all gone rather still, and they all begin to shake their heads and say "No-o-o." The nurses cajole them, and finally a little boy is brave enough to declare, "I'll be second if somebody else will be first." Following that bold statement, a father, who was standing with the parents behind the children, came forward and said he would be the first. After the parent and the little boy accepted their shots, the rest of the children fell in line and everyone was inoculated . . . except the teacher.

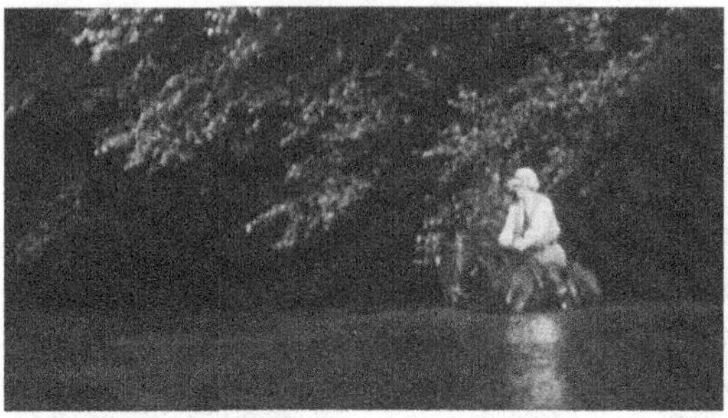

Fording the River • Still from *The Forgotten Frontier,* 1931 • *National Library of Medicine #8600028A*

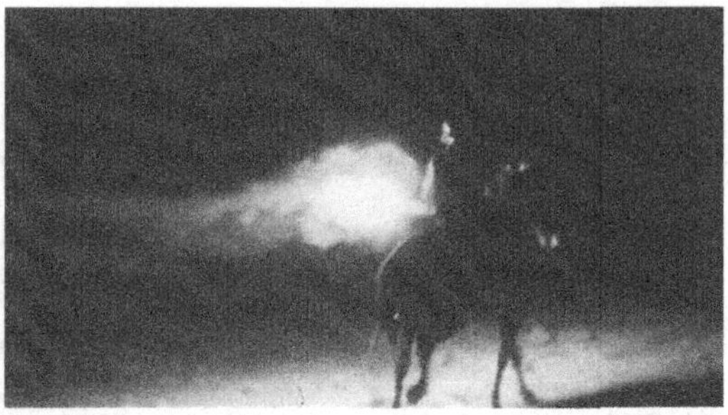

Riding at Night • Still from *The Forgotten Frontier,* 1931 • *National Library of Medicine #8600028A*

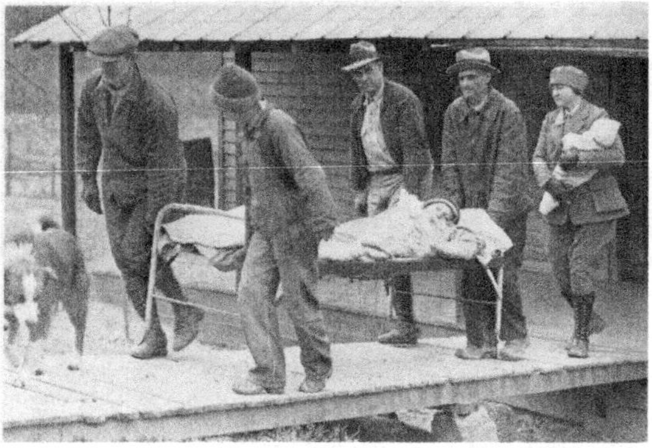

Moving a Patient, 1937 • Published in *Wide Neighborhoods: A Story of the Frontier Nursing Service,* by Mary Breckinridge. Lexington KY: The University Press of Kentucky, 1981. Original edition 1952. • *Photo by Marvin Breckinridge, National Library of Medicine #8211678*

The extraordinary abilities of the nurses were shown throughout the film. The women had to ride in rough, mountainous terrain during all kinds of weather. They had to ford rivers—horses swimming through water up to their necks. They rode at night with torches by their sides, the only way to light the path to a family in need. *The Forgotten Frontier* shows it all, and the dedication of the Frontier Nursing Service to its work and patients is evident throughout the reels. The stirring story of their service made it to the big screen, premiering in New York City in 1931. The film would go on to play for the rest of the decade until 1939, when it was last shown in a private viewing. *The Forgotten Frontier* is a wonderful, moving piece of cinema that demonstrates the care and skill the FNS offered to the people of Kentucky. These fortunate people had one person to thank above all for this beloved service, and her name was Mrs. Mary Breckinridge.

CHAPTER 6

UNEXPECTED STORIES

INTRODUCTION • SUSAN L. SPEAKER

In essence, history is about people—what they have thought and done, how they have lived, and the roles they have played in humanity's collective story. *Circulating Now* has been—and continues to be—a fine venue for telling the diverse individual stories embedded in the historical collections of the National Library of Medicine (NLM). In the blog, authors have been able to fill out some of medicine's well-known "heroic" narratives, but also reveal the little-recognized, unexpected, and even quirky stories discovered in the archives that add richness and depth to our understanding of the past.

Oftentimes, just a few documents or photos, or chance encounters with people and projects, can open up important but hidden stories. Jill L. Newmark, an Exhibition Program registrar and curator, in "A Civil War Surgeon's Books Rediscovered," wrote of her discovery of three books owned by Dr. Alexander Augusta, the first Black medical officer commissioned in the Civil War, donated to the NLM by his widow. Black physicians were rare in the mid nineteenth century; only a dozen served officially in the Civil War. And like many African Americans of the period, they were socially and economically marginalized and therefore they often left behind few documents or artifacts. Augusta's books, then, beyond being unique, are a particularly rare and precious part of this group's historical record.

The historical voices of women physicians are likewise often muted, especially during wartime, when they are working in the intensely male context of military medicine. Like physicians of color, they may not leave a lot of historical records because they rarely belong to the social, political, and professional elites who have typically generated, valued, and preserved such documents. Women and African Americans who entered medicine occupied distinct second and third professional tiers. They were rarely admitted to the best medical schools or residency programs, and seldom taught in them; they did not hold hospital or research privileges at leading institutions and were denied membership in influential state and national medical associations. Outside of the elite networks of medicine and working in demanding (if not lucrative) general practices, women and Black doctors did not publish much, either. Fortunately, oral histories can capture some of their stories. Psychiatrist Lucy Ozarin was one of the first women physicians commissioned by the U.S. Navy in World War II, and one of only seven women naval psychiatrists who served during that conflict. We at the NLM learned about her pioneering medical career when, in retirement, she became a volunteer in the NLM History of Medicine Division. Her projects here included curating an exhibit on diseases of the mind and writing biographies of American psychiatrists. The 2014 oral history interview (part of a project by the U.S. Navy Bureau of Medicine and Surgery) featured on *Circulating Now*, "A Remarkable Career in Psychiatry," tells her personal story in her own voice while it illuminates the challenges faced by women physicians in the second half of the twentieth century.

Contributions to the historical record come in a variety of forms, and from a variety of sources. As archivist John Rees shows us in "A Pharmacist's Mate First Class," Charles H. Stevens, a pharmacist's mate serving on a hospital ship between 1945 and 1952, took photographs that illustrated life on board, and collected a set of professional photos of the ship and the hospital staff. These, together with other memorabilia, form a small collection that gives a us a window into an unusual wartime hospital experience. The collection is also notable because it was given to the NLM by the American Veterans for Equal Rights. As a gay veteran, Stevens participated for many years in that group's campaign against the U.S. military's "don't ask, don't tell" policy on LGBT service members.

Roy Bard Sheetz took photographs for his scrapbook and collected other keepsakes as he served at a Red Cross Military Hospital in France during the last year of the Great War. Like many other officers, he then went home, put his wartime memories away, and got on with his life. Many years later, as Katherine Akey relates in "Hidden Faces of WWI: Maxillofacial Portraits Preserved," Sheetz's "ordinary" wartime collection came to the NLM, and proved to be an extraordinary record, in part because it includes portraits of patients with severe maxillofacial injuries, which are rare in American WWI collections.

When physicians and scientists become eminent and well-known, their public stories focus mainly on their publications, accomplishments, awards, and other acknowledgements of their success. Yet archival collections often include materials that reveal their early experiences and formative influences, as seen in "One Medical Officer's Armistice Day." Stanhope Bayne-Jones, during his long career, made diverse contributions to military medicine, public health administration, and medical education, but as a young man he served as a medical officer during World War I. His letters to his family mark him as a thoughtful writer and careful observer of events. He didn't have to work at the front; indeed, his training at Johns Hopkins had focused much more on bacteriology and hygiene, and the Army wanted to post him to its central laboratory near Paris, but he chose to forego the safety of the lab and support the troops in the trenches. His direct experience with trying to prevent or control disease in both the wounded and the well, and dealing with the logistics of medical transport, shaped his life's work. His Armistice Day letter captured both the surreal atmosphere when the guns stopped, and the bizarre military thinking that kept both sides shooting at each other for several hours after the armistice agreement had been signed (so that Bayne-Jones himself was nearly killed while trying to evacuate a wounded soldier minutes before the scheduled cease-fire took effect).

Michael E. DeBakey's papers likewise hold stories that didn't figure in his later "legend" but that shaped his approach to his later career. The legend often mentions that DeBakey invented a transfusion device that used a roller pump—but not that he and two colleagues attempted, unsuccessfully, to work with a medical equipment manufacturer to put the device on the market at a reasonable price. Like many surgeons, DeBakey was also an inventor (or tinkerer), designing instruments and devices he needed when they didn't exist. His early experience with the transfusion device, as historian Heidi Morefield notes in "Tinkering with Profitability: DeBakey and the Affordable Blood Transfusion Instrument," informed his more successful venture with Dacron vascular grafts twenty years later.

The stories of the professional careers of "minority" physicians are always entwined with their efforts to overcome cultural limitations such as racism and sexism. Leonidas Berry's papers chronicle an impressive career in gastroenterology and community health; they are also a record of a larger American cultural context that included routinized, pervasive racism. Abigail Porter's post, "Leonidas H. Berry and the Fight to Desegregate Medicine," highlights that context, showing Berry's lifelong efforts to protest segregation in the South, and racial discrimination in hospital staffing and in-patient care. Berry had to battle against racism not just in the lives of his patients, but as a Black physician denied full professional acknowledgment by his White peers.

Historians may be among the most frequent users of the NLM collections, but biographers and other researchers also find them valuable. A physician's papers, for example, might contain correspondence and other materials from friends, family, business associates, or patients who are themselves subjects of interest. Robert Gottlieb's post on Sarah Bernhardt, "The Divine Sarah and Her Divine Doctor," draws from the Emanuel Libman collection. Libman, an eminent New York diagnostician, attended the famous actress in 1917, and she corresponded with him in her typically dramatic style. Gottlieb, a biographer of Bernhardt, describes the shocking truth revealed by these letters, namely, that Bernhardt (contrary to all knowledge) knew enough English to write to Libman!

The papers of Howard Bishop are rather unusual in the collections, as he was not a medical practitioner, researcher, or public health administrator. He was instead a self-styled advocate for health reform in the mid twentieth century. An analytical chemist, he believed he had found the three greatest threats to human health—caffeine, nicotine, and alcohol—and conducted a campaign to enlist business leaders and celebrities in his effort to raise awareness and eliminate those hazards. The correspondence featured in James Labosier's post, "Hot Spots of Human Destruction," will seem at least a little nutty to most readers; yet Bishop, sincerely concerned about health, and trying to help improve it, is an example of a "people's medicine" tradition that has always existed side by side with professional medicine.

People in general love stories, and historical collections contain vast numbers of them, if one knows where and how to look. Still, historical tales (to the great puzzlement of historians, archivists, librarians, and conservators) don't always sell themselves, possibly because many readers think history is boring or irrelevant. During *Circulating Now's* first few years, authors highlighted the historical collections of the NLM by connecting them to things that are attractive and relatable to general readers. As the blog has evolved, we have also used a look-behind-the-scenes approach to demonstrate—in myriad, engaging ways—how the historical enterprise is carried out, and the collaborative, inclusive nature of our work. We show how historical accounts, both large stories and small vignettes, are put together. Readers can see history's raw materials—its primary source documents, films, or images—and learn how researchers discover and extract historical meaning from them. Each author's interpretation reveals different layers, colors, textures in the historical fabric, along with new perspectives, drawn from new evidence, or old evidence seen in new ways, using new tools. *Circulating Now's* diverse group of contributors, together with its broad range of topics, show that "history" is a living discipline, and that its stories belong to us all.

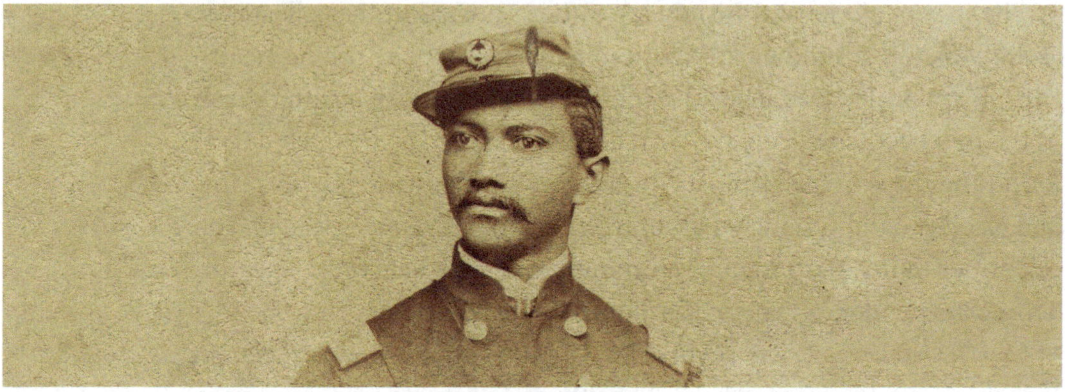

A CIVIL WAR SURGEON'S BOOKS REDISCOVERED

https://circulatingnow.nlm.nih.gov/2014/04/04/a-civil-war-surgeons-books-rediscovered/

April 4, 2014 • Rare Books & Journals, Exhibitions

JILL L. NEWMARK

". . . the sight of his uniform stirred the faintest heart to faith in the new destiny of the race, for Dr. Augusta wore the oak leaves of a major on his shoulders."

On the eve of the anniversary celebration of the signing of the D.C. Emancipation Act, April 16, 1863, the crowd that gathered at the Fifteenth Street Presbyterian Church in Washington, DC, could not help but notice the presence of a distinguished Black soldier wearing a military officer's uniform. The oak leaves on the epaulettes of Alexander T. Augusta's uniform were newly received as he had been given an appointment as surgeon in the Union Army earlier in the month, on April 4th, becoming the first African American commissioned medical officer in the U.S. Army. His appearance at the anniversary gathering was cause for celebration and

TOP Lt. Colonel Alexander T. Augusta, Civil War Surgeon, c. 1863 • *Courtesy Oblate Sisters of Providence Archives, Baltimore*

was acknowledged in the next issue of Washington, DC's daily newspaper, The *Evening Star,* describing Dr. Augusta's appearance as an "occasion of much applause and gratulation."

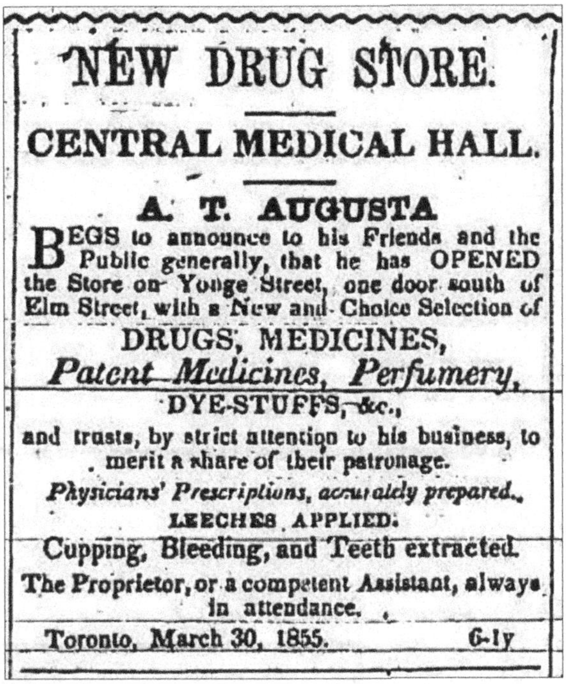

Ad for Augusta's drug store, in *The Provincial Freedmen*, October 13, 1855. • *Courtesy Knowledge Ontario and Our Digital World*

Alexander T. Augusta is among thirteen known African Americans that served as surgeons during the American Civil War and one of only two that were commissioned officers in the U.S. Army. Augusta was free born in Norfolk, Virginia in 1825 and became interested in a medical education and career as a physician. His desire and determination to become a physician was not deterred by the prevailing prejudice and discrimination in the United States that created obstacles for Black people pursuing careers as professionals. Augusta was forced to leave his native country and immigrate to Canada to obtain a medical degree, which he received from Trinity Medical College, Toronto in 1856. He established a medical practice and was the proprietor of a drug store in Toronto before applying for a position as surgeon with the United States Colored Troops (U.S.C.T.) through a letter of application to President Abraham Lincoln and Secretary of War Edwin Stanton in January 1863.

Augusta's application was accepted and after successfully passing the Army Medical Board's rigorous three-day examination, Augusta was appointed surgeon with the U.S. Army and given the rank of Major. He was assigned duty at the Contraband Hospital in Washington, DC, in May 1863, before mustering in with the 7th Regiment of the U.S.C.T. at Camp Stanton in Benedict, Maryland in October as its regimental surgeon and the ranking medical officer among four U.S.C.T. regiments there.

Surgeons serving during the war, including Augusta, owned a copy of the *Hand-book for the Military Surgeon,* a compendium of all aspects of the duties of a medical officer including hospital administration, sanitary

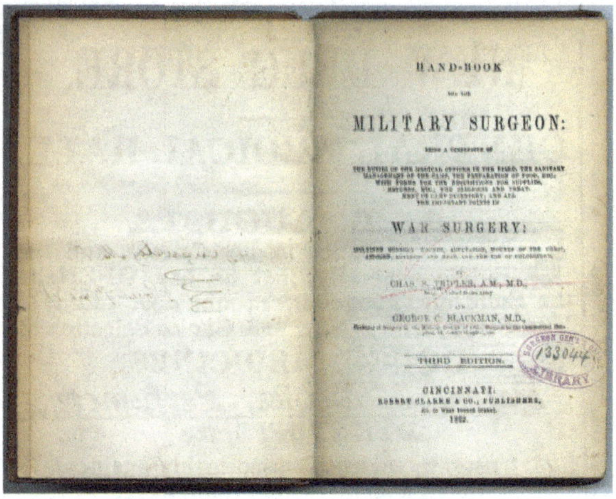

Hand-book for the Military Surgeon by Charles S. Tripler, MD, and George C. Blackman, MD, 1862 • Being a Compendium of the duties of the medical officer in the field, the sanitary management of the camp, the preparation of food, etc. . . • *National Library of Medicine #46920340R*

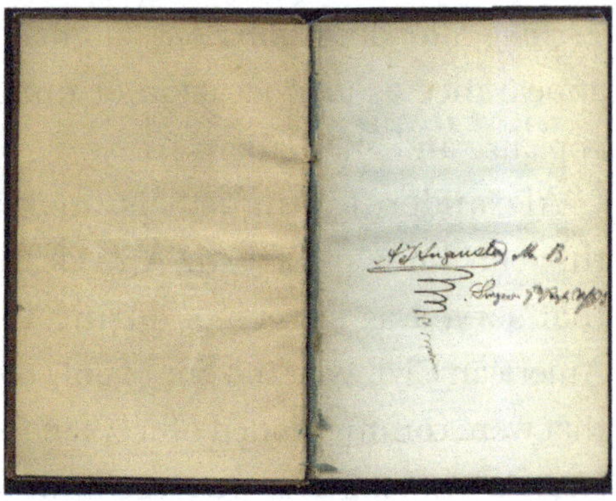

Inscription page from Augusta's personal copy of the *Hand-book for the Military Surgeon* by Charles S. Tripler, MD and George C. Blackman, MD, 1862 • *National Library of Medicine #46920340R*

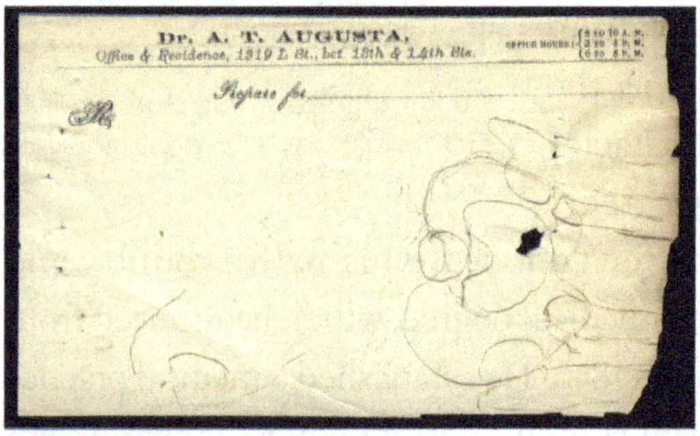

A page from Augusta's prescription pad, with drawing • *National Library of Medicine #46920340R*

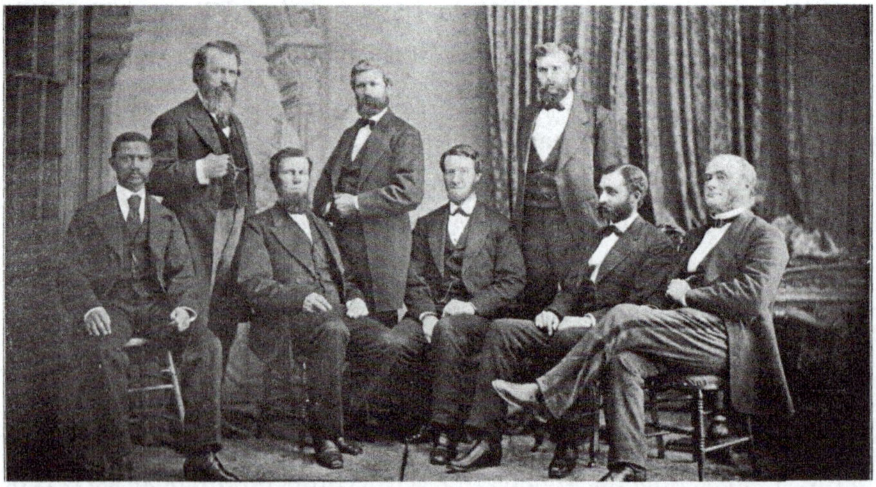

Faculty of Howard University, Medical Department, 1869–70 • A.T. Augusta (seated at far left), S.L. Loomis, G.S. Palmer, O.O. Howard, R. Reyburn, J.T. Johnson, C.B. Purvis, P.H. Strong

management, food preparation, and war surgery. Augusta's personal copy of this important military publication is a treasure among the Civil War collections in the History of Medicine Division of the National Library of Medicine. Uncovered recently during the ongoing digitization project of library materials, Augusta's copy of the *Hand-book* was identified among three books from his personal collection donated to the Surgeon General's Library by Augusta's wife, Mary O. Augusta, after her husband's death in 1890. Hidden within one of these books was a rare page from Augusta's prescription pad used in his private medical practice while living and working in Washington, DC. It was likely slipped into the book by Augusta after he drew an illustration of a pelvis, perhaps as part of a teaching moment with a student or to provide a description of anatomy to a patient.

The significance of these personal possessions of Alexander T. Augusta is made more noteworthy not only by the fact that Augusta was one of only a handful of African Americans that served as surgeons during the Civil War, but by the rarity of identifying and locating personal possessions from these African American Civil War surgeons.

• • •

For more information on Alexander T. Augusta and African American Surgeons in the Civil War, please visit the Binding Wounds, Pushing Boundaries: African Americans in Civil War Medicine *exhibition website.*

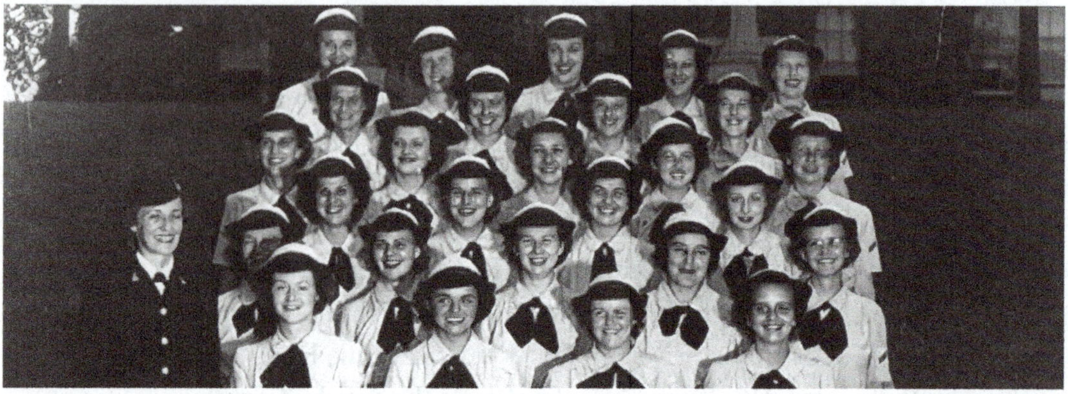

A REMARKABLE CAREER IN PSYCHIATRY

https://circulatingnow.nlm.nih.gov/2014/08/18/a-remarkable-career-in-psychiatry/

August 18, 2014 • About Us, News

ELIZABETH A. MULLEN

In 2012 Dr. Lucy Ozarin was interviewed at the National Library of Medicine (NLM) as part of an oral history project related to the U.S. Navy Bureau of Medicine and Surgery (BUMED). In honor of our remarkable friend and colleague, Circulating Now *offers excerpts from that interview today on the occasion of her 100th birthday. Lucy volunteered at the NLM from 2004 to 2013 researching and writing biographies of notable American psychiatrists and curating the NLM's* Diseases of the Mind *website. Before her service with us as a medical historian, Lucy earned a living as a psychiatrist. From 1943 to 1946, she served in the Navy where she earned the distinction of being one of the first women psychiatrists commissioned in the Navy (and only one of seven women Navy psychiatrists in World War II). Happy Birthday, Lucy.*

• • •

BUMED: Before we delve into your remarkable career I want to capture a bit of your early life. Where were you born?

Lucy Ozarin: I was born in Brooklyn in 1914. We left there when I was about seven and moved to a small town on Long Island and I was there throughout my childhood and education. I went to Lawrence High School in the next town, since we did not have a high school in my town. Then I went to New York University. . . . Then I went to medical school at New York Medical College. . . . I graduated from medical school in 1937. After that I interned at Harlem Hospital for two years. . . . I got out of Harlem in 1939 while the Depression was still going on. I had no money. We weren't wealthy and I couldn't go into practice. The choices were to work in a hospital, either tuberculosis or a mental hospital. I thought psychiatry would be less "catching." I got a job as a resident in Westchester County. The Westchester County Hospital had a small psychiatric unit. I was there for about seven months and then my father had a stroke. I then left Westchester and got a job at the Gowanda State Hospital, 35 miles from Buffalo where my family was living. I stayed there for three years and saw what a state hospital was like.

BUMED: What were your impressions of Gowanda?

LO: It was rural. We drew patients from Western New York. State hospitals were not very good in 1940. After the war broke out and the men on the staff left, I was the only physician for a thousand patients. Which is impossible of course.

In 1943, when legislation for women physicians in the Navy was passed I decided I was going to go into the Navy. In [August] 1943 I did. I resigned even though the superintendent would not let me go. I got a temporary job as Assistant to the Superintendent at Metropolitan Hospital in New York. I was there for about six months and then I was sworn in. I was amused because the Navy used the same form for the men and I'm referred to as a "him."

BUMED: After being sworn in did you go through an indoctrination course?

LO: I had no indoctrination. I put on a uniform one day and went to Washington. My father had died the same week I was sworn, and it was a very emotional time. But as I say, I put on the uniform and reported to Bethesda. I didn't know how to salute.

I came to Bethesda and was assigned to psychiatry. The man in charge of psychiatry was CAPT [Forrest] Harrison. He was an older man and he was very warm-hearted. I stayed in Bethesda at that time from October 1943 until February 1944. The hospital was a beautiful structure and on the land around they began to build the temporary wards. There were lines of wards on both sides of the hospital . . . after four months I got orders to go to Camp Lejeune. I was there for about six weeks. It was very unsatisfying. . . .

There were two women physicians on base and they had been assigned to the dependents clinic located outside the base. I don't think the commander of the hospital knew what to do with me. I got the feeling that he wasn't sympathetic to psychiatry. You have to realize that in the forties psychiatry was still something that meant state hospitals and "crazy people" to most of the population. . . . I was told to examine laborers who had applied for jobs at the hospital. Here I was doing physical examinations. I already had four years of experience in psychiatry and this job did not seem appropriate. . . . After a few weeks I wrote to one of the fellows I met at Bethesda and I'm sure he took my letter to CAPT Harrison because I got orders to go to the WAVES training station at Hunter College in New York. That was an interesting experience.

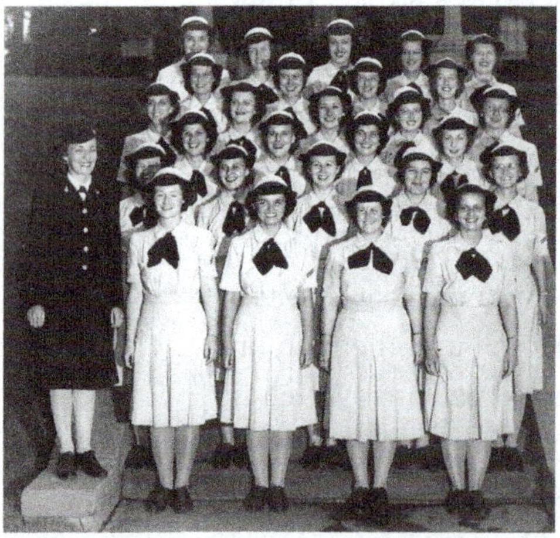

Graduation Photograph, ca. Summer 1943 • WAVE Yeoman Class, Naval Training Center, Women's Reserve, The Bronx, New York (Hunter College) • *Courtesy of PO3c Chris E. Donley, USN*

BUMED: What were you doing at Hunter College?

LO: Well, every two weeks we got 1,500 recruits. There were a number of doctors there including two women. . . . When the WAVES came every two weeks we had to examine them. And there I was doing the psychiatric part of the examination. It was good duty and I was comfortable [at Hunter

College]. When I wasn't on duty I could go shop or do whatever in New York. That worked fine, but it didn't last. I was there until February 1945. . . .

I moved back to Bethesda and found a room. It was hard work. One month I had seventy-seven admissions. By that time George Raines was in charge of psychiatry at Bethesda. He was very strict and I don't think he knew how to deal with women psychiatrists. One day Francis Braceland came in. He was the head of psychiatry at the Surgeon General's office. George went around the room and introduced every single physician on his staff until he came to me and then he skipped me completely. This amused me. He didn't pay much attention to me until one day when he said at a staff meeting that he had looked at the admissions and saw that I was handling more than any of the men. In time, I became a friend of George and we became fond of each other and he was supportive of me. . . .

There were many WAVES in Washington. We got a lot of admissions, especially from those from the Communications Bureau. One of the big problems was that they functioned around the clock with three shifts and it was difficult for some of the girls to adjust. They became anxious. They became irritable. They didn't feel good so they landed in Bethesda. I would talk to each of them. Some would go back to duty and overtly some wanted out. These were very young women and some could not adjust to the living quarters. . . .

BUMED: Did you finish your service at Bethesda?

LO: I stayed at Bethesda until 1946 when they were beginning to discharge the physicians. I got time to study at St. Elizabeth's when I was in service. I took my boards in 1945 and passed them for the first time. The boards for psychiatry and neurology was established in 1934. . . . It was a terrible ordeal and I vowed I would never again take an examination. . . . I went down to the VA's central office and met Harvey Tompkins. He was head of Hospital Psychiatry then. . . . I talked to Harvey for about ten minutes then he took me into his boss, Dan Blain and I got hired by the VA, just like that. . . .

I then went on to become Chief of Hospital Psychiatry for the VA. Now I had absolutely no authority. It was a staff job. I don't know if I had a job description, but they let me do what I wanted. I used to read every

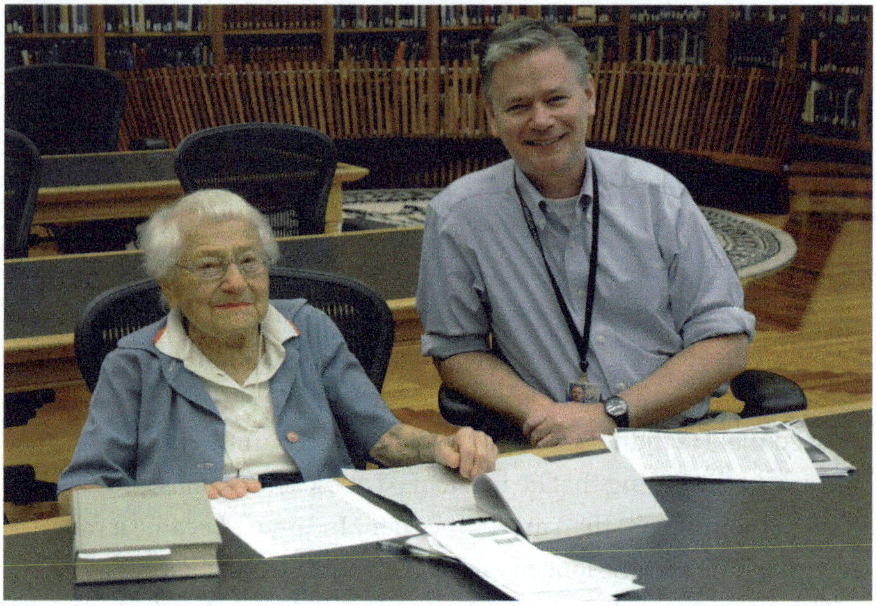

Lucy Ozarin and Michael J. North in the History of Medicine Division reading room, ca. 2010

report that came across my desk. One day I realized that one thing I was seeing was that half the people at VA mental hospitals had been there between five to ten years. . . . I went to Harvey and asked him "Why is this happening?" And he said, "Go and find out." So I began to visit the hospitals. . . . The [state] mental hospitals back then were "hell holes."

At that time the VA was a growing concern with all the thousands of veterans being admitted. Yet the hospital had all this backlog of chronic patients. I think there were more psychiatric casualties at the VA than any other diagnoses. The VA had forty-one mental hospitals all across the country. And in time I visited every one. . . . I had a very satisfactory stay in the VA. . . .

I decided to pursue a career in Public Health, which was very important in those days. I came back to Washington to the Public Health Division of Psychiatry and stayed there until I retired. In the Navy, I met all of the big names. Right now, one of my assignments here is to write brief biographies of psychiatrists for Wikipedia. This has been going on for two years and I have written fifty-three. I hope they will make it to Wikipedia eventually. Now I have just done a draft on Larry Kolb. . . . He was in the Navy and had the ward next to mine. . . . I must tell you about one incident. . . . One day a young sailor came to see me. This was in Ward 137. That was the WAVES NP Ward. He came because his girlfriend had been admitted to my ward. She was one who didn't want to be in the Navy. But she was upset because she found herself engaged to two sailors. I recognized this young sailor was very tense and upset. I was upset because of seeing him. I got up and went next door to talk to Larry, but he didn't help me much. And I let this sailor go. Well, a week or two or three later his father came to see me. This boy had drowned himself. And it's one of my regrets of my life. I wish I could have done something for him. He wasn't anyway connected to a medical situation, but I regret it. . . .

I'll tell you another incident I remember. Ward 137 was over the patients' laundry. In summer, when the dryers were on, it got incredibly hot. Well, we got inspection every week and one day the commanding officer came to the ward. He was a very nice fella. I went around with him and said put your hand on the floor. The laundry got shut down the next day. That was a wonderful example of taking action. But it took a commanding officer to do something. We didn't have air conditioning in those days, and it was hot.

BUMED: Overall you have fond memories of your service in the Navy.

LO: The Navy was an instructive place for me because I rubbed shoulders with the greats in psychiatry. That was my real introduction to the field. I had a very good experience in the Navy, except for Camp Lejeune.

• • •

Read the full interview here.

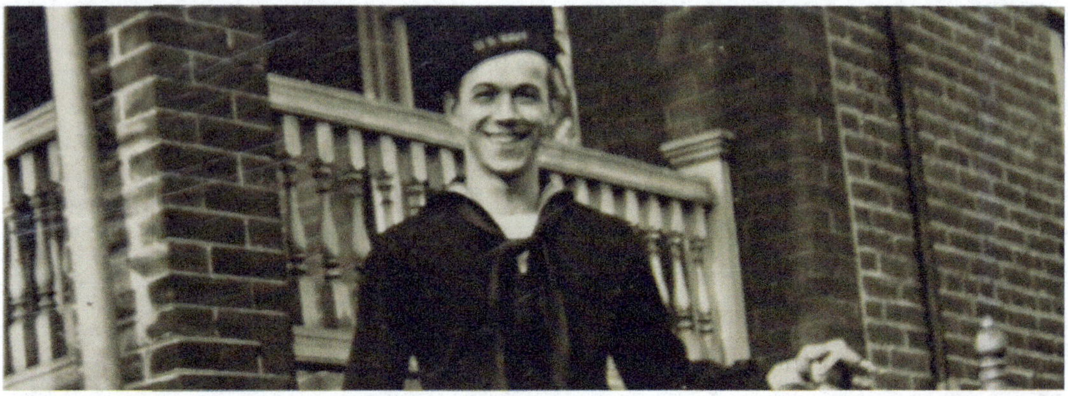

A PHARMACIST'S MATE FIRST CLASS

https://circulatingnow.nlm.nih.gov/2015/11/10/a-pharmacists-mate-first-class/

November 10, 2015 • Archives & Manuscripts

JOHN REES

In celebration of Veteran's Day, the Archives and Modern Manuscripts program highlights the recent acquisition of the Charles Henry Stevens Papers, 1945–1946, selections of which are currently on display in our reading room at the National Library of Medicine in Bethesda, Maryland. The collection was generously donated by his nephew via the American Veterans for Equal Rights.

Stevens, from Philadelphia, Pennsylvania, was a Pharmacist's Mate First Class. He served on the Navy hospital ship USS *Repose* during the last days of World War II combat in the Pacific and continued his service during the Korean Conflict. As a gay man, he later helped in the battle to repeal the military's "don't ask, don't tell" policy. He was active in lesbian,

TOP Charles Henry Stevens, ca. 1945 • *Charles Henry Stevens Papers, National Library of Medicine #101671161*

gay, bisexual, transgender, and queer (LGBTQ) issues during his civilian life living in Atlanta, Georgia, and a member of American Veterans for Equal Rights.

> Pharmacist's mates are petty officers who, under the direction of medical officers, administer medical assistance, treatment, and services to naval personnel. They may serve in the sick bay or dispensary of a ship or shore station, at a naval hospital, or on a hospital ship. When assigned to a marine landing party, they render first aid to the injured on a battle field, or at a dressing station. Many pharmacist's mates in addition to skill, training and experience acquired in the performance of general hospital duties, take specialized training and through practical experience become competent medical technicians in such fields as X-ray, clinical laboratory, pharmacy, epidemiology and sanitation, fever-therapy, etc. Those pharmacist's mates who are employed as technicians are required to attend regular classes in general medicine to maintain skills and knowledge previously acquired. —*United States Navy Rating Description for the Pharmacist Mate, Second Class, NAVPERS 15386, Navy Department Bureau of Naval Personnel, 1945*

His papers are small in size, but rich in content. Included is a nearly complete set of standard professional photographs taken during the ship's commissioning day. There are also several crowd photos of the ship's crew, perhaps taken just before a departure. In addition, there are several personal photographs taken by Stevens of the ship and harbor while deployed to Shanghai, China, and soldiers recuperating at a shore hospital. There are also a few of Stevens himself at home and around Philadelphia on shore leave.

The collection also contains a ship's newsletter from 1946, Stevens's dog tags, and his Pharmacist's Mate uniform insignia. Below are a few items from the collection, which provides a portal into the life and service of Pharmacist's Mate Charles Henry Stevens.

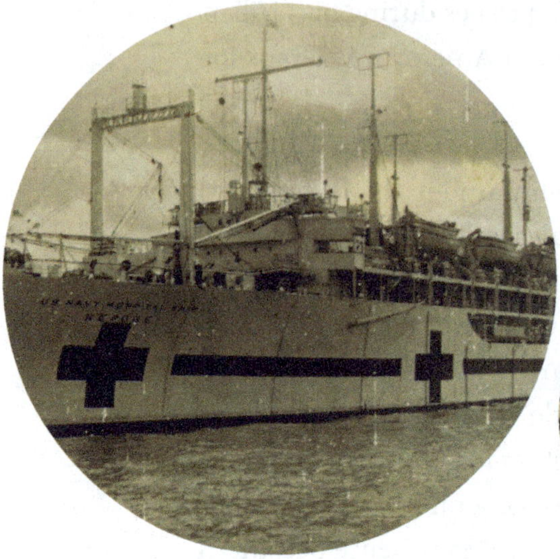
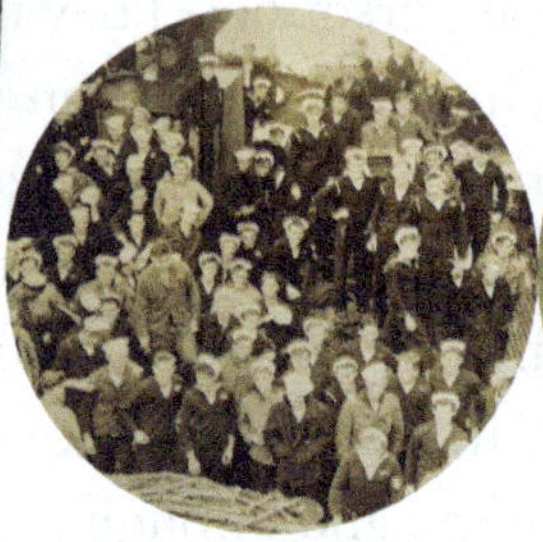
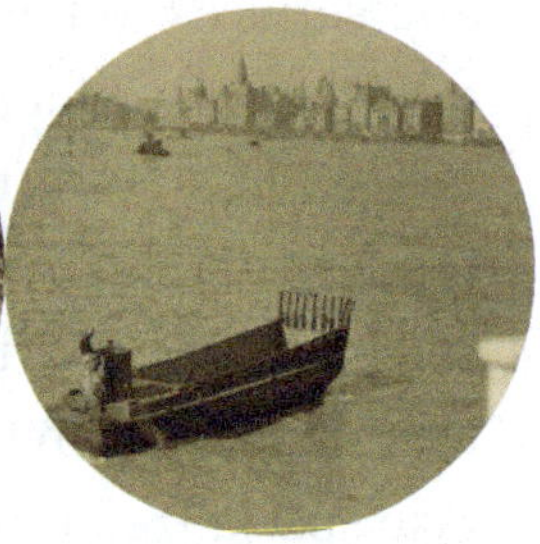

LEFT TO RIGHT **(1)** USS *Repose* anchored in Shanghai Harbor • *Charles Henry Stevens Papers, National Library of Medicine #101671161* **(2)** Crew of the USS *Repose* • *Charles Henry Stevens Papers, National Library of Medicine #101671161* **(3)** View of Shanghai, China, taken from the bow of the USS *Repose* • *Charles Henry Stevens Papers, National Library of Medicine #101671161*

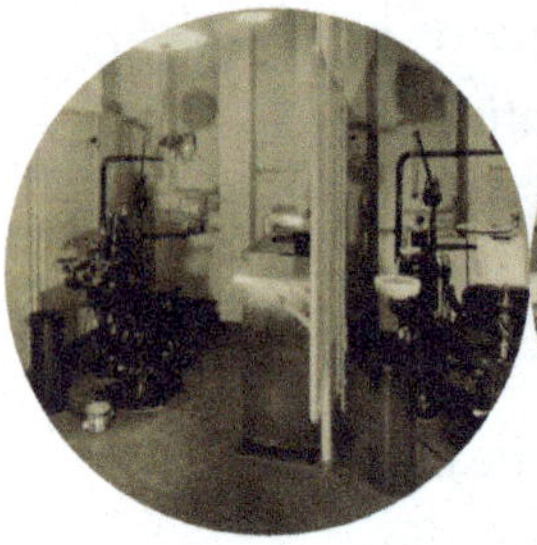
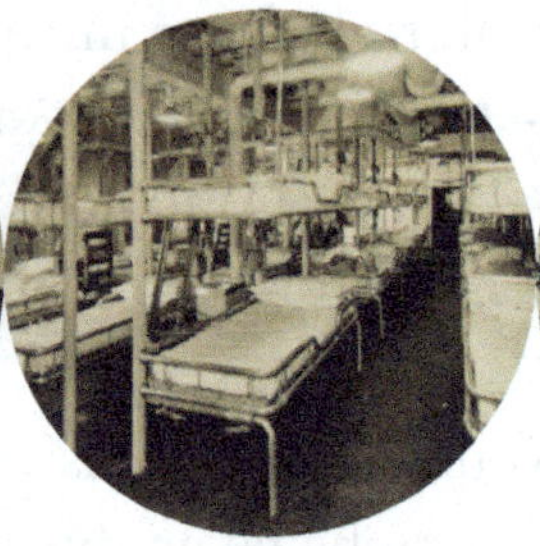
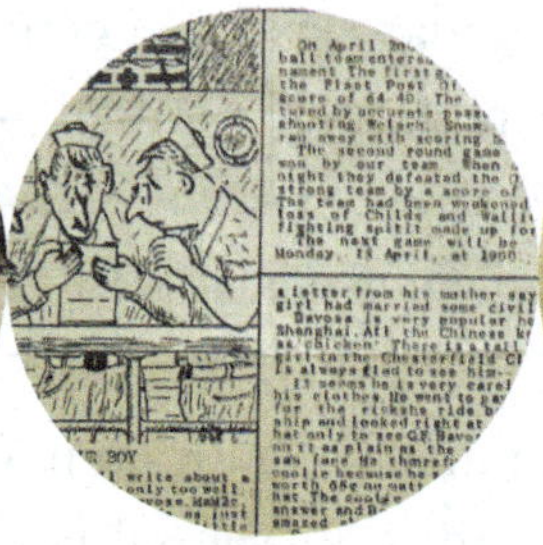
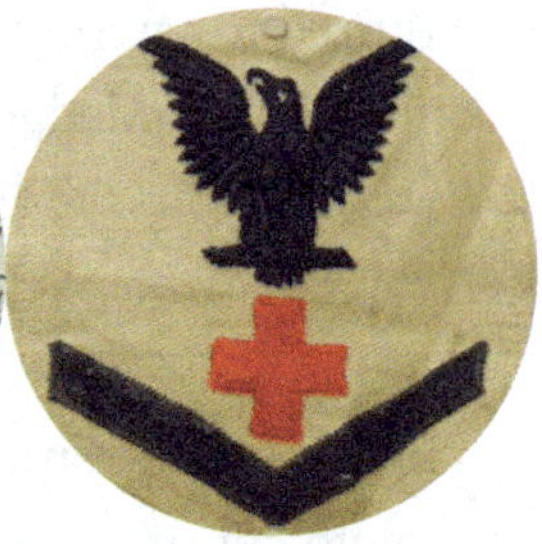

LEFT TO RIGHT **(1)** Dental clinic area aboard the USS *Repose* • *Charles Henry Stevens Papers, National Library of Medicine #101671161* **(2)** Fifty-two-bed patient's ward aboard the USS *Repose* • *Charles Henry Stevens Papers, National Library of Medicine #101671161* **(3)** Issue of the *Repose Review*, the ship newsletter, April 13, 1946 • *Charles Henry Stevens Papers, National Library of Medicine #101671161* **(4)** Stevens' Naval Pharmacist's Mate uniform insignia • *Charles Henry Stevens Papers, National Library of Medicine #101671161*

• • •

These materials are currently on display in the History of Medicine Reading Room at the National Library of Medicine, visit us M–F 8:30 to 5:00 EST. For questions about these materials, including how to consult them, please contact the History of Medicine Division reference staff via NLM Customer Support.

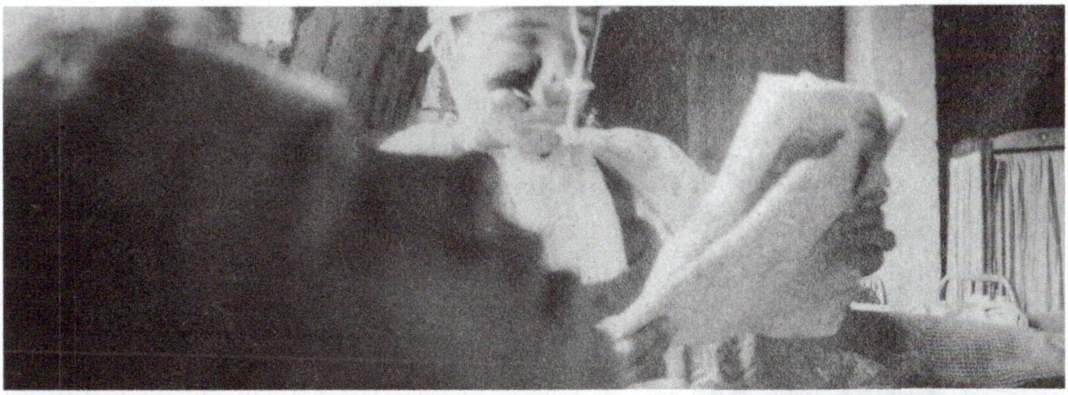

HIDDEN FACES OF WW1: MAXILLOFACIAL PORTRAITS PRESERVED

https://circulatingnow.nlm.nih.gov/2018/08/02/hidden-faces-of-ww1-maxillofacial-portraits-preserved/

August 2, 2018 • Prints & Photographs, Guests

KATHERINE AKEY

Circulating Now *welcomes guest blogger* Katherine Akey*. Ms. Akey is Adjunct Professor of Photography in the Corcoran School of the Arts and Design at the George Washington University and Fellow in the Living Legacy of the First World War project at the Carnegie Council for Ethics in International Affairs. She is also the* line producer *for the United States World War One Centennial Commission weekly* WW1 Centennial News Podcast*. Today she employs her considerable expertise to give us insight into a private and profound photographic collection of an American surgeon in the Great War, now held in the public trust at the National Library of Medicine (NLM).*

• • •

Roy Bard Sheetz was born on Halloween, 1892. He left his small hometown in Lancaster, Pennsylvania for Camp Meade after being called up in the draft in the summer of 1917; like so many other Americans at

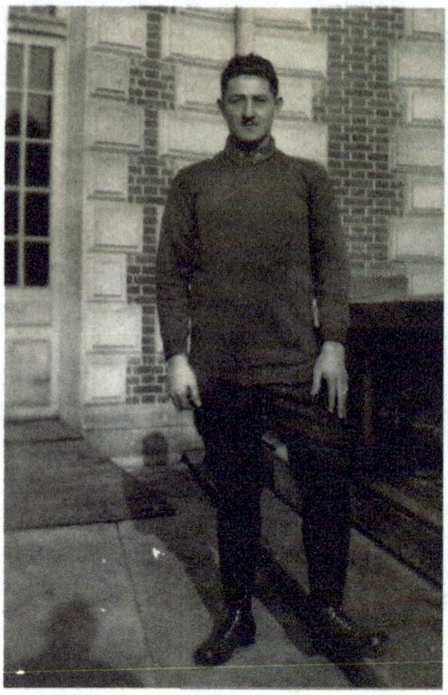

Roy Bard Sheetz at the American Red Cross Military Hospital #1 in Neuilly-sur-Seine, Paris, 1918–19 • *Roy Bard Sheetz Collection, National Library of Medicine*

the time, he would have found himself thrown into an Army that was just starting to flex its muscles, expanding and growing to accommodate the world's first modern, global war.

And like so many other Americans of his time, Sheetz was trained, he was shipped out across the Atlantic, and he served—and upon returning home, he did his best to return to his previous life, taking over the family business and raising a family of his own. Like most veterans of the era, he spoke little of his experiences and kept what physical evidence he had of it tucked away.

His stripes, his tourist map of Paris, his photo albums and ticket stubs lay in the dark of his bedroom closet decade after decade. Like so many other collections of life during wartime, these odds and ends gathered dust and could very easily have ended up in the local antiques store, the trash, or continued to languish in an attic. Instead, thanks to his family, Sheetz's belongings were donated to the National Library of Medicine.

The Roy Bard Sheetz collection traces his service during World War I from his training at Camp Meade, Maryland to his tour around the fighting front of France and his service at the American Red Cross Hospital #1 in Neuilly-sur-Seine, Paris. Through additional research, I was able to piece together a patchy timeline of his service in France. After undergoing officer training at Camp Meade in the winter of 1917, Roy Sheetz was assigned as an assistant to First Lieutenant Frank Leonard of Indianapolis, who had spent the previous nine months training as a dentist for the Dental Reserve Corps. They arrived in France in May, 1918 and went on to serve together at the American Red Cross Hospital #1 in Neuilly-sur-Seine from then until January, 1919.

Sheetz served near the front at the Aisne Marne in July and at Chateau Thierry in August, 1918—and looking at images in Sheetz's photo albums, we can trace his movements as he traveled around the St. Mihiel salient that summer. One image in particular features the town of Flirey, the town name worn but legible on a sign aloft in a building's ruins. There is

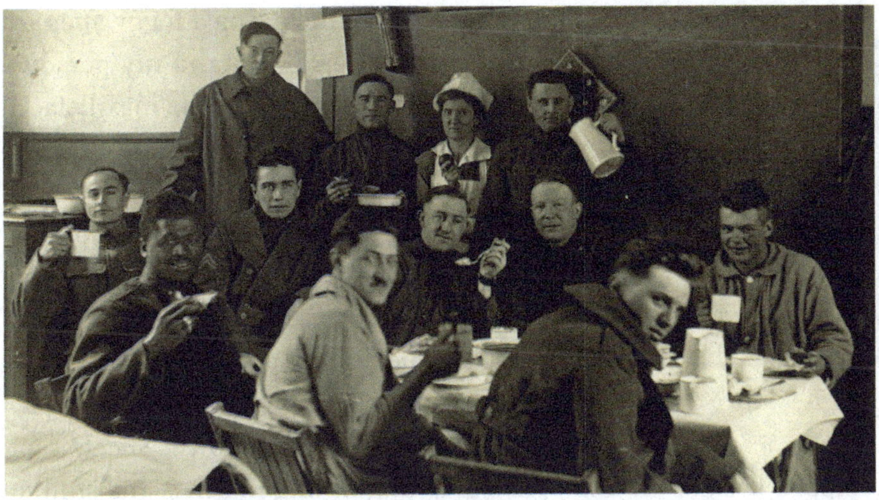

A group photo including Roy Sheetz (center front row) • *Roy Bard Sheetz Collection, National Library of Medicine*

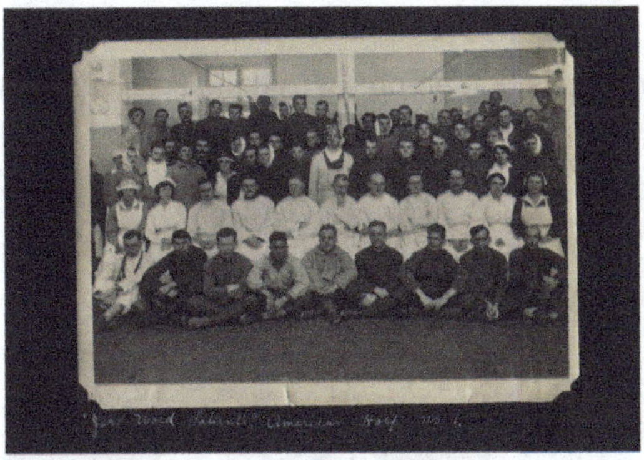

"Jaw Ward Patients," American Hospital No. 1 • Medical staff and patients of the jaw ward at the American Red Cross Military Hospital #1 in Neuilly-sur-Seine, Paris • *Roy Bard Sheetz Collection, National Library of Medicine*

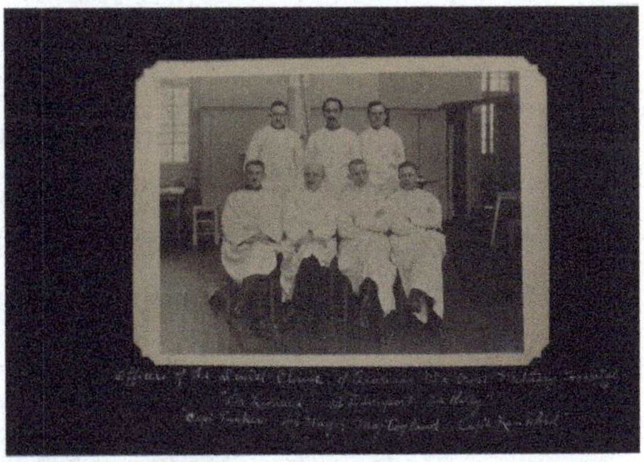

Officers of the Dental Clinic of American Red Cross Military Hospital #1 • "Dr. Leonard, Fr. Davenport, Lt. Kelly." "Capt Tucker, Dr. Hays, Maj. Cogland, Capt. Lankford" • *Roy Bard Sheetz Collection, National Library of Medicine*

also a photograph of a destroyed railway bridge that was well documented in Flirey. Another snapshot of Sheetz's features what is likely the Hotel in Chateau Thierry, and yet another the damaged but regal Cathedral at Reims.

His albums then turn into an intimate and beautiful documentation of life in Neuilly-sur-Seine: shots of sunlight streaming into the wards of the American Red Cross Military Hospital #1; group photos of the officers, the surgeons, and the patients; snapshots of the sights to see in Paris during

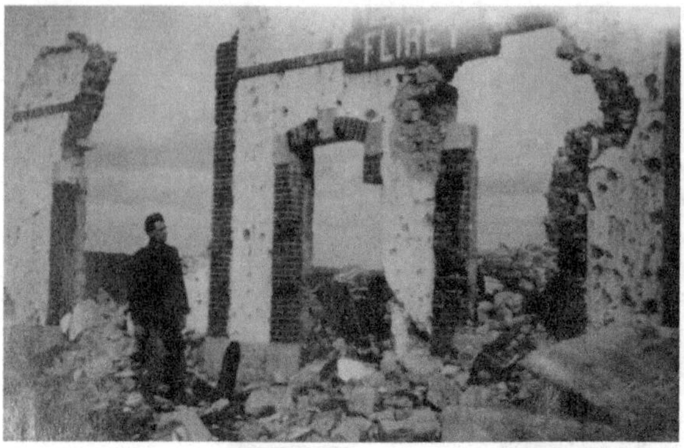

Ruins in the town of Flirey, 1918 • *Roy Bard Sheetz Collection, National Library of Medicine*

wartime, including a foggy, magical trip to Versailles; and my personal favorites, images of the maxillofacial patients sitting together, reading the newspaper. The end of Sheetz's time in France was marked with some loss and sadness; the dentist he was assisting, First Lieutenant Frank Leonard, died of influenza and pneumonia in January 1919, and shortly thereafter the hospital was quickly shut down. Sheetz soon shipped back to the U.S., photographing boxing matches and smiling nurses aboard his transport ship as he headed home.

Every collection of photographs, especially those made in wartime, is remarkable. But Sheetz's has something particularly remarkable for an American sergeant—official medical photographs of maxillofacial surgical patients, displaying in vivid clarity their wounds and their progress toward recovery. In the Sheetz collection are thirty-five portraits, stark images of maxillofacial patients like those that he and the team of dentists and surgeons in Neuilly-sur-Seine would have been treating. Whether or not the

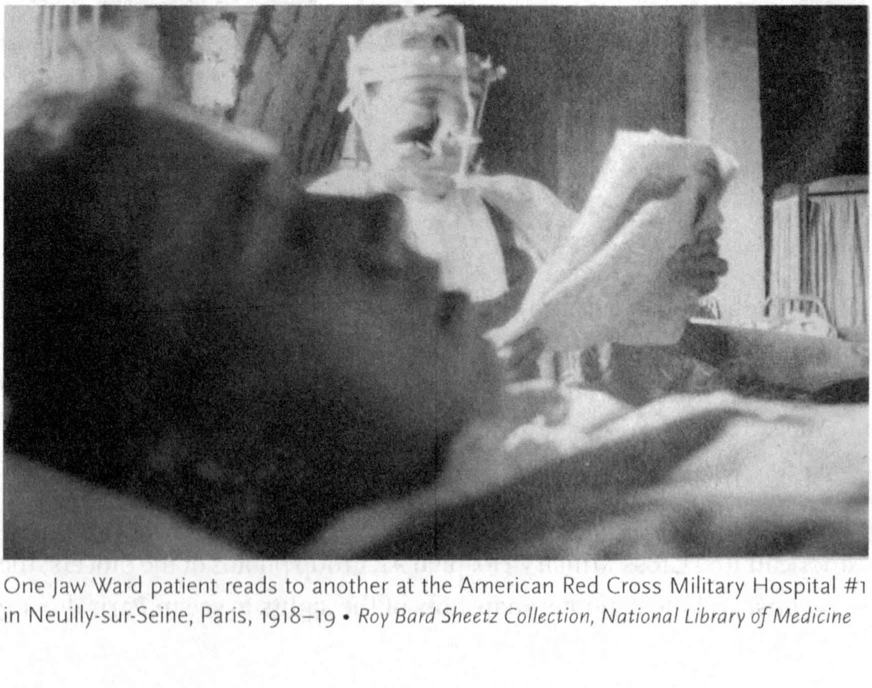

One Jaw Ward patient reads to another at the American Red Cross Military Hospital #1 in Neuilly-sur-Seine, Paris, 1918–19 • *Roy Bard Sheetz Collection, National Library of Medicine*

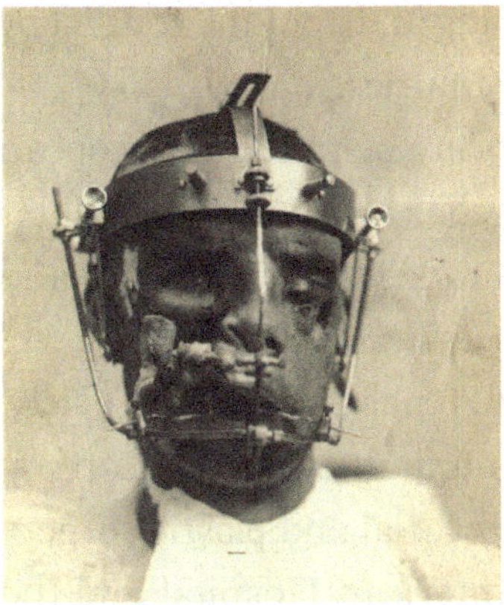

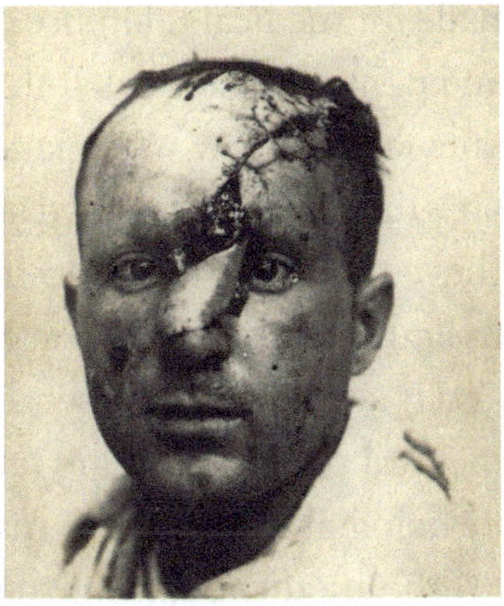

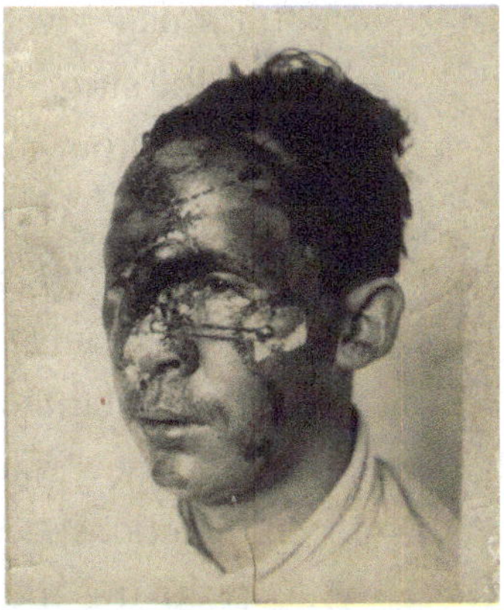

LEFT TO RIGHT (1) Photographic Record of Treatment • One of the maxillofacial patients, here shown with a stabilizing halo • *Roy Bard Sheetz Collection, National Library of Medicine #101662717* **(2)** Photographic Record of Treatment • One of the maxillofacial patients with a skin graft • *Roy Bard Sheetz Collection, National Library of Medicine #101616382* **(3)** Photographic Record of Treatment • One of the maxillofacial patients in the midst of treatment with surgical pins and stitches • *Roy Bard Sheetz Collection, National Library of Medicine #101616385*

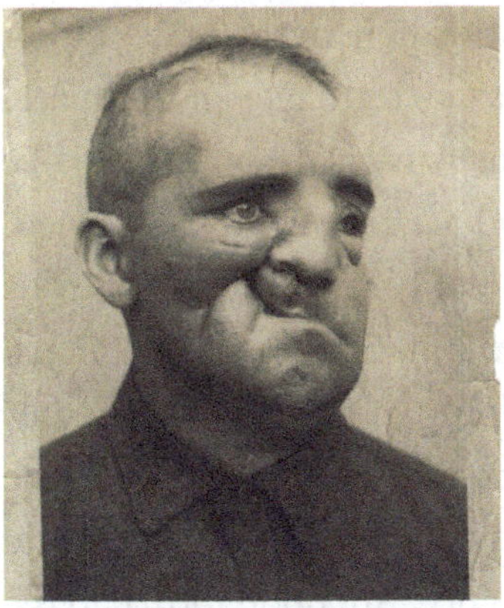

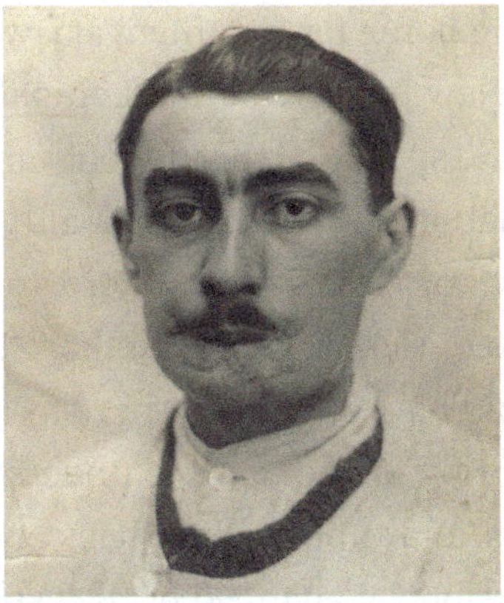

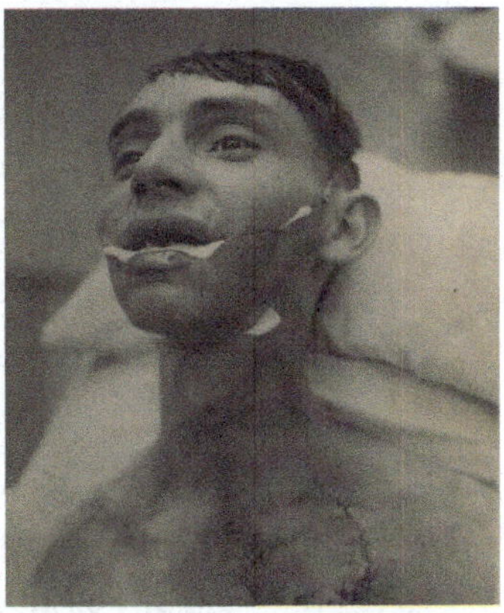

LEFT TO RIGHT (1) Photographic Record of Treatment • One of the maxillofacial patients toward the end of treatment • *Roy Bard Sheetz Collection, National Library of Medicine #101616380* **(2)** Photographic Record of Treatment • One of the maxillofacial patients toward the end of treatment • *Roy Bard Sheetz Collection, National Library of Medicine #101616381* **(3)** Photographic Record of Treatment • One of the maxillofacial patients wearing a prosthetic • *Roy Bard Sheetz Collection, National Library of Medicine #101614665*

men in the images are in fact patients of Sheetz and Dr. Leonard remains unclear—but it is very likely they were treated at the American Red Cross Military Hospital #1 and were photographed there for medical reference.

How Roy Sheetz came to take these images home with him remains foggy—but they represent some of very, very few such images in the national public archives of the United States. The wounds they depict—some of the most gruesome ever to be inflicted upon humankind, no doubt—were quite common during the war, and thousands of similar images were made for medical reference during and after the conflict by the surgeons and dentists who treated these injuries.

Other portraits taken of jaw ward patients are plentiful in European public collections; the efforts of talented surgeons like Dr. Harold Gillies in the UK or those at the Val De Grace in France are well-known and documented. In France in particular, the *gueules cassées* as they're known, maintain to this day a very public presence in French culture and society. But jaw ward medical photographs are few in number in American collections; despite being at the center of maxillofacial and plastic surgery during the war, the medical staff of the American Hospital and the American Red Cross Military Hospital #1 did not bring back images of these injuries en masse, rather these archives of medical technique were kept within the institutions that produced them.

Some American soldiers suffered these types of wounds—many of them returning home for treatment at jaw wards here in the States either at Cape May, New Jersey or in St. Louis, Missouri. Images of them and their injuries are sprinkled throughout various American collections, like those at the National Museum of Health and Medicine at Walter Reed. But the images of American soldiers are notably few and the injuries depicted markedly less severe than those from the European collections.

Sheetz would have spent day after day helping men with these deeply impactful injuries; it's not hard to understand that the experience of the nurses, doctors, and support staff that worked with the wounded in World War I would be forever changed by the experience. But upon return to the United States, what reminders would there be of that service that Sheetz had undertaken? The presence of the *gueules cassées* in America during and after the War was insignificant, bordering on nonexistent. There were occasional newspaper articles at the time, most of which lauded the surgeons and hailed the miraculous transformation the soldiers underwent—often overlooking the difficult reality of reconstructive surgery at the time and the psychological aspect to the trauma.

Essentially, these wounds and their lingering trauma seem to have been treated as exclusively private matters. Universally, the men in the jaw wards were sequestered from other patients so as not to bring down morale; they weren't even permitted to see their own reflection until the surgeons felt they could bear it. And, in America, soldiers with facial

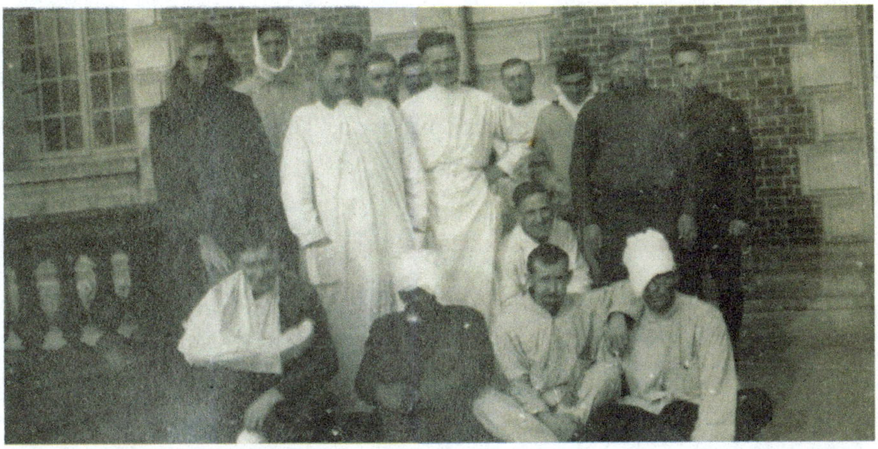

Jaw Ward patients getting some fresh air at the American Red Cross Military Hospital #1 in Neuilly-sur-Seine, Paris, 1918–19 • *Roy Bard Sheetz Collection, National Library of Medicine*

injuries had little public presence at all; once these men left their sequestration in the Army hospitals, they took on their disfigurements and traumas alone or within the small circle of their family and loved ones. Perhaps this is just reflective of statistics; France, followed by Britain and Germany, had more *gueules cassées* than any other country, so the need to confront these injuries and their effect on society at large would have been a much more pressing issue in Europe than here in the United States.

Yet here is Roy Sheetz, who spent a year as a young man in the service of these wounded soldiers and made the effort to keep that experience close to him through photography. Perhaps these portraits are images of particular patients he helped care for, or perhaps he just couldn't bear to see duplicate copies of any portrait of these men thrown away as the American Red Cross Military Hospital #1 was emptied out and shuttered after the Armistice. No matter his reason, Sheetz managed to give an American institution, and now us, its own glimpse at the face of modern warfare, of the horror and destruction wrought in Europe for years before American involvement—a view of the wrenching disfigurement that was so well hidden from American eyes for the last century.

• • •

For questions about this collection and other historical collections, including how to consult them, please contact the History of Medicine Division reference staff via NLM Customer Support.

• • •

Through 2018, Circulating Now *will periodically publish posts featuring NLM collections that illuminate the medical history of* The Great War, *which lasted from August 1914 to November 1918.*

Reflection

The ethical dilemmas surrounding images of conflict are as old as photography itself, but they take on new importance in this era of seemingly boundless image production and proliferation. The immediacy of new images coming out of the conflict of Ukraine, just a few weeks old as I write this, is unprecedented. Photographs and videos can be captured, captioned, and spread worldwide nearly instantly, many of them graphically depicting the effects of war on the human body.

How are we, the public, to navigate this flood? Who is producing these images, why, and in what context are they being presented, re-shared, and consumed? How will our understanding of the human body, of disfigurement, and of photography change in its wake? Will we become further desensitized, or increasingly empathetic? Do we open the floodgates of image consumption, or close our eyes and turn away?

In the face of this onslaught, perhaps the study of one soldier's photographs seems like a small, insignificant step toward better understanding the impact of these difficult images. No one set of photographs can tell the whole story of trauma, of war, can make clear to us the truth of human experience of carnage and catastrophe; however, they can tell us one story, one point of view, one set of moments in time carefully contained through the magic of the camera. From there, perhaps we can find a lodestar by which to navigate the floodwaters, a framework with which we can critically and empathetically navigate our way forward. —Katherine Akey, 2023

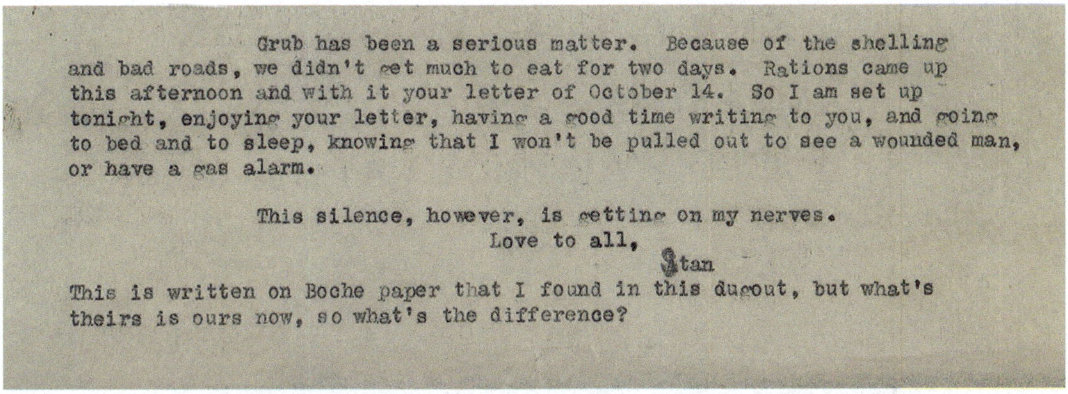
Grub has been a serious matter. Because of the shelling and bad roads, we didn't get much to eat for two days. Rations came up this afternoon and with it your letter of October 14. So I am set up tonight, enjoying your letter, having a good time writing to you, and going to bed and to sleep, knowing that I won't be pulled out to see a wounded man, or have a gas alarm.

This silence, however, is getting on my nerves.

Love to all,

Stan

This is written on Boche paper that I found in this dugout, but what's theirs is ours now, so what's the difference?

ONE MEDICAL OFFICER'S ARMISTICE DAY

https://circulatingnow.nlm.nih.gov/2018/11/09/one-medical-officers-armistice-day/

November 9, 2018 • Archives & Manuscripts, The Great War

SUSAN L. SPEAKER

The newspaper headlines on November 11, 1918 were exultant: after more than four long years, the Great War was over!

For those close to the front lines, however, the cease-fire at 11:00 AM that day was almost surreal. Stanhope Bayne-Jones, an American medical officer who had been working at the front since mid-1917, wrote to his sister Marian that evening and noted,

> "Our guns had stopped—and no shells were coming on us. It seemed mysterious, queer, unbelievable. All the men knew what the silence meant, but nobody shouted or threw his hat in the air."

The last few months of the war were marked by fierce battles, as Allied forces moved to reverse Germany's successful March offensive. The eastward push took the armies back over territory littered with remains from the early years of the conflict. Bayne-Jones' letters from that autumn

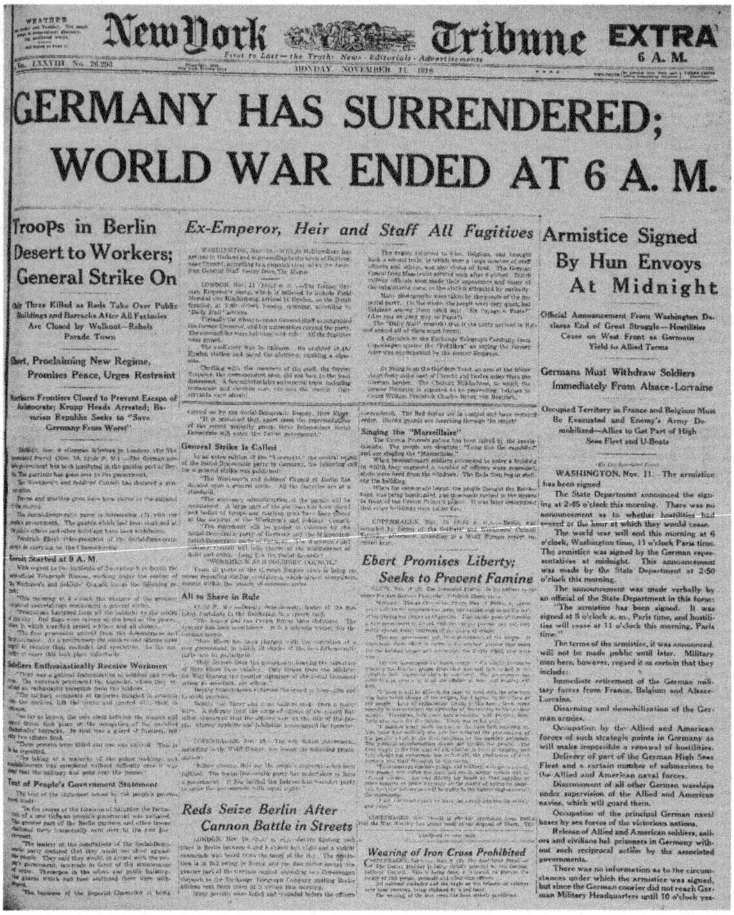

New York Tribune EXTRA 6 A. M.

First to Last—the Truth: News · Editorials · Advertisements

Vol. LXXVIII No. 26,293 MONDAY, NOVEMBER 11, 1918

GERMANY HAS SURRENDERED; WORLD WAR ENDED AT 6 A. M.

Troops in Berlin Desert to Workers; General Strike On

Three Killed as Reds Take Over Public Buildings and Barracks After All Factories Are Closed by Walkout—Rebels Parade Town

Ebert, Proclaiming New Regime, Promises Peace, Urges Restraint

Northern Frontiers Closed to Prevent Escape of Aristocrats; Krupp Heads Arrested; Bavarian Republic Seeks to "Save Germany From Worst"

Ex-Emperor, Heir and Staff All Fugitives

General Strike Is Called

Singing the "Marseillaise"

All to Share in Rule

Ebert Promises Liberty; Seeks to Prevent Famine

Reds Seize Berlin After Cannon Battle in Streets

Wearing of Iron Cross Prohibited

Armistice Signed By Hun Envoys At Midnight

Official Announcement From Washington Declares End of Great Struggle—Hostilities Cease on West Front as Germans Yield to Allied Terms

Germans Must Withdraw Soldiers Immediately From Alsace-Lorraine

Occupied Territory in France and Belgium Must Be Evacuated and Enemy's Army Demobilized—Allies to Get Part of High Seas Fleet and U-Boats

WASHINGTON, Nov. 11. The armistice has been signed.

The State Department announced the signing at 2:45 o'clock this morning. There was no announcement as to whether hostilities had ceased or the hour at which they would cease.

The world war will end this morning at 6 o'clock, Washington time, 11 o'clock Paris time. The armistice was signed by the German representatives at midnight. This announcement was made by the State Department at 2:50 o'clock this morning.

The announcement was made verbally by an official of the State Department in this form: "The armistice has been signed. It was signed at 5 o'clock a. m., Paris time, and hostilities will cease at 11 o'clock this morning, Paris time."

The terms of the armistice, it was announced, will not be made public until later. Military men here, however, regard it as certain that they include:

Immediate retirement of the German military forces from France, Belgium and Alsace-Lorraine.

Disarming and demobilization of the German armies.

Occupation by the Allied and American forces of such strategic points in Germany as will make impossible a renewal of hostilities.

Delivery of part of the German High Seas Fleet and a certain number of submarines to the Allied and American naval forces.

Disarmament of all other German warships under supervision of the Allied and American navies, which will guard them.

Occupation of the principal German naval bases by sea forces of the victorious nations.

Release of Allied and American soldiers, sailors and civilians held prisoners in Germany without such reciprocal action by the associated governments.

There was no information as to the circumstances under which the armistice was signed, but since the German courier did not reach German Military Headquarters until 10 o'clock yes-

Armistice headline in the *New York Tribune* • *Chronicling America, Library of Congress*

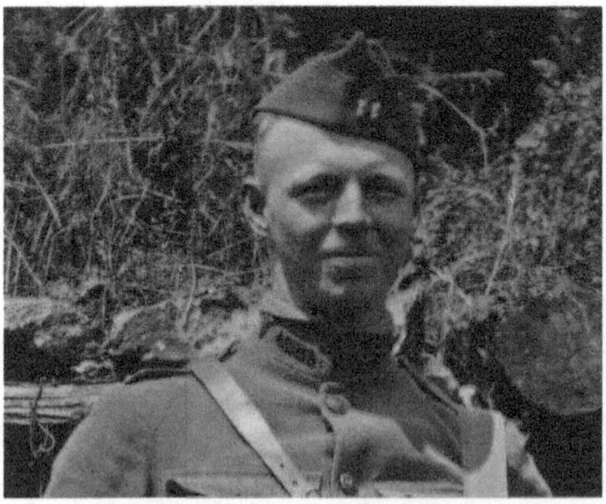

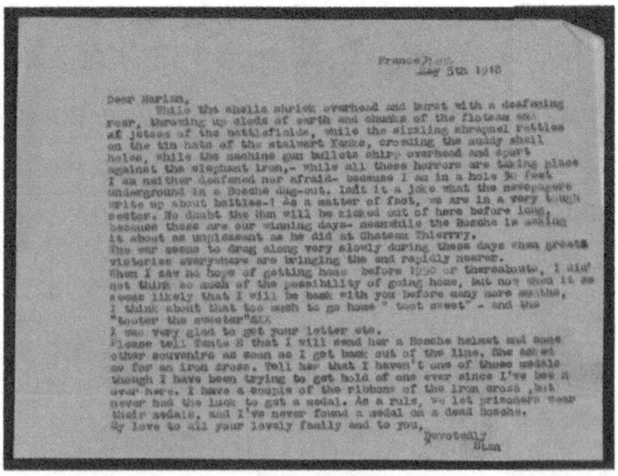

France,
Nov 5th 1918

Dear Marian,

While the shells shriek overhead and burst with a deafening roar, throwing up clods of earth and chunks of the flotsam and of jetsam of the battlefields, while the sizzling shrapnel rattles on the tin hats of the stalwart Yanks, crowding the muddy shell holes, while the machine gun bullets chirp overhead and spurt against the elephant iron,- while all these horrors are taking place I am neither deafened nor afraid- because I am in a hole 30 feet underground in a Bosche dug-out. Isn't it a joke what the newspapers write up about battles-! As a matter of fact, we are in a very tough sector. No doubt the Hun will be kicked out of here before long, because these are our winning days- meanwhile the Bosche is making it about as unpleasant as he did at Chateau Thierry.
The war seems to drag along very slowly during these days when great victories everywhere are bringing the end rapidly nearer.
When I saw no hope of getting home before 1950 or thereabouts, I did not think so much of the possibility of going home, but now when it seems likely that I will be back with you before many more months, I think about that too much to go home " toot sweet" - and the "tooter the sweeter"
I was very glad to get your letter etc.
Please tell Tante E that I will send her a Bosche helmet and some other souvenirs as soon as I get back out of the line. She asked me for an iron cross. Tell her that I haven't one of those medals though I have been trying to get hold of one ever since I've been over here. I have a couple of the ribbons of the iron cross, but never had the luck to get a medal. As a rule, we let prisoners wear their medals, and I've never found a medal on a dead Bosche.
My love to all your lovely family and to you,

Devotedly
Stan

LEFT TO RIGHT (1) Stanhope Bayne-Jones, ca. 1918 • "Our guns had stopped—and no shells were coming on us. It seemed mysterious, queer, unbelievable. All the men knew what the silence meant, but nobody shouted or threw his hat in the air." • *Stanhope Bayne-Jones Papers, National Library of Medicine MS C 155* **(2)** Typewritten letter to Marian, Nov. 5, 1918 • *Stanhope Bayne-Jones Papers, National Library of Medicine MS C 155*

describe camping in the remaining dugouts and seeing bones, equipment, shells, and boots left from the Battle of Verdun (February–December 1916); the weary medical officer was confident that the Allies would soon conquer the Germans. But though there were rumors of peace overtures from the Germans, and talk of an armistice, Bayne-Jones felt that such news was "bad for the troops, as it may make them relax their efforts. We must whip the Boche—and then our diplomats may talk. The best principle I know is—'leave it to [Marshal Ferdinand] Foch.'"

Marshal Foch, commander of the French forces, and other Allied leaders felt the same way. German representatives met with the Allies from November 8 to November 11 to discuss an armistice. They requested a cease-fire while the negotiations were in process, but Marshal Foch, who headed the Allied delegation and dictated the peace terms, refused. Allied officers were told to step up attacks for those last days. The peace agreement was signed by 5:00 AM on 11/11, with a cease-fire ordered for 11:00 AM. Officers got the news hours before that, as it traveled quickly

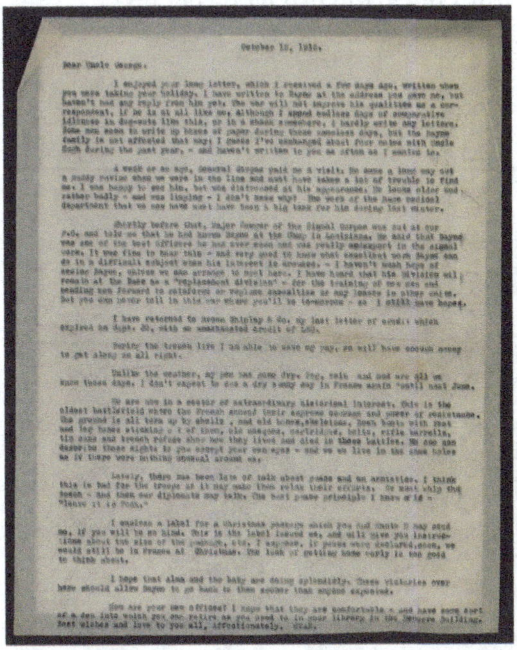

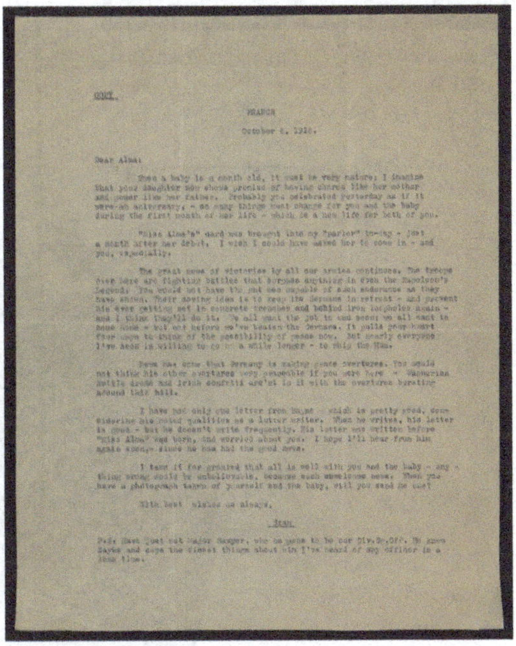

LEFT TO RIGHT (1) Typewritten letter to Uncle George, October 15, 1918 • ". . . Fog, rain and mud are all we know these days. I don't expect to see a dry sunny day in France again until next June . . ." • *Stanhope Bayne-Jones Papers, National Library of Medicine MS C 155* **(2)** Typewritten letter to Alma, October 6, 1918 • ". . .The great news of victories by all our armies continues. The troops over here are fighting battles that surpass anything in even the Napoleon's Legend . . ." • *Stanhope Bayne-Jones Papers, National Library of Medicine MS C 155*

through the lines via radio and telephone; many of them were incredulous when they received orders to continue attacking until the last minute. The decision to go on fighting after peace talks started meant that 6,750 more were killed and 15,000 wounded on both sides, many of them on the morning of the armistice.

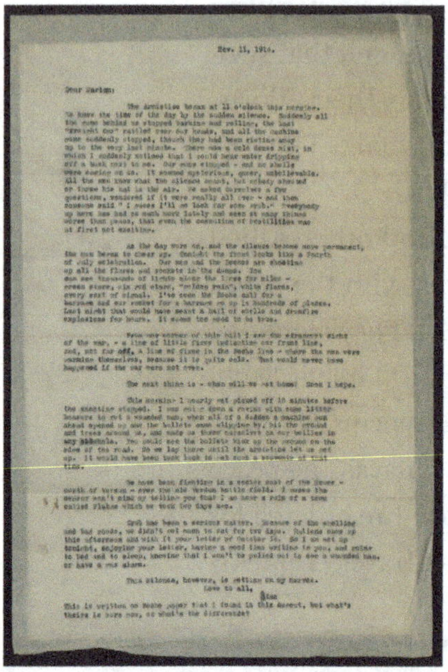

Typewritten letter to Marian, November 11, 1918 • *Stanhope Bayne-Jones Papers, National Library of Medicine MS C 155*

Bayne-Jones was nearly one of those, as he told his sister,

> "This morning I nearly got picked off 15 minutes before the shooting stopped. I was going down a ravine with some litter bearers to get a wounded man, when all of a sudden a machine gun ahead opened up and the bullets came clipping by, hit the ground and trees around us, and made us throw ourselves on our bellies in any old hole. You could see the bullets kick up the ground on the edge of the road. So we lay there until the armistice let us get up."

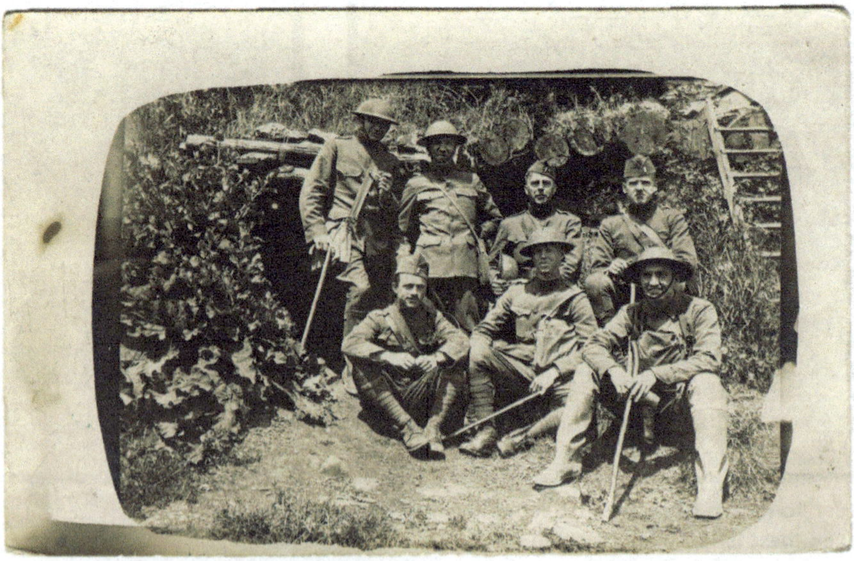

Stanhope Bayne-Jones in a group of soldiers, ca. 1918 • *Stanhope Bayne-Jones Papers, National Library of Medicine MS C 155*

Like most of the soldiers, Bayne-Jones was eager to finish the war and go home. Alas, the army kept him for another six months and sent him to Germany as a sanitation officer. But that's a story for another post!

• • •

Through 2018, Circulating Now *will periodically publish posts featuring National Library of Medicine collections that illuminate the medical history of* The Great War, *which lasted from August 1914 to November 1918.*

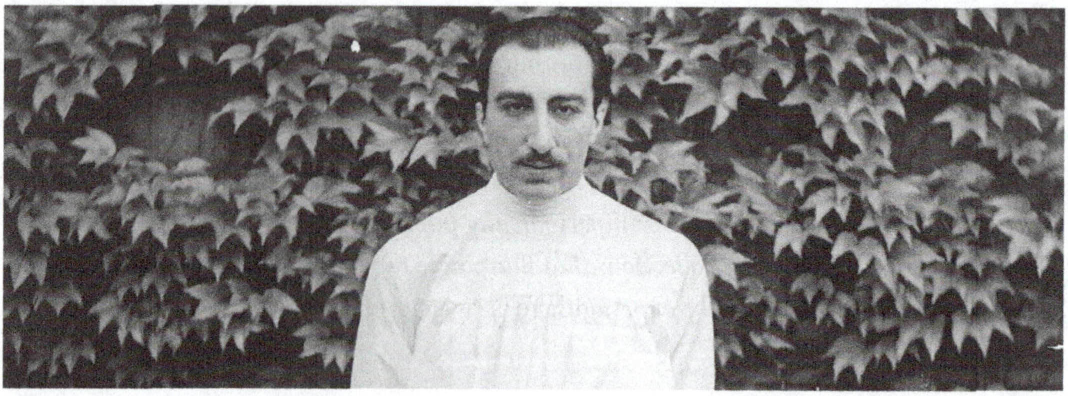

TINKERING WITH PROFITABILITY: DEBAKEY AND THE AFFORDABLE BLOOD TRANSFUSION INSTRUMENT

https://circulatingnow.nlm.nih.gov/2017/09/12/tinkering-with-profitability-debakey-and-the-affordable-blood-transfusion-instrument/

September 12, 2017 • Archives & Manuscripts

HEIDI MOREFIELD

Dr. Michael E. DeBakey was one of the most visible American surgeons of the late twentieth century: he pioneered surgeries, published extensively, advised presidents, and tended to many celebrity patients. The hands-on and innovative approach he took to surgery extended beyond the operating theater—ever since his early training under the direction of Dr. René Leriche he styled himself as a tinkerer as well. One of the lesser known of DeBakey's early prototypes—a collaboration with Dr. George Lilly, a former colleague from the Tulane University School of Medicine, and Mr. Charles "Ernest" Schmidt, a mechanical engineer and his former roommate at Tulane—was a blood transfusion apparatus that the pair hoped to design as a new model of affordable medical technology.

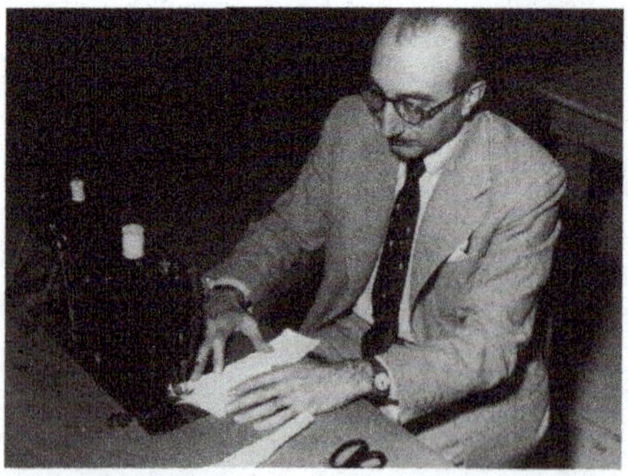

Michael DeBakey at home sewing a Dacron Artificial Artery, 1955 • *Baylor College of Medicine,* Profiles in Science, *National Library of Medicine*

"Affordable" in this case meant keeping the price below twenty dollars (still a fair amount of money in 1935) in order to achieve wide distribution. DeBakey wrote that he thought it was "most important to keep the price of the instrument as low as possible. In planning the instrument this was one of my primary objects. The other was to make it as simple as possible."

Yet both of these goals were complicated by the transition to mass production for the market. At the outset, it seemed that the manufacturing company that they contracted with, the A. S. Aloe Company of St. Louis, Missouri, was in agreement with their target price range. In a letter, the company's president wrote that he was primarily concerned about sales volume and that keeping the retail price to "considerably less than $25.00" would be essential to make the device profitable. DeBakey's simple design played a key role in realizing this, as it kept manufacturing costs low.

By the time the manufacturer had perfected the mass-market prototype and was ready to proceed with selling the instrument, however, the planned retail price had soared to $39.50—nearly twice the original goal. Minor improvements, such as adding a cc. counter and a ratchet to prevent the handle from being turned the wrong way, had driven the manufacturing costs up considerably. At the same time, Aloe wanted to be sure that the device remained profitable even after their advertising and royalty costs were covered.

Royalties also proved a particular sticking point for the three patent holders. After initially agreeing to a 10 percent royalty rate, Aloe informed Drs. DeBakey and Lilly that the best they could do would be to pay royalties on the basis of 10 percent of the manufacturing cost, which was just $22.50. The need for profitability prevented them from being able to offer royalties on the full retail price, which the company and inventors all agreed they absolutely had to keep below $40.00.

Aloe's president played on medical ethics and the presumed altruism of doctors to try to make his lower offer seem generous. He wrote to Debakey:

> "I know that the question in your mind, is not how much royalty you should take, but whether you should take any. This is such an important matter with us that I have tried to look into the oath of Aesculapius [sic.] from an ethical and philosophical background and I cannot interpret that oath to mean that any man is not entitled to the fruits of his inventive genius."

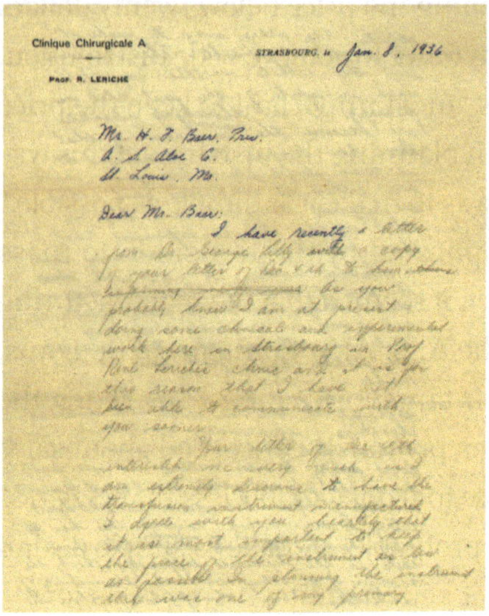
Clinique Chirurgicale A

STRASBOURG, le Jan. 8, 1936

PROF. R. LERICHE

Mr. H. F. Baer, Pres.

Dear Mr. Baer:

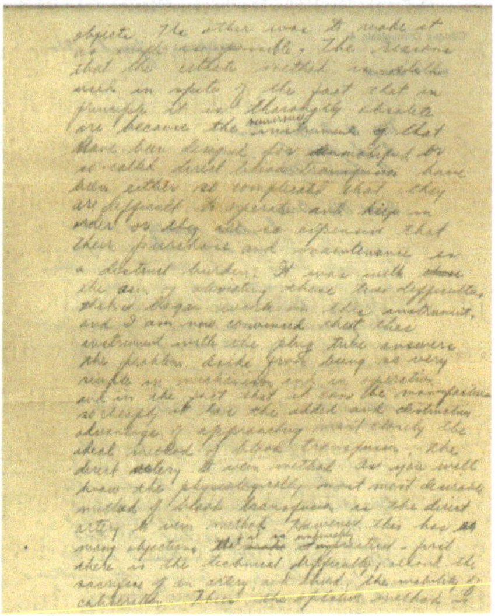

LEFT TO RIGHT **(1)** Keep the Price as Low as Possible • Michael DeBakey to H.F. Baer, January 8, 1936, page 1 • *Michael E. DeBakey Papers, National Library of Medicine MS C 582* **(2)** Make it as Simple as Possible • Michael DeBakey to H.F. Baer, January 8, 1936, page 2 • *Michael E. DeBakey Papers, National Library of Medicine MS C 582*

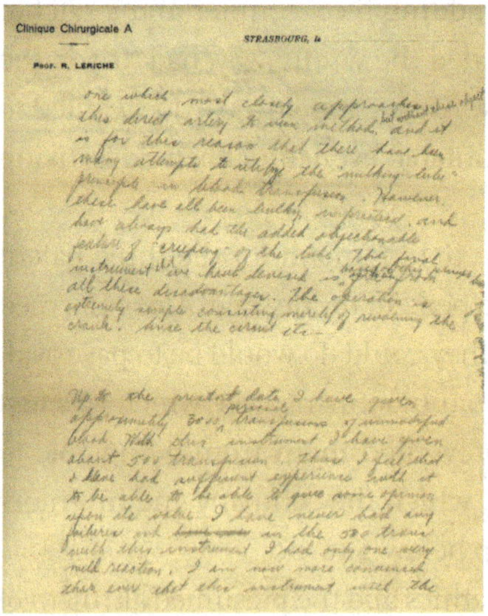
Clinique Chirurgicale A

STRASBOURG, le

PROF. R. LERICHE

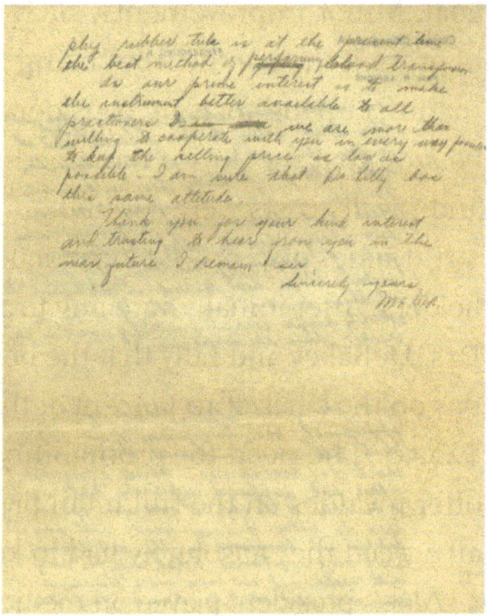

LEFT TO RIGHT **(1)** Personal Testimony of Value • Michael DeBakey to H.F. Baer, January 8, 1936, page 3 • *Michael E. DeBakey Papers, National Library of Medicine MS C 582* **(2)** Prime Interest is to Make Available to All Practitioners • Michael DeBakey to H.F. Baer, January 8, 1936, page 4 • *Michael E. DeBakey Papers, National Library of Medicine MS C 582*

If Dr. DeBakey had never expressed reservations about accepting royalty payments for his inventions, the royalty dispute troubled his two co-patent holders considerably. DeBakey had given the instrument his name and was far more concerned with perfecting its operation and getting it into as many hands as possible than with arguing over profits and royalty contracts. They therefore proceeded with the deal, and the Aloe Company sold just 108 DeBakey transfusion instruments between July 1936 and the end of February 1937. Sales tapered off throughout the rest of that year.

Despite the best of intentions, Dr. DeBakey could not find a way to mass produce a simple and affordable blood transfusion instrument. The manufacturer's demand for profit and marketability ran counter to his vision of an accessible instrument that individual physicians could afford. Mr. Schmidt, the engineer, suggested simplifying the device further and lowering the price. Dr. Lilly, upset over the royalty sharing agreement and particularly with a perceived slight over reimbursement for a patent attorney's fees by Mr. Schmidt, would soon pull out of the deal. Dr. DeBakey, for his part, continued to tinker with the transfusion instrument in his own medical practice.

This early experience laid the foundations for his persistence in inventing other longer-lived and much lauded devices including the Dacron graft, a left ventricular assist device (LVAD), and the artificial heart. Throughout his career, Dr. DeBakey saw himself as a technological innovator committed to improving surgical practice, even if the realities of manufacture often proved a challenge.

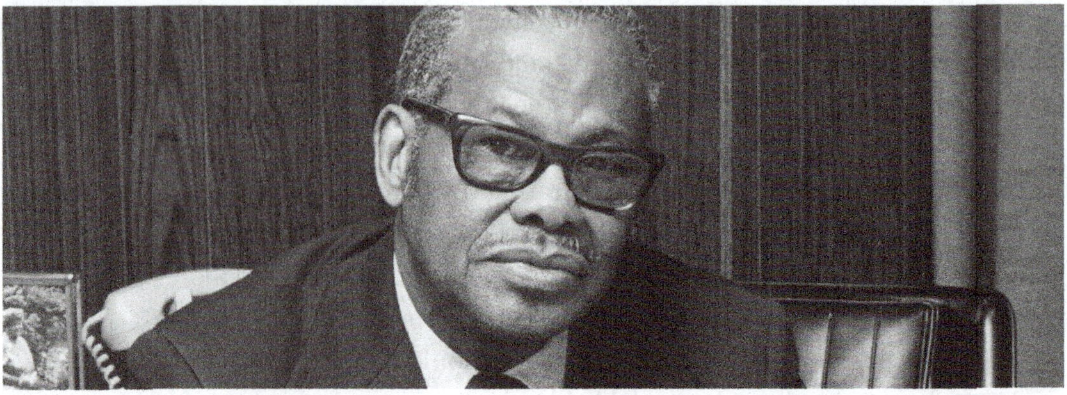

LEONIDAS H. BERRY AND THE FIGHT TO DESEGREGATE MEDICINE

https://circulatingnow.nlm.nih.gov/2018/07/17/leonidas-h-berry-and-the-fight-to-desegregate-medicine/

July 17, 2018 • Archives & Manuscripts, Exhibitions

ABIGAIL PORTER

The National Library of Medicine (NLM) announces new public access to more than 1,600 materials selected and digitized from the Leonidas H. Berry Papers, 1907–1982 manuscript collection including letters, photographs, and ephemera documenting the career and personal life of the trailblazing physician and civil rights advocate. His work is recognized in the NLM traveling banner exhibition For All the People: A Century in Citizen Action in Health Care Reform*; the online adaptation of the exhibition features 1,686 digitized items in a digital gallery. Stay tuned this week as* Circulating Now *features materials from the collection in honor of what would be Dr. Berry's 116th birthday—July 16, 2018.*

• • •

When Leonidas H. Berry (1902–1995) graduated from Rush Medical College in 1929, racial segregation was a harsh and codified reality in

America. Along with racially segregated schools, restaurants, and buses, medicine was subject to an enforced racial order and characterized by a vast inequality. Medical practices and clinics were segregated by race, few medical schools admitted Black students, and many hospitals would not hire Black doctors or admit Black patients.

Many of Dr. Berry's papers housed at the National Library of Medicine lay bare the contours of this system of segregated and unequal healthcare in America in the mid twentieth century. This blog showcases four items that highlight Dr. Berry's multi-pronged, vigorous efforts to fight discrimination in medicine, as well as the impact of racial bias on his career and outlook.

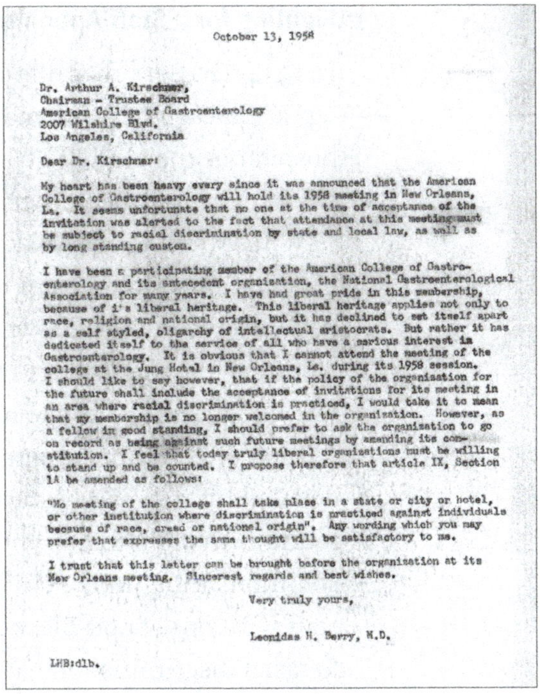

October 13, 1958

Dr. Arthur A. Kirschner,
Chairman - Trustee Board
American College of Gastroenterology
2007 Wilshire Blvd.
Los Angeles, California

Dear Dr. Kirschner:

My heart has been heavy every since it was announced that the American College of Gastroenterology will hold its 1958 meeting in New Orleans, La. It seems unfortunate that no one at the time of acceptance of the invitation was alerted to the fact that attendance at this meeting must be subject to racial discrimination by state and local law, as well as by long standing custom.

I have been a participating member of the American College of Gastroenterology and its antecedent organization, the National Gastroenterological Association for many years. I have had great pride in this membership, because of i's liberal heritage. This liberal heritage applies not only to race, religion and national origin, but it has declined to set itself apart as a self styled, oligarchy of intellectual aristocrats. But rather it has dedicated itself to the service of all who have a serious interest in Gastroenterology. It is obvious that I cannot attend the meeting of the college at the Jung Hotel in New Orleans, La. during its 1958 session. I should like to say however, that if the policy of the organisation for the future shall include the acceptance of invitations for its meeting in an area where racial discrimination is practiced, I would take it to mean that my membership is no longer welcomed in the organization. However, as a fellow in good standing, I should prefer to ask the organization to go on record as being against such future meetings by amending its constitution. I feel that today truly liberal organizations must be willing to stand up and be counted. I propose therefore that article IX, Section 1A be amended as follows:

"No meeting of the college shall take place in a state or city or hotel, or other institution where discrimination is practiced against individuals because of race, creed or national origin". Any wording which you may prefer that expresses the same thought will be satisfactory to me.

I trust that this letter can be brought before the organisation at its New Orleans meeting. Sincerest regards and best wishes.

Very truly yours,

Leonidas H. Berry, M.D.

LHB:dlb.

Letter from Dr. Berry objecting to a medical society meeting being held in segregated New Orleans, 1958 • "I feel that today, truly liberal institutions must be willing to stand up and be counted." • *Leonidas H. Berry Papers, National Library of Medicine MS C 423*

1958: A Meeting in Segregated New Orleans

In 1954, in a landmark ruling, the U.S. Supreme Court unanimously ruled that racial segregation of children in public accommodations was unconstitutional, and that "separate-but-equal" education and services were not equal at all. The ruling was a key turning point in the Civil Rights Movement.

In many southern states, however, the ruling was met with stiff resistance. When the American College of Gastroenterology scheduled its 1958 annual meeting in New Orleans, Dr. Berry concluded he would not be able to attend due to continued racial discrimination there and "long standing custom."

In a letter to the society's chairman, Berry objected to the choice of a meeting location where racial segregation continued to be practiced. He asked that the organization go on record against segregation, pointing out that organizations "must be willing to stand up and be counted." Berry's willingness to speak out against discrimination was a hallmark of his life.

Fighting for a Staff Appointment

In 1934, Dr. Berry became a junior attending physician in gastroenterology at Chicago's Provident Hospital, the first Black-owned and -operated hospital in the United States. A year later he became chairman of the Division of Gastroenterology, a position he held for thirty-five years.

While working at Provident, Berry also joined Chicago's Michael Reese Hospital in 1946, becoming the first Black physician to do so. For the next seventeen years, however, Berry fought to advance from a limited "courtesy" appointment to the attending staff, being told repeatedly he was not qualified, despite being known worldwide in his field.

In a letter of appeal sent to a Michael Reese official in 1960, Berry detailed his extensive career accomplishments and his concern that he found himself still confined to the "fringes." Berry's experience was common at the time. Few Black physicians were named to permanent staff positions at non-Black hospitals well into the twentieth century due to racial discrimination.

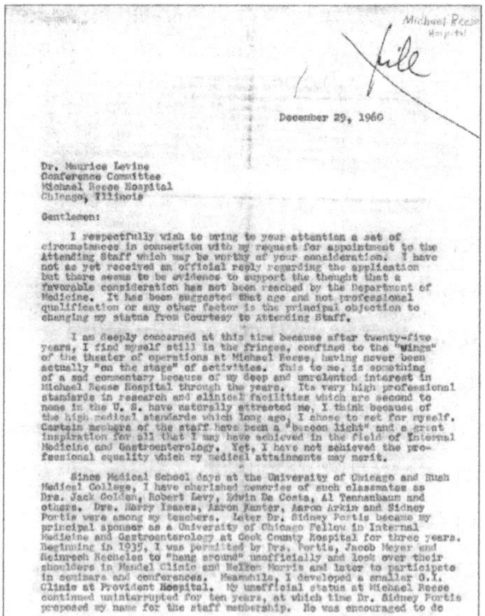

Michael Reese Hospital

File

December 29, 1960

Dr. Maurice Levine
Conference Committee
Michael Reese Hospital
Chicago, Illinois

Gentlemen:

I respectfully wish to bring to your attention a set of circumstances in connection with my request for appointment to the Attending Staff which may be worthy of your consideration. I have not as yet received an official reply regarding the application but there seems to be evidence to support the thought that a favorable consideration has not been reached by the Department of Medicine. It has been suggested that age and not professional qualification or any other factor is the principal objection to changing my status from Courtesy to Attending Staff.

I am deeply concerned at this time because after twenty-five years, I find myself still in the fringes, confined to the "wings" of the theater of operations at Michael Reese, having never been actually "on the stage" of activities. This to me, is something of a sad commentary because of my deep and unrelented interest in Michael Reese Hospital through the years. Its very high professional standards in research and clinical facilities which are second to none in the U. S. have naturally attracted me, I think because of the high medical standards which long ago, I chose to set for myself. Certain members of the staff have been a "beacon light" and a great inspiration for all that I may have achieved in the field of Internal Medicine and Gastroenterology. Yet, I have not achieved the professional equality which my medical attainments may merit.

Since Medical School days at the University of Chicago and Rush Medical College, I have cherished memories of such classmates as Drs. Jack Golden, Robert Levy, Edwin De Costa, Al Tennenbaum and others. Drs. Harry Isaacs, Aaron Kanter, Aaron Arkin and Sidney Portis were among my teachers. Later Dr. Sidney Portis became my principal sponser as a University of Chicago Fellow in Internal Medicine and Gastroenterology at Cook County Hospital for three years. Beginning in 1935, I was permitted by Drs. Portis, Jacob Meyer and Heinreich Necheles to "hang around" unofficially and look over their shoulders in Mandel Clinic and Nelson Morris and later to participate in seminars and conferences. Meanwhile, I developed a smaller G.I. Clinic at Provident Hospital. My unofficial status at Michael Reese continued uninterrupted for ten years, at which time Dr. Sidney Portis proposed my name for the staff membership. He was encouraged to do

Letter from Dr. Berry appealing his denial of an appointment to the attending staff at a hospital, 1960 • ". . . after twenty-five years, I find myself still in the fringes . . . confined to the 'wings'. . . " • *Leonidas H. Berry Papers, National Library of Medicine MS C 423*

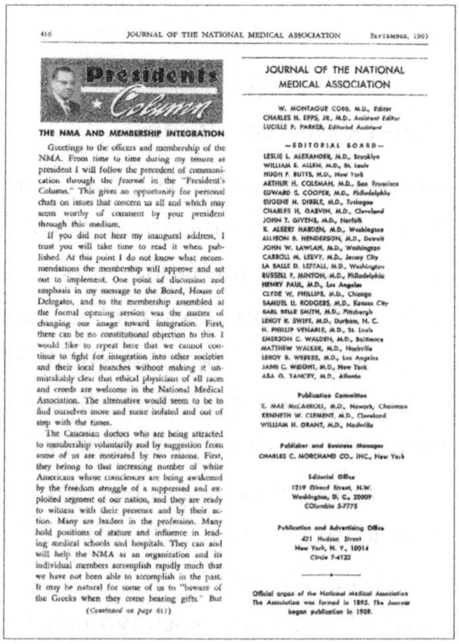

416 JOURNAL OF THE NATIONAL MEDICAL ASSOCIATION September, 1965

THE NMA AND MEMBERSHIP INTEGRATION

Greetings to the officers and membership of the NMA. From time to time during my tenure as president I will follow the precedent of communication through the *Journal* in the "President's Column." This gives an opportunity for personal chats on issues that concern us all and which may seem worthy of comment by your president through this medium.

If you did not hear my inaugural address, I trust you will take time to read it when published. At this point I do not know what recommendations the membership will approve and set out to implement. One point of discussion and emphasis in my message to the Board, House of Delegates, and to the membership assembled at the formal opening session was the matter of changing our image toward integration. First, there can be no constitutional objection to this. I would like to repeat here that we cannot continue to fight for integration into other societies and their local branches without making it unmistakably clear that ethical physicians of all races and creeds are welcome in the National Medical Association. The alternative would seem to be to find ourselves more and more isolated and out of step with the times.

The Caucasian doctors who are being attracted to membership voluntarily and by suggestion from some of us are motivated by two reasons. First, they belong to that increasing number of white Americans whose consciences are being awakened by the freedom struggle of a suppressed and exploited segment of our nation, and they are ready to witness with their presence and by their action. Many are leaders in the profession. Many hold positions of stature and influence in leading medical schools and hospitals. They can and will help the NMA as an organization and its individual members accomplish rapidly much that we have not been able to accomplish in the past. It may be natural for some of us to "beware of the Greeks when they come bearing gifts." But

(*Continued on page 417*)

JOURNAL OF THE NATIONAL MEDICAL ASSOCIATION

W. MONTAGUE COBB, M.D., *Editor*
CHARLES H. EPPS, JR., M.D., *Assistant Editor*
LUCILLE P. PARKER, *Editorial Assistant*

—EDITORIAL BOARD—
LESLIE L. ALEXANDER, M.D., Brooklyn
WILLIAM E. ALLEN, M.D., St. Louis
HUGH P. BUTTS, M.D., New York
ARTHUR H. COLEMAN, M.D., San Francisco
EDWARD S. COOPER, M.D., Philadelphia
EUGENE H. DIBBLE, M.D., Tuskegee
CHARLES H. GARVIN, M.D., Cleveland
JOHN T. GIVENS, M.D., Norfolk
K. ALBERT HARDEN, M.D., Washington
ALLISON B. HENDERSON, M.D., Detroit
JOHN W. LAWLAH, M.D., Washington
CARROLL M. LEEVY, M.D., Jersey City
LA SALLE D. LEFFALL, M.D., Washington
RUSSELL F. MINTON, M.D., Philadelphia
HENRY PAUL, M.D., Los Angeles
CLYDE W. PHILLIPS, M.D., Chicago
SAMUEL U. RODGERS, M.D., Kansas City
EARL BELLE SMITH, M.D., Pittsburgh
LEROY R. SWIFT, M.D., Durham, N. C.
H. PHILLIP VENABLE, M.D., St. Louis
EMERSON C. WALDEN, M.D., Baltimore
MATTHEW WALKER, M.D., Nashville
LEROY R. WEEKES, M.D., Los Angeles
JANE C. WRIGHT, M.D., New York
ASA G. YANCEY, M.D., Atlanta

Publication Committee
E. MAE McCARROLL, M.D., Newark, *Chairman*
KENNETH W. CLEMENT, M.D., Cleveland
WILLIAM H. GRANT, M.D., Nashville

Publisher and Business Manager
CHARLES C. MORCHAND CO., INC., New York

Editorial Office
1219 Girard Street, N.W.
Washington, D. C., 20009
COlumbia 5-7775

Publication and Advertising Office
421 Hudson Street
New York, N. Y., 10014
Circle 7-4122

Official organ of the National Medical Association
The Association was formed in 1895. The *Journal* began publication in 1909.

Dr. Berry's column on the importance of integrating the National Medical Association, 1965 • *Leonidas H. Berry Papers, National Library of Medicine MS C 423*

Integrating the National Medical Association

In 1965, Berry became president of the National Medical Association (NMA). African American doctors, excluded by race from the American Medical Association (AMA), established the NMA in 1895 to fight discrimination in medical societies, as well as medical schools and hospitals. Berry had been a member for thirty years.

When the NMA was formed, White physicians were excluded. During his NMA presidency, Berry launched an ambitious program to integrate the NMA, convinced that it was needed to be effective and "in step with the times." In the 1960s, constituent member societies of the AMA, particularly in the South, continued to deny African American doctors membership.

Berry appointed a special NMA committee to solicit membership of outstanding White doctors. In 1966, Berry proudly reported that 100 White doctors from places like Yale, Harvard, and Columbia had joined the NMA. The AMA finally agreed to end its practice of racial exclusion of members in 1968.

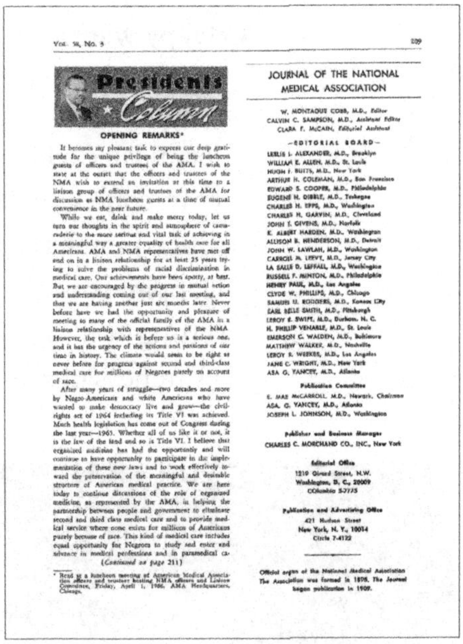

VOL. 58, NO. 3

209

Presidents Column

OPENING REMARKS*

It becomes my pleasant task to express our deep gratitude for the unique privilege of being the luncheon guests of officers and trustees of the AMA. I wish to state at the outset that the officers and trustees of the NMA wish to extend an invitation at this time to a liaison group of officers and trustees of the AMA for discussion as NMA luncheon guests at a time of mutual convenience in the near future.

While we eat, drink and make merry today, let us turn our thoughts in the spirit and atmosphere of camaraderie to the more serious and vital task of achieving in a meaningful way a greater equality of health care for all Americans. AMA and NMA representatives have met off and on in a liaison relationship for at least 25 years trying to solve the problems of racial discrimination in medical care. Our achievements have been spotty, at best. But we are encouraged by the progress in mutual action and understanding coming out of our last meeting, and that we are having another just six months later. Never before have we had the opportunity and pleasure of meeting so many of the official family of the AMA in a liaison relationship with representatives of the NMA. However, the task which is before us is a serious one, and it has the urgency of the actions and passions of our time in history. The climate would seem to be right as never before for progress against second and third-class medical care for millions of Negroes purely on account of race.

After many years of struggle—two decades and more by Negro-Americans and white Americans who have wanted to make democracy live and grow—the civil-rights act of 1964 including its Title VI was achieved. Much health legislation has come out of Congress during the last year—1965. Whether all of us like it or not, it is the law of the land and so is Title VI. I believe that organized medicine has had the opportuntiy and will continue to have opportunity to participate in the implementation of these new laws and to work effectively toward the preservation of the meaningful and desirable structure of American medical practice. We are here today to continue discussions of the role of organized medicine, as represented by the AMA, in helping the partnership between people and government to eliminate second and third class medical care and to provide medical service where none exists for millions of Americans purely because of race. This kind of medical care includes equal opportunity for Negroes to study and enter and advance in medical professions and in paramedical ca-

(Continued on page 211)

* Read at a luncheon meeting of American Medical Association officers and trustees hosting NMA officers and Liaison Committee, Friday, April 1, 1966, AMA Headquarters, Chicago.

JOURNAL OF THE NATIONAL MEDICAL ASSOCIATION

W. MONTAGUE COBB, M.D., *Editor*
CALVIN C. SAMPSON, M.D., *Assistant Editor*
CLARA F. McCAIN, *Editorial Assistant*

—EDITORIAL BOARD—

LESLIE L. ALEXANDER, M.D., Brooklyn
WILLIAM E. ALLEN, M.D., St. Louis
HUGH F. BUTTS, M.D., New York
ARTHUR H. COLEMAN, M.D., San Francisco
EDWARD S. COOPER, M.D., Philadelphia
EUGENE H. DIBBLE, M.D., Tuskegee
CHARLES H. EPPS, M.D., Washington
CHARLES H. GARVIN, M.D., Cleveland
JOHN I. GIVENS, M.D., Norfolk
K. ALBERT HARDEN, M.D., Washington
ALLISON B. HENDERSON, M.D., Detroit
JOHN W. LAWLAH, M.D., Washington
CARROLL M. LEEVY, M.D., Jersey City
LA SALLE D. LEFFALL, M.D., Washington
RUSSELL F. MINTON, M.D., Philadelphia
HENRY PAUL, M.D., Los Angeles
CLYDE W. PHILLIPS, M.D., Chicago
SAMUEL U. RODGERS, M.D., Kansas City
EARL BELLE SMITH, M.D., Pittsburgh
LEROY R. SWIFT, M.D., Durham, N. C.
H. PHILLIP VENABLE, M.D., St. Louis
EMERSON C. WALDEN, M.D., Baltimore
MATTHEW WALKER, M.D., Nashville
LEROY R. WEEKES, M.D., Los Angeles
JANE C. WRIGHT, M.D., New York
ASA G. YANCEY, M.D., Atlanta

Publication Committee

E. MAE McCARROLL, M.D., Newark, *Chairman*
ASA G. YANCEY, M.D., Atlanta
JOSEPH L. JOHNSON, M.D., Washington

Publisher and Business Manager
CHARLES C. MORCHAND CO., INC., New York

Editorial Office
1219 Girard Street, N.W.
Washington, D. C., 20009
COlumbia 5-7775

Publication and Advertising Office
421 Hudson Street
New York, N. Y., 10014
Circle 7-4122

Official organ of the National Medical Association. The Association was formed in 1895. The Journal began publication in 1909.

Dr. Berry's remarks about ending racial discrimination in medicine, 1966 • "making it unmistakably clear that ethical physicians of all races and creeds are welcome in the National Medicine Association" • *Leonidas H. Berry Papers, National Library of Medicine MS C 423*

Pressing the Medical Profession to End Discrimination

When Berry became NMA president in 1965, significant social and political change was occurring nationwide. In 1964, Congress passed the landmark Civil Rights Act. A year later, Congress approved Medicare.

Berry, along with civil rights leaders, believed these new laws would be crucial tools for ending racial discrimination in hospitals and medicine. Berry reinvigorated a joint NMA-AMA "Liaison Committee" to push for an end to discrimination in medicine. Mindful that the AMA had officially opposed Medicare's passage, Berry publicly declared that the AMA had a "moral obligation" to aggressively lead the way in implementing the new laws.

In addition to exhorting the AMA to deliver healthcare equality, Berry met and corresponded with federal officials responsible for assessing any continued discrimination in medical facilities receiving federal funds. As Berry noted in correspondence, "We will serve as a national force to implement the law with justice at the local level."

A Happy Warrior

> Happiness is unremitting zeal to achieve and faith to overcome formidable odds. Happiness is outwitting your adversary when you have done it with honesty and fairness. Happiness is measuring your triumph attained by sharpened intellect and hard-earned skills. Happiness is standing alone by the sea and watching a beautiful setting sun cast the lengthening shadow of a man and having the awareness of self-identity.
>
> —Leonidas H. Berry, 1971

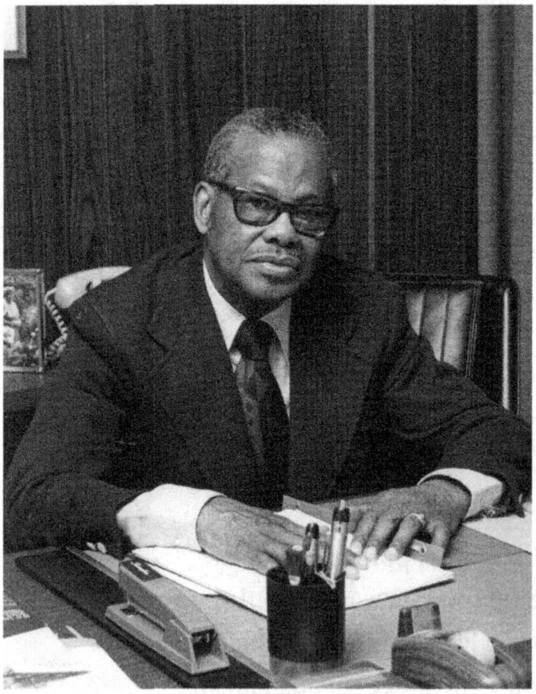

Leonard H. Berry, MD, prominent physician and president of the National Medical Association 1965–66, was a leader of campaigns against racial discrimination in hospitals. • "Happiness is unremitting zeal to achieve and faith to overcome formidable odds . . . " —Leonidas H. Berry, 1971 • *Leonidas H. Berry Papers, National Library of Medicine MS C 423*

Bound by a belief that doctors must participate in civic affairs in a democratic society, Berry deeply engaged in fighting the institutionalized racism that marked America during his lifetime. Skillfully and tirelessly, he pressed the medical profession and government leaders to extend to all "the necessities of life in reasonable and just proportions."

In some instances, Berry's papers hint at the toll his activism took, with him noting he was "battled-scared and weary" and regretful that he would never see "the sunlit vistas of the mountaintop."

In a 1971 dinner speech, Berry pondered, at age sixty-nine, whether he should be bitter for the discrimination that "beset the ambitions of his youth and up to the present day." Instead, he stated he preferred to label himself a "Happy Warrior," declaring that happiness comes from having a goal in life and aiming for the stars.

Berry's papers housed at the National Library of Medicine tell a compelling story of how much he did, in fact, accomplish in life both himself and for others.

Reflection

In 2017, a colleague and I at the National Library of Medicine were tasked with processing items from the Leonidas H. Berry Papers to make them publicly accessible in a digital gallery. We quickly learned that such work on a large scale can be slow and demanding. The work was estimated to take a few months. Instead it took a year.

Looking back, it is clear that this slow, day-by-day work is representative of what it can take for archival collections to come to light and yield gems. As we examined Berry's letters, speeches, and memos, a picture of a man and his actions, spirit, and passions emerged. He was a caring physician and mentor, but also a fierce civil rights advocate. In 2020, when Black Lives Matter protests broke out in the United States, I found myself remembering Berry's exhortation from a 1966 speech: "Let us turn our thoughts . . . to the serious and vital task of achieving in a meaningful way greater equality of care for all Americans."

After my immersion in this project, my colleague and I both reflected that we wished we could have met Berry. In a way, working with this collection, we did. Writing a blog post after completing the project was a rewarding way to dive deep into several documents and the stories they tell. The Library is fortunate to have this collection in its holdings. It lays bare aspects of medicine, public health, and civil rights in America that are significant and still reverberating. —Abigail Porter, 2023

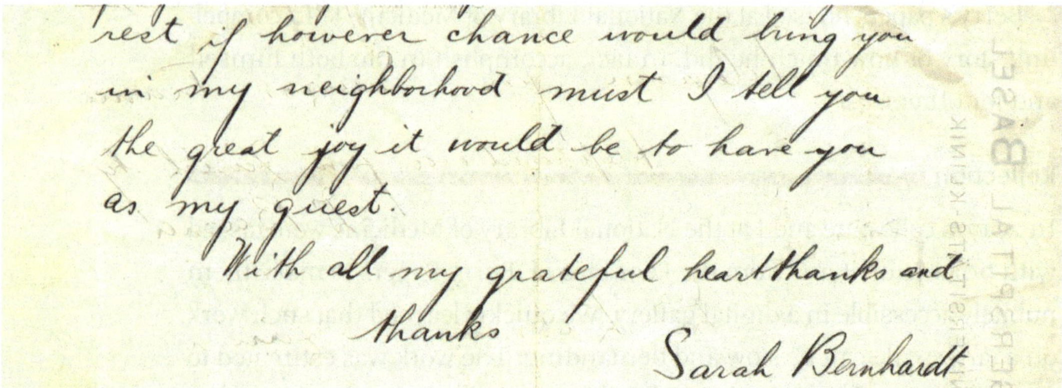
rest if however chance would bring you
in my neighborhood must I tell you
the great joy it would be to have you
as my guest.
With all my grateful heartthanks and
thanks
Sarah Bernhardt

THE DIVINE SARAH AND HER DIVINE DOCTOR

https://circulatingnow.nlm.nih.gov/2014/04/17/the-divine-sarah-and-her-divine-doctor/

April 17, 2014 • Archives & Manuscripts, Guests

ROBERT GOTTLIEB

Circulating Now *welcomes guest blogger Robert Gottlieb. Robert is a writer and editor, and the author of* Sarah: The Life of Sarah Bernhardt*;* George Balanchine: The Ballet Maker*;* Great Expectations: The Sons and Daughters of Charles Dickens*; and* Lives and Letters. *From 1987 to 1992 he was the editor of* The New Yorker. *Before that, he served as editor-in-chief of Simon & Schuster and Alfred A. Knopf, and he has edited some of the most significant books of the twentieth century, from* Catch-22 *to Toni Morrison's* Beloved *to Bill Clinton's autobiography.*

• • •

When I was working on my biography of the great French stage actress Sarah Bernhardt (1844–1923) several years ago, I was startled to find on the web a series of headlined stories in the *New York Times* charting her progress as she struggled to recover from the severe case of uremia that had landed her in New York's Mt. Sinai hospital:

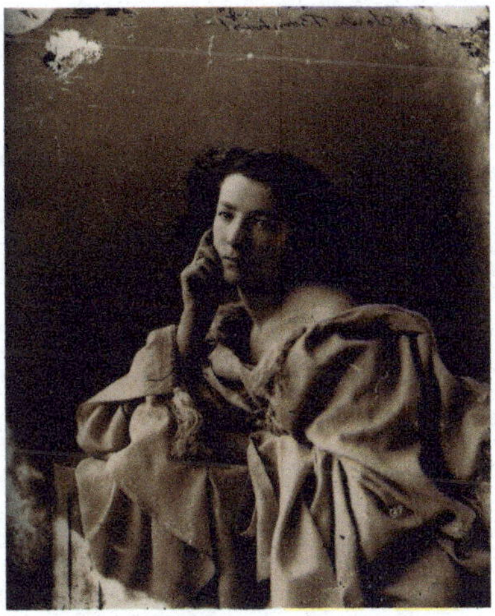

Actress Sarah Bernhardt at the height of her fame • *Wikimedia Commons*

> April 17, 1917: SARAH BERNHARDT MAY GO UNDER KNIFE
>
> April 18: SARAH BERNHARDT IS OPERATED ON—SURGEONS RESORT TO ONLY HOPE OF SAVING LIFE OF ACTRESS SUFFERING FROM INFECTED KIDNEY—RESTS EASILY AFTERWARDS
>
> April 20: MME. BERNHARDT BETTER—Actress's Marvelous Vitality Gives Hope of Her Recovery April 21: MME. BERNHARDT GAINS—Hope Now for Her Recovery—Queen Alexandra Sends Message

And so on, until April 28th, by which time she's clearly out of danger. It's the kind of coverage only a president or a pope would receive. But then she was more famous—and was famous longer—than mere presidents and popes.

Now, from the historical collections of the National Library of Medicine, comes a clutch of notes and telegrams and hospital records from and about Sarah, and we learn that on April 17th, her temperature went up to 103°F and that during the operation "six ounces of foul smelling pus obtained. Large irregular calculus in the pelvis, which was removed." Sarah exaggerated about a lot of things (*most* things?) but not about the seriousness of her medical condition.

Equally fascinating is the series of notes and telegrams she dashed off during the ensuing years to her doctor of choice, the famous Emanuel Libman (1872–1946). Whenever she was in danger, or thought she was, she bombarded him with accounts of her condition and pleas that he rush to her side. "I know that you are resting from your great work and great devouement [devotion]. I am very ill in great need of your diagnosting [sic]. I will respect your rest if however chance would bring you in my neighborhood must I tell you of the great joy it would be to have you as my guest. With all my grateful heart and thanks." A mistake-ridden telegram from her vacation home off the coast of Brittany:

> OH MY DEAR Y HAVE GREAT TROUBLE IMPOSSIBLE TO TAKE BOT [sic] NORD BECAUSE THE SEA IS EURIOUS [sic] Y HOPE TO MORROW THAT SHALL BE POSSIBLE ALL MY LOVE.

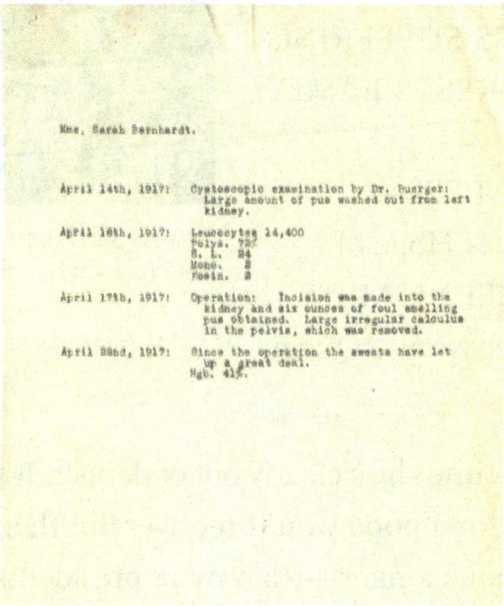

Mme. Sarah Bernhardt.

April 14th, 1917: Cystoscopic examination by Dr. Buerger: Large amount of pus washed out from left kidney.

April 16th, 1917: Leucocytes 14,400
Polys. 72%
S. L. 24
Mono. 2
Eosin. 2

April 17th, 1917: Operation: Incision was made into the kidney and six ounces of foul smelling pus obtained. Large irregular calculus in the pelvis, which was removed.

April 22nd, 1917: Since the operation the sweats have let up a great deal.
Hgb. 41%.

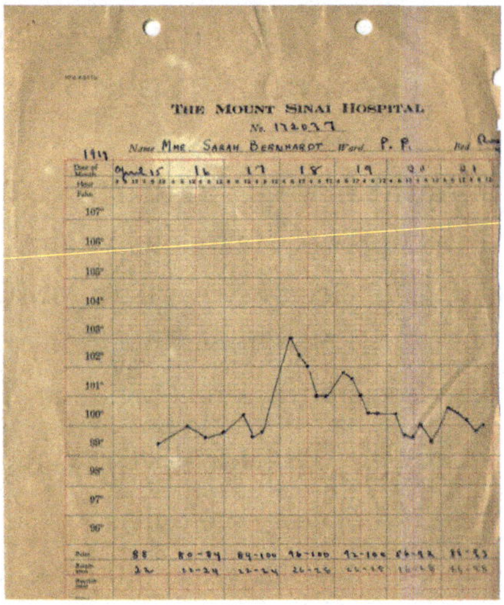

LEFT TO RIGHT (1) Page from Sarah Bernhardt's medical records • *Emanuel Libman Papers, National Library of Medicine MS C 406* **(2)** Sarah Bernhardt's medical chart • *Emanuel Libman Papers, National Library of Medicine MS C 406*

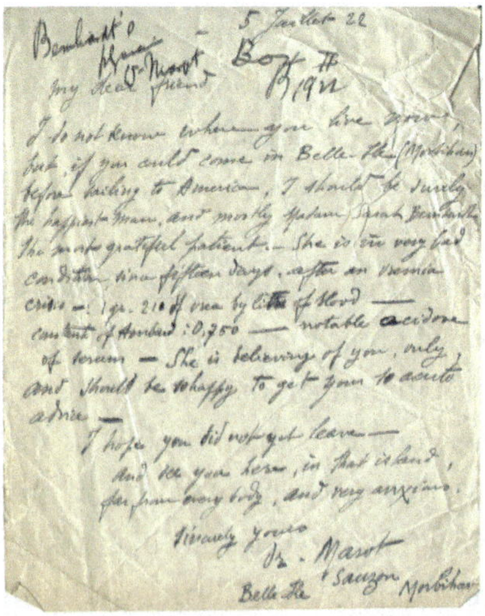

5 Juillet 22

Bernhardt's [illegible] Dr. Marot Box # B 1922

My dear friend

I do not know where you live now, but if you could come in Belle Ile (Morbihan) before [illegible] to America, I should be surely the happiest man, and mostly Madame Sarah Bernhardt the most grateful patient.— She is in very bad condition since fifteen days, after an uremia crisis — [illegible] 2,10 of urea by litre of blood — content of [illegible] : 0,750 — notable acidosis of serum — She is believing of you, only and should be so happy to get your [illegible] advice —

I hope you did not yet leave — and see you here, in that island, far from every body, and very anxious.

Sincerely yours
Dr. Marot
Belle Ile Sauzon Morbihan

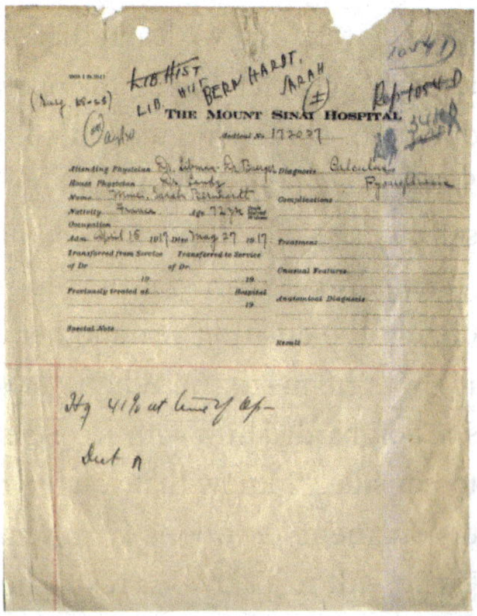

THE MOUNT SINAI HOSPITAL

Attending Physician Dr. Libman – Dr. Buerger
Name Mme. Sarah Bernhardt
Nativity France
Occupation
Adm. April 16 1917 Disc. May 27 1917
Diagnosis Calculus Pyonephrosis
Complications
Treatment
Transferred from Service
Transferred to Service
Unusual Features
Previously treated at
Anatomical Diagnosis
Special Notes
Result

Hg 41% at time of op—

LEFT TO RIGHT (1) Physician's letter to Dr. Libman about Sarah's case • *Emanuel Libman Papers, National Library of Medicine MS C 406* **(2)** Sarah Bernhardt's hospital records • *Emanuel Libman Papers, National Library of Medicine MS C 406*

If she wasn't demanding his presence, she was sending him Happy New Year telegrams. When Sarah wanted a man, or something from a man, she pulled out all the stops.

Fortunately, the doctor was equally devoted to her. Among the portraits of famous colleagues and patients that hung in his home, two stood out: one of Sarah, signed with a florid acknowledgment in French; and one of Albert Einstein, signed in German, "To the noble-minded Dr.

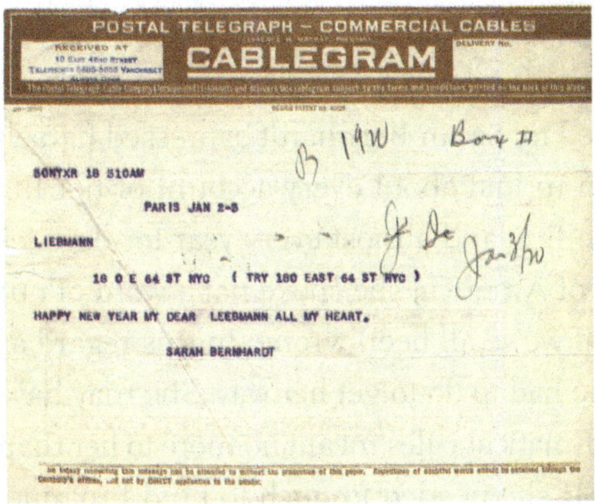
POSTAL TELEGRAPH – COMMERCIAL CABLES
CABLEGRAM
B 1920 Box II
8ONYXR 18 510AM
PARIS JAN 2-8
LIEBMANN
10 0 E 64 ST NYC (TRY 180 EAST 64 ST NYC)
HAPPY NEW YEAR MY DEAR LEEBMANN ALL MY HEART.
SARAH BERNHARDT

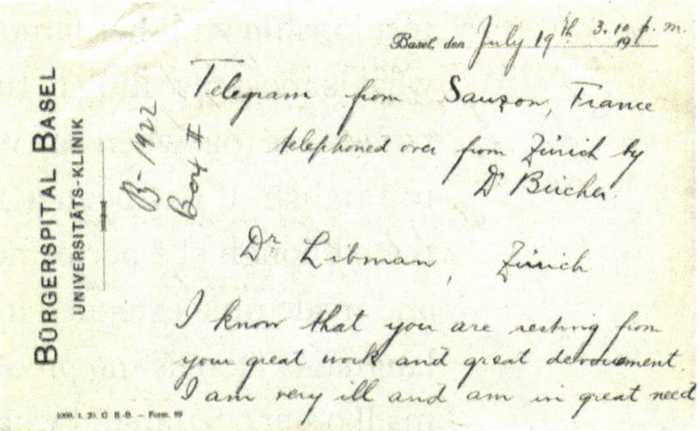
BÜRGERSPITAL BASEL
UNIVERSITÄTS-KLINIK
B-1922 Box II
Basel, den July 19th 3.10 p.m.
Telegram from Sauzon, France
telephoned over from Zürich by
Dr Büchi
Dr Libman, Zürich
I know that you are resting from
your great work and great devotement.
I am very ill and am in great need

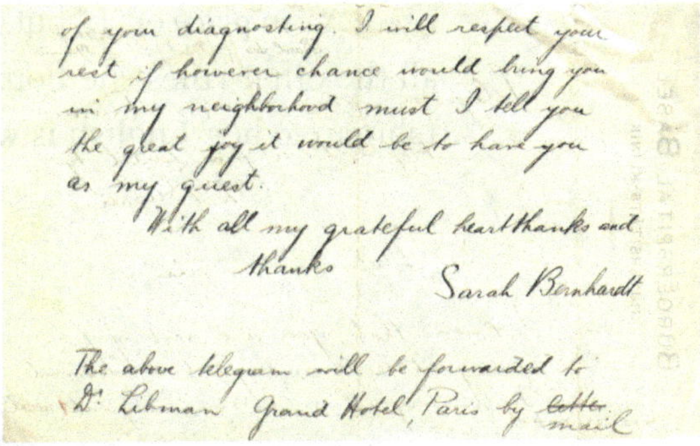
of your diagnosting. I will respect your
rest if however chance would bring you
in my neighborhood must I tell you
the great joy it would be to have you
as my guest.
With all my grateful heartthanks and
thanks
Sarah Bernhardt
The above telegram will be forwarded to
Dr Libman Grand Hotel, Paris by ~~letter~~ mail

ABOVE (1) A telegram from Sarah Bernhardt to Dr. Libman • *Emanuel Libman Papers, National Library of Medicine MS C 406* **TOP RIGHT (2)** A telegram from Sarah Bernhardt to Dr. Libman • *Emanuel Libman Papers, National Library of Medicine MS C 406* **BOTTOM RIGHT (3)** A telegram from Sarah Bernhardt to Dr. Libman • *Emanuel Libman Papers, National Library of Medicine MS C 406*

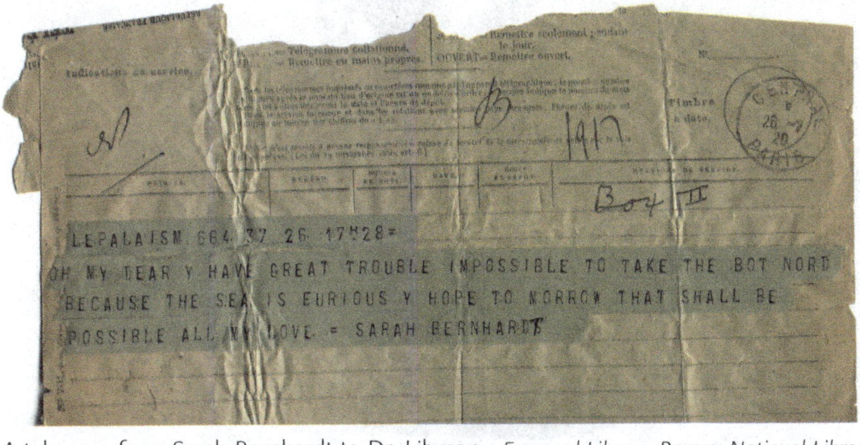
1917
Box II
LEPALAISM 664 37 26 17H28 =
OH MY DEAR Y HAVE GREAT TROUBLE IMPOSSIBLE TO TAKE THE BOT NORD
BECAUSE THE SEA IS FURIOUS Y HOPE TO MORROW THAT SHALL BE
POSSIBLE ALL MY LOVE = SARAH BERNHARDT

A telegram from Sarah Bernhardt to Dr. Libman • *Emanuel Libman Papers, National Library of Medicine MS C 406*

Libman with the secret-divining eyes." As someone with no knowledge of medical history, I was fascinated to learn about this amazing doctor, whose diagnostic powers were world-famous and who was not only on the cover of *Time* magazine in 1935 but was the subject of a fascinating profile in *The New Yorker* (April 9, 1939) by the famous playwright and biographer S.N. Behrman. Libman, it turns out, was as eccentric as he was brilliant. It's time for a biography.

But if it is the insights into Bernhardt's medical condition and her relationship with her famous doctor that are the focus of these papers, what is most revealing to the lay person—and, in particular, to the biographer—is that when she wanted to, Sarah Bernhardt expressed herself in English. It has been a given in just about every account of her life that although she performed in England almost every year for decades and made nine extended tours of America, she spoke not a word of our language. Here is the proof that we've all been wrong: in this regard as in all others, Sarah did what she had to do to get her way. She may have used "Y" in place of "I," but grammatical rules meant no more to her than all the other rules she flouted. If she needed English to bind Emanuel Libman to her, English is what she gave him.

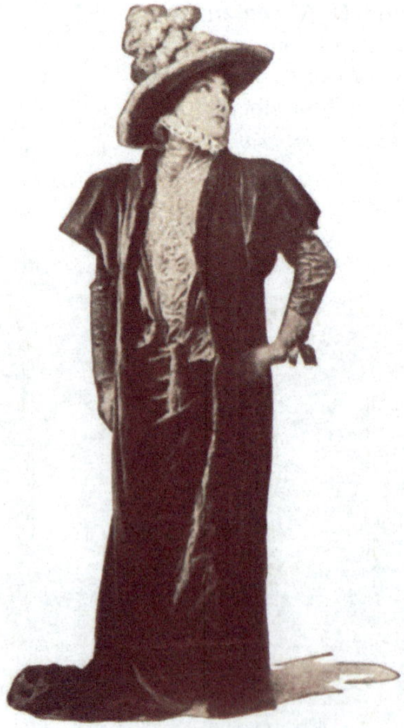

Mme. Sarah Bernhardt • *National Library of Medicine #101461518*

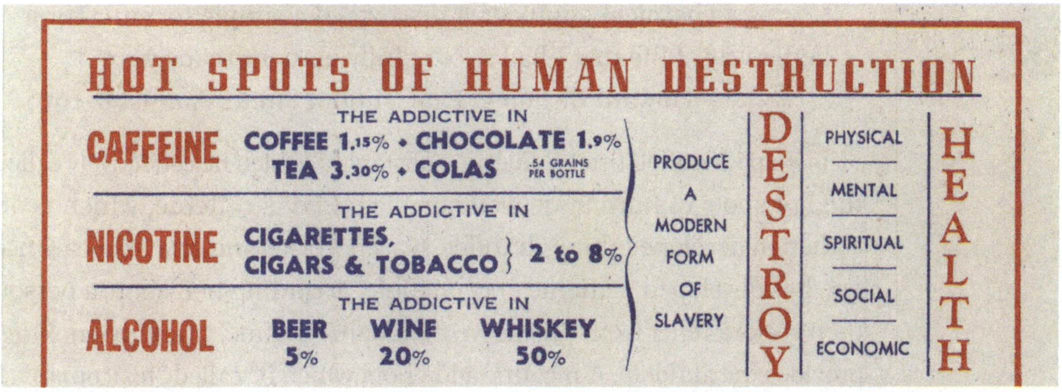

HOT SPOTS OF HUMAN DESTRUCTION: THE HOWARD BISHOP PAPERS

https://circulatingnow.nlm.nih.gov/2019/05/30/hot-spots-of-human-destruction-the-howard-bishop-papers/

May 30, 2019 • Archives & Manuscripts

JAMES LABOSIER

Howard Bishop was confident that he knew what was best for people and that people needed to be told. In the 1940s and 1950s, Bishop sent thousands of letters to celebrities, businessmen, politicians, companies of all sorts, and anyone else he identified in the act of encouraging unhealthy habits.

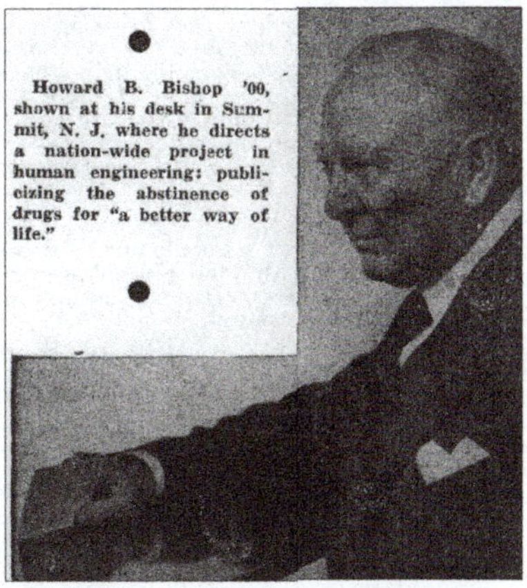

Howard Bishop, ca. 1945 • *Howard Bishop Papers, National Library of Medicine MS C 562*

From his own personal experience and training, Bishop had researched and lived the healthier lifestyle he encouraged. Born in 1878, (just over fifty years after the American Temperance Society was founded in 1826) Howard Berkey Bishop spent forty years as an analytical chemist, eventually owning the Sterling Products Company of Easton, Pennsylvania. He believed that three regularly ingested substances were most responsible for human ailments and premature death.

"... as a chemical engineer, I discovered a simple formula for a better way of life that I had successfully used for many years."
—Howard Bishop to Paul Clifford Smith, August 8, 1956

Bishop identified three addictive substances, which he collectively called the hot spots of human destruction. The first is caffeine, which is an addiction developed through coffee, tea, chocolate, and cola drinks. Once one has developed "caffeine encephalitis," according to Bishop, a person then seeks a relief from this nerve irritation. Nicotine, through smoking, provides the antidote. A nicotine addiction, which he called "toxicomania," then results, leaving people in a never-ending cycle of caffeine and nicotine. The addition of alcohol generally follows.

In 1939 he retired, sold his company, and a year later founded the Human Engineering Foundation. Through this non-profit institution he

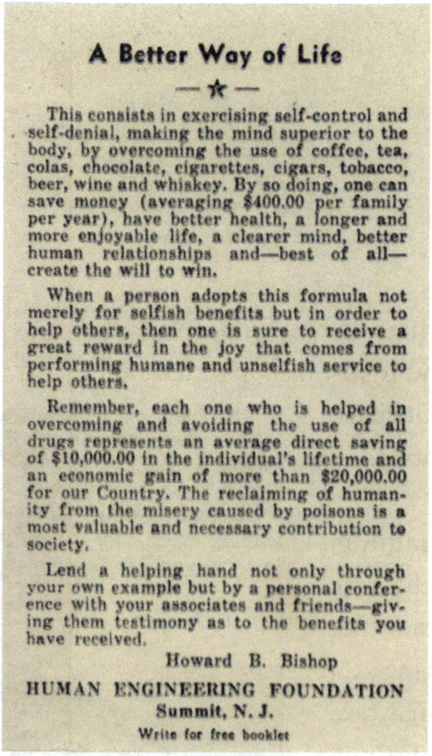

A Better Way of Life

—★—

This consists in exercising self-control and self-denial, making the mind superior to the body, by overcoming the use of coffee, tea, colas, chocolate, cigarettes, cigars, tobacco, beer, wine and whiskey. By so doing, one can save money (averaging $400.00 per family per year), have better health, a longer and more enjoyable life, a clearer mind, better human relationships and—best of all—create the will to win.

When a person adopts this formula not merely for selfish benefits but in order to help others, then one is sure to receive a great reward in the joy that comes from performing humane and unselfish service to help others.

Remember, each one who is helped in overcoming and avoiding the use of all drugs represents an average direct saving of $10,000.00 in the individual's lifetime and an economic gain of more than $20,000.00 for our Country. The reclaiming of humanity from the misery caused by poisons is a most valuable and necessary contribution to society.

Lend a helping hand not only through your own example but by a personal conference with your associates and friends—giving them testimony as to the benefits you have received.

Howard B. Bishop

HUMAN ENGINEERING FOUNDATION
Summit, N. J.
Write for free booklet

A Better Way of Life, ca. 1940 • Some of the literature Bishop usually enclosed with his letters • *Howard Bishop Papers, National Library of Medicine MS C 562*

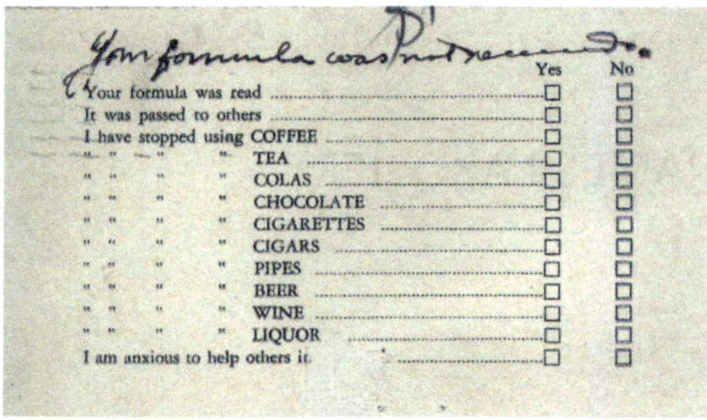

	Yes	No
Your formula was read	☐	☐
It was passed to others	☐	☐
I have stopped using COFFEE	☐	☐
" " " " TEA	☐	☐
" " " " COLAS	☐	☐
" " " " CHOCOLATE	☐	☐
" " " " CIGARETTES	☐	☐
" " " " CIGARS	☐	☐
" " " " PIPES	☐	☐
" " " " BEER	☐	☐
" " " " WINE	☐	☐
" " " " LIQUOR	☐	☐
I am anxious to help others it	☐	☐

Leaders in Business and Industry Survey, ca. 1945 • Some of the literature Bishop usually enclosed with his letters • *Howard Bishop Papers, National Library of Medicine MS C 562*

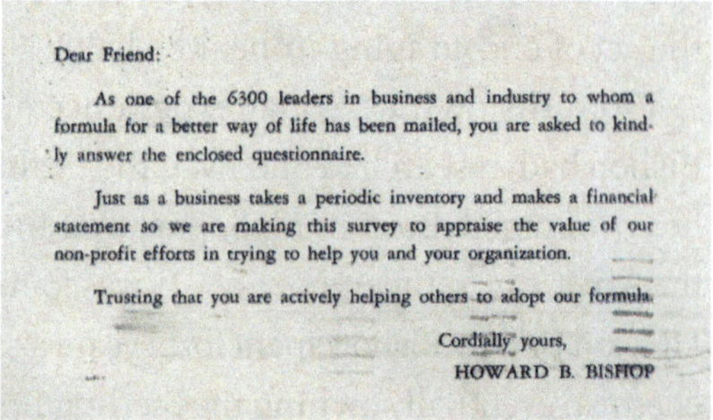

Dear Friend:

As one of the 6300 leaders in business and industry to whom a formula for a better way of life has been mailed, you are asked to kindly answer the enclosed questionnaire.

Just as a business takes a periodic inventory and makes a financial statement so we are making this survey to appraise the value of our non-profit efforts in trying to help you and your organization.

Trusting that you are actively helping others to adopt our formula.

Cordially yours,
HOWARD B. BISHOP

Leaders in Business and Industry Survey Card, ca. 1945 • Some of the literature Bishop usually enclosed with his letters • *Howard Bishop Papers, National Library of Medicine MS C 562*

devoted the remainder of his life to his cause, which resonates globally today in the World Health Organization's World No Tobacco Day.

> "... helping to save the lives of millions of people who are dying premature deaths on account of the habitual use of various addictives."
> —Howard Bishop to Alden Emery, January 22, 1952

The main problem with this effort was his style of persuasion. Perhaps it resulted from years of giving orders as head of his company or was just the way he personally communicated with everybody; whatever the case, his chosen method for informing and helping people was direct and blunt confrontation.

Bishop pored over newspapers and magazines for photographs and advertisements illustrating the use of the "hot spots of human destruction." Then he would write to the person or party responsible to inform them that they were hurting mankind.

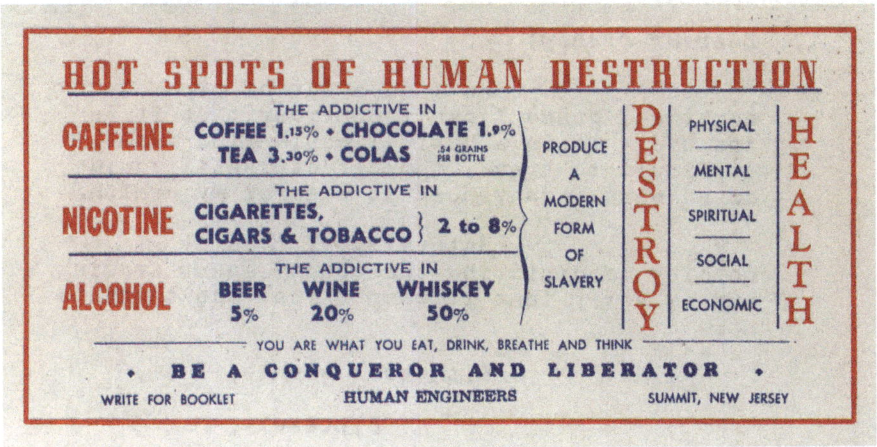

Hot Spots of Human Destruction, 1949 • Some of the literature that Bishop usually enclosed in his letters • *Howard Bishop Papers, National Library of Medicine MS C 562*

Celebrities and politicians were regular recipients. To Edward R. Murrow he said, "It has been on my mind for some time to write to you and tell you how ridiculous it appears for a famous man like yourself... to smoke a cigarette on every program . . . " Baseball commissioner Ford Frick was told that the " . . . cigarette smoking morons and others are naturally lead to believe that since those famous ballplayers smoke Chesterfield cigarettes it is quite the thing to do." Winston Churchill received the helpful advice that " . . . by overcoming the use of tobacco and all caffeine and alcoholic drinks, your mind will be clearer, your health will be better, you will live longer and enjoy life more." He was particularly aggrieved by advertising companies that showed incidental smoking in ads for other products. One particularly incendiary expression he used in letters to them was: "Josef Stalin must be well pleased with the enclosed advertisements that undermines and pollutes the life blood of our Nation."

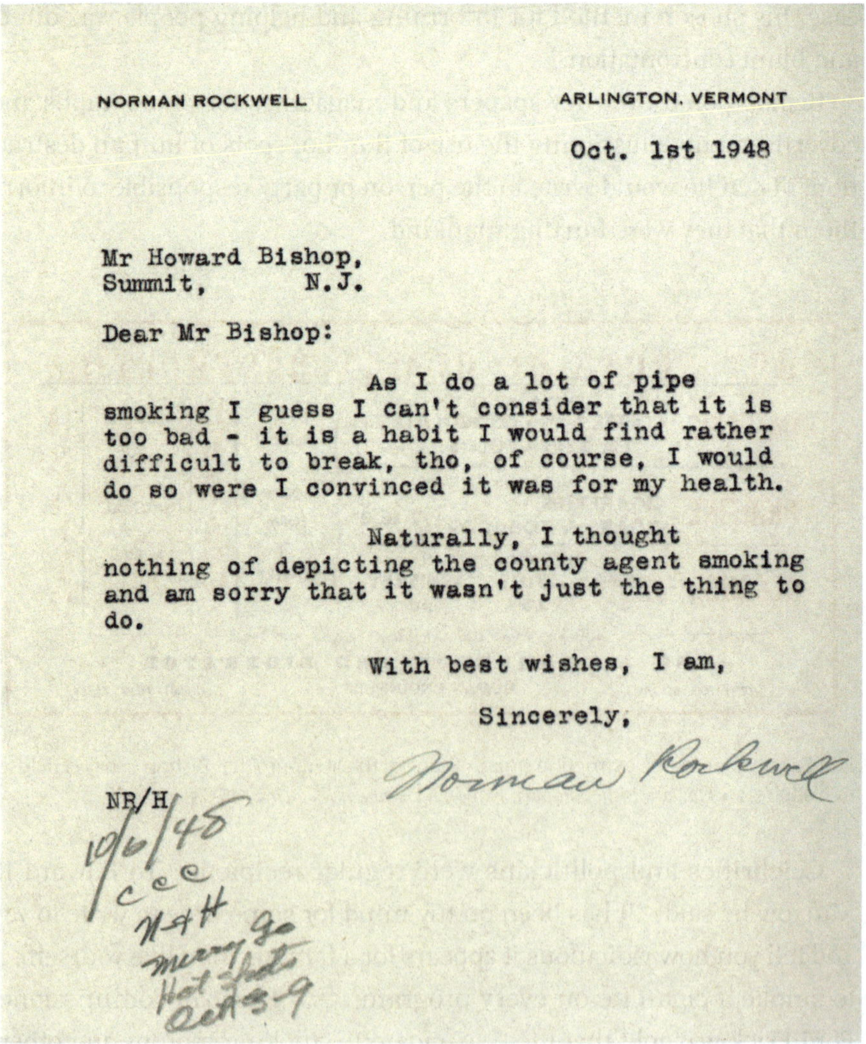

NORMAN ROCKWELL ARLINGTON, VERMONT

Oct. 1st 1948

Mr Howard Bishop,
Summit, N.J.

Dear Mr Bishop:

As I do a lot of pipe smoking I guess I can't consider that it is too bad - it is a habit I would find rather difficult to break, tho, of course, I would do so were I convinced it was for my health.

Naturally, I thought nothing of depicting the county agent smoking and am sorry that it wasn't just the thing to do.

With best wishes, I am,

Sincerely,

Norman Rockwell

NR/H

Letter from Norman Rockwell to Howard Bishop, October 1, 1948 • Norman Rockwell honestly defended his painting. • *Letter courtesy of the Norman Rockwell Family Agency, Howard Bishop Papers, National Library of Medicine MS C 562*

The correspondence in the Howard Bishop papers at the National Library of Medicine shows that, despite Bishop's tone-deaf style, many correspondents such as hotels and businesses asked for more of his literature and signage to distribute. Many of his letters, preserved as copies in the files, appear to have gone unanswered. A good number of

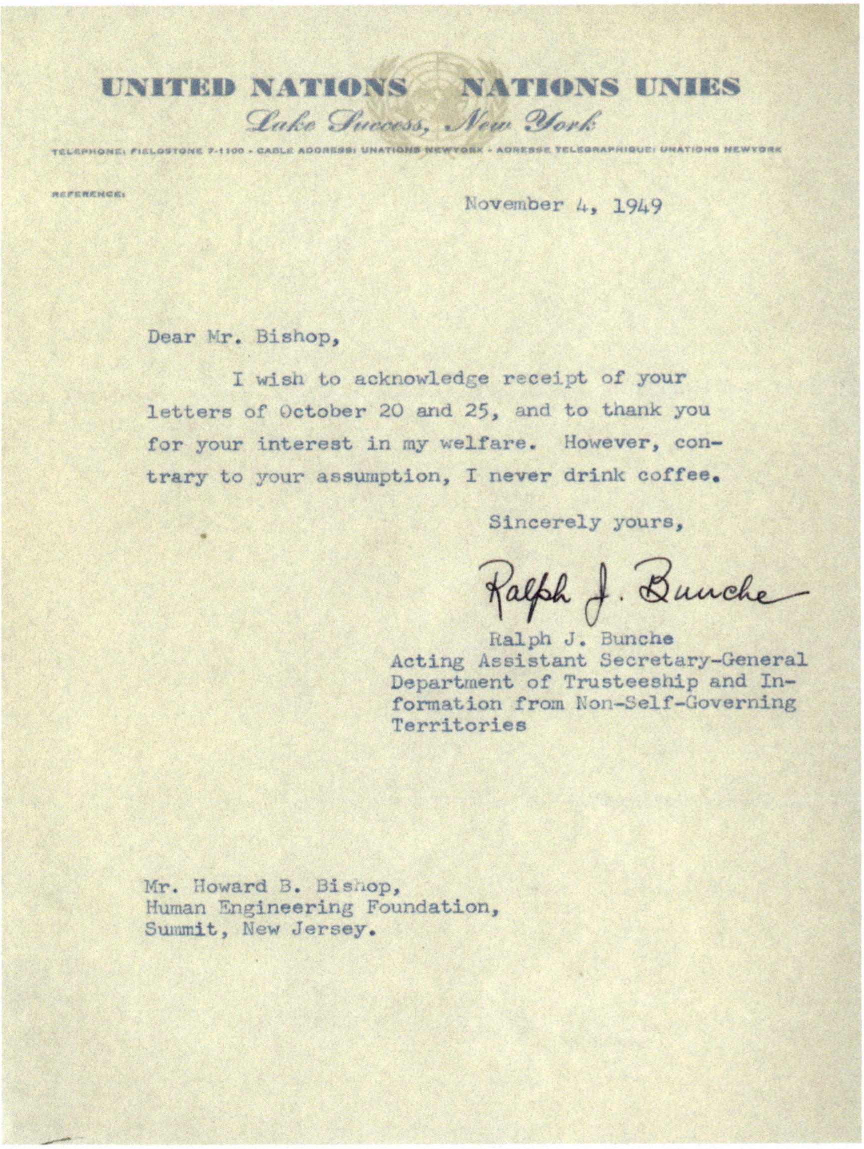

UNITED NATIONS NATIONS UNIES

Lake Success, New York

TELEPHONE: FIELDSTONE 7-1100 · CABLE ADDRESS: UNATIONS NEWYORK · ADRESSE TELEGRAPHIQUE: UNATIONS NEWYORK

REFERENCE:

November 4, 1949

Dear Mr. Bishop,

I wish to acknowledge receipt of your letters of October 20 and 25, and to thank you for your interest in my welfare. However, contrary to your assumption, I never drink coffee.

Sincerely yours,

Ralph J. Bunche

Ralph J. Bunche
Acting Assistant Secretary-General
Department of Trusteeship and Information from Non-Self-Governing Territories

Mr. Howard B. Bishop,
Human Engineering Foundation,
Summit, New Jersey.

Ralph J. Bunche: "I never drink coffee." • Bunche's response to Bishop is curiously worded. Bishop had written about a photograph of Bunche smoking and drinking coffee; Bunche denied only the coffee drinking. • *Howard Bishop Papers, National Library of Medicine MS C 562*

the negative replies fall into three categories: honest reactions to Bishop's style and purpose, indignation at his presumption, and outright ridicule.

•••

Learn more about Howard Bishop and explore the finding aid for the Howard B. Bishop Papers 1921–1961 in the History of Medicine Division at the National Library of Medicine.

CONTRIBUTOR BIOGRAPHIES: THEN & NOW

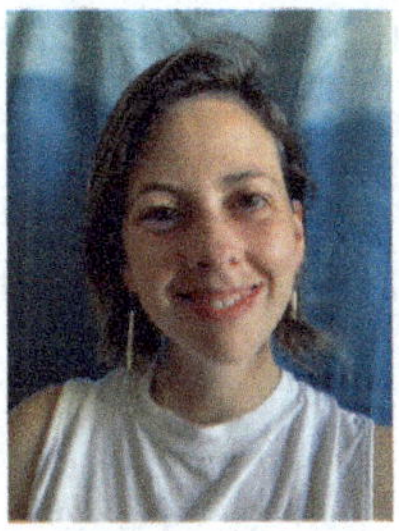

KATHERINE AKEY, MFA, authored "Hidden Faces of WWI: Maxillofacial Portraits Preserved" in 2018 when she was an artist living in Washington, DC, and working for the US WW1 Centennial Commission. Today, she lives in San Francisco, California, where she makes artwork about polar exploration, World War I, love, and memory. Her practice includes photography, printmaking, fiber arts, and creative writing. She holds her MFA from the International Center of Photography, was a Fellow with the Carnegie Council for Ethics in International Affairs, was the Visiting Assistant Professor in Studio Arts at Corcoran School of the Arts and Design at GWU from 2018–2020, and produced the WW1 Centennial News podcast for the US WW1 Centennial Commission from 2018–2020. Her work has been exhibited internationally, and she has participated in several artist residencies including The Arctic Circle, Bonfire Walk&Talk, and An Artist Residency in Motherhood.

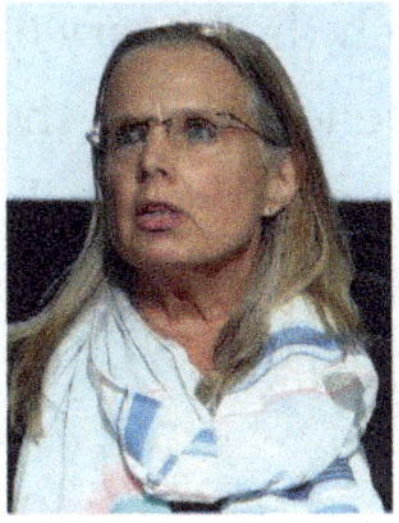

ANNE ARMSTRONG, JD, DLS, co-authored "Power to the People: Washington Gives Back" in 2016 with Jennifer Brier, Julie Kutruff, Erin Carlson Mast, and Patricia Tuohy, when she was deputy director of the National Guard Educational Foundation and director of the National Guard Memorial Museum, Archive, and Library. Today, she serves as the Chief Historian for the Defense Information Systems Agency in Ft. Meade, Maryland.

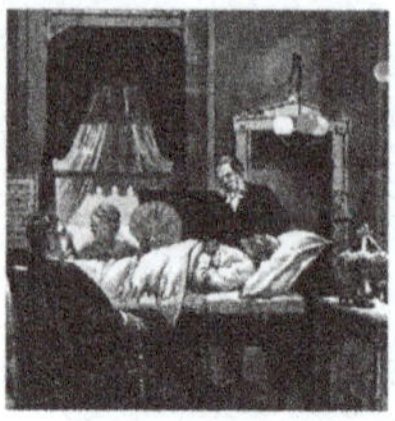

LENORE BARBIAN, PHD, co-authored "'The President Is Somewhat Restless...'" with Jeffrey S. Reznick in 2013 when she was Associate Professor and Anthropology Program Director at Edinboro University of Pennsylvania. Today, she is Professor of Anthropology at Pennsylvania Western University Edinboro. In addition, she serves as the head of the university's Honors Program and a fellow of the Institute for Forensic Sciences. She is currently part of a multidisciplinary team investigating the optimal presentation of forensic facial reconstructions in missing persons cases. She is author of numerous articles, including "Remains of War: Walt Whitman, Civil War Soldiers, and the Legacy of Medical Collections," co-authored with Jeffrey S. Reznick and Paul Sledzik, which received the 2013 best article award from the Archivists and Librarians in the History of the Health Sciences (ALHHS), now called Librarians, Archivists, and Museum Professionals in the History of the Health Sciences (LAMPHHS).

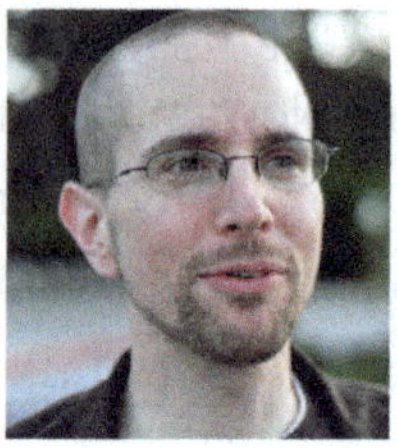

DAN BOUK, PHD, authored "Revealing Data: The Color of Their Eyes" in 2017 when he was Associate Professor of History at Colgate University and author of *How Our Days Became Numbered: Risk and the Rise of the Statistical Individual* (University of Chicago Press, 2015). This post was inspired by research he did for an article on the history and political economy of personal data over the last 200 years, which was published in late 2017 in the History of Science Society's annual journal *Osiris*. Today, Bouk continues to teach the history of quantification at Colgate and recently completed a fellowship at the Data & Society Research Institute. He is the author of a new book, published by Farrar, Straus and Giroux, titled *Democracy's Data: The Hidden Stories in the U.S. Census and How to Read Them.*

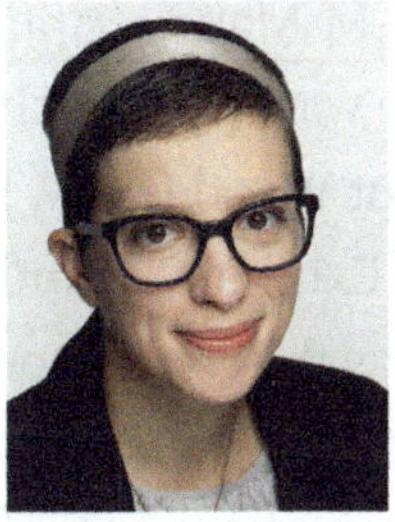

ASHLEY BOWEN, PHD, authored "Revealing Data: Rain, Epidemics, and Life on the Docks in 1918" and "Finding Hope: A Woman's Place Is in the Lab" in 2018 when she was a contract collections researcher in the Exhibition Program at the NLM. Today, she is Creative Execution Manager for Heritage Werks, Inc., a heritage services company based in Atlanta, Georgia. Prior to joining Heritage Werks, she worked as a guest curator in the Exhibits Program at the National Library of Medicine and as editor of the American Historical Association's newsmagazine *Perspectives on History*. Her general research interests include nineteenth-century public health and medicine, the material culture of medicine, and representations of patient experience.

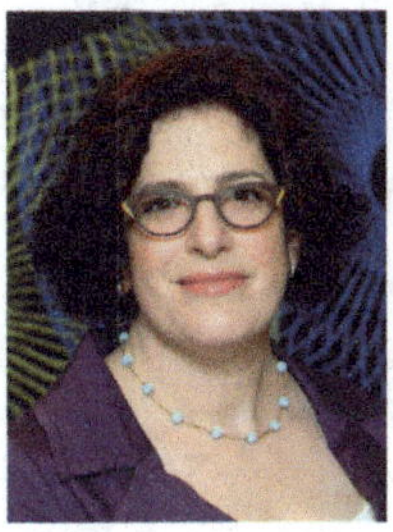

JENNIFER BRIER, PHD, co-authored "Power to the People: Washington Gives Back" in 2016 with Anne Armstrong, Julie Kutruff, Erin Carlson Mast, and Patricia Tuohy, when she moderated the panel described in the post and was professor at University of Illinois Chicago, a position she holds today. Dr. Brier runs a project called History Moves that encourages community members to think of themselves and act as history makers. History Moves has just completed a transmedia history project called, "I'm Still Surviving: A Living Women's History of HIV/AIDS." This project engaged almost forty women living with HIV to produce a history of HIV/AIDS with women at its center.

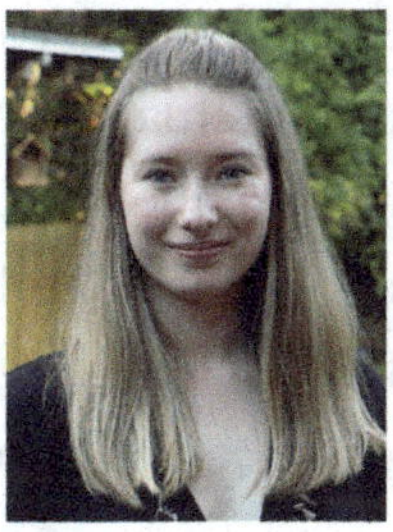

EMMA CARTER, MIS, authored "The Forgotten Frontier: Nursing Done in Wild Places" in 2018 when she was a junior at Millsaps College in Jackson, Mississippi, majoring in history with a museum studies minor. She interned in the Historical Audiovisuals program during summer 2018. Today, she is still interested in working in a library or archive. In the fall of 2022, she graduated from the University of Tennessee, Knoxville with her master's degree in information science and earned the Best Project Award for her outstanding work on a digital library group project with community partner, the Girl Scout Museum at Daisy's Place. She is currently working as an Intellectual Property Rights Researcher at the Indianapolis Museum of Art at Newfields.

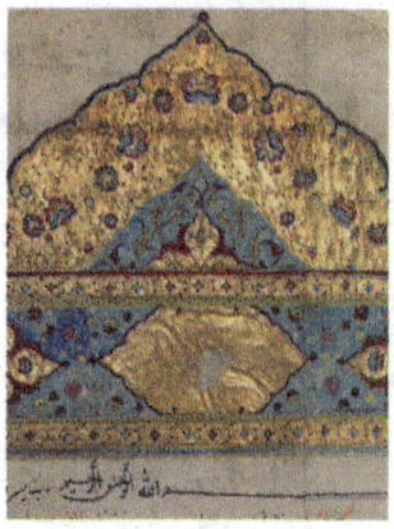

ROBERTA CASAGRANDE-KIM, PHD, authored "NLM Manuscripts on Loan to Romance and Reason" in 2018 when she was a Research Associate at the Institute for the Study of the Ancient World (ISAW) at New York University and Assistant Manager of Exhibitions and Publications at the Onassis Foundation USA. She was the co-curator of the 2018 exhibition *Romance and Reason: Islamic Transformations of the Classical Past* at ISAW. Today, Roberta continues her work of Research Associate at ISAW, focusing primarily on the archeological exploration of the Late Antique site of Amheida (Egypt) and the Hellenistic phases of Niğde Kınık Höyük (Turkey) and the publication of the finds associated with these excavations.

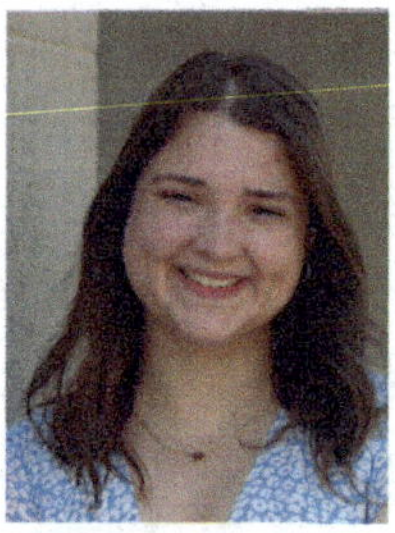

MARY CULLER, MA, co-authored the preface of this book with E. Thomas Ewing while she was completing her master's degree in history with a certificate in public history from Virginia Tech. She is currently working as the Museum Projects Coordinator at the International Tennis Hall of Fame in Newport, Rhode Island.

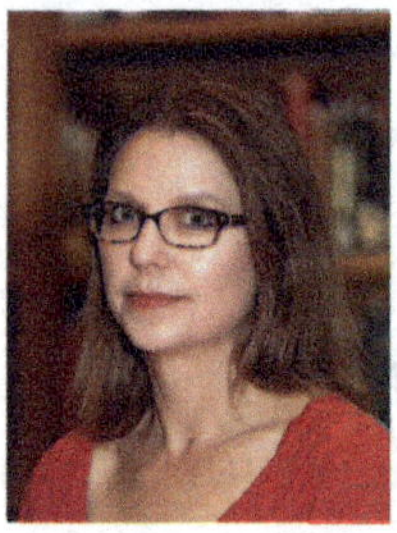

SARAH EILERS, MA, MLS, authored "Winter Wounds, Paper Dressing" in 2015 while working as a contract archivist for the Historical Audiovisuals program in the History of Medicine Division at the NLM, and "Revealing Data: Concepts and Controversies in Modern Medicine, 1969–70" in 2018, having become the fulltime manager of the program, a position she held until her departure from the NLM in 2023 after overseeing preservation and access workflows for several hundred global health and family planning film titles and working with colleagues both inside and outside of the NLM to further develop the curated film site *Medicine on Screen.*

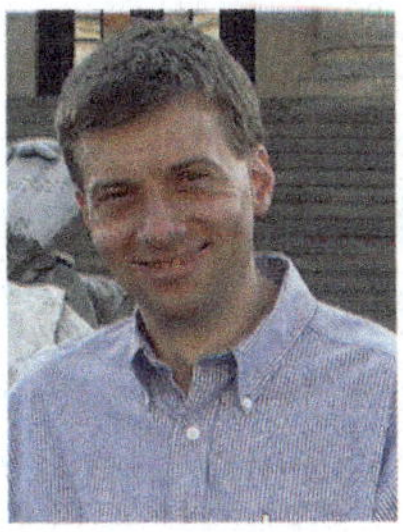

E. THOMAS EWING, PHD, co-author of the preface of this book with Mary Culler, co-authored "Revealing Data: Measuring Mortality during an Epidemic" in 2018, with Ian Hargreaves, Jessica King, Andrew Pregnall, and Tyler Talnagi, when he was a professor of history at Virginia Tech, a position he holds today, and director of the Tracking the Russian Flu project supported by the National Endowment for the Humanities and a 4-VA research grant. Today, his study of Russian influenza continues, with an article published in *Public Health Reports* in 2022. In the spring of 2020, students in his course presented on their research on the 1918 influenza pandemic in a webinar hosted by the National Library of Medicine. During the COVID-19 pandemic, he led a collaborative project examining the use of face masks during the 1918 influenza epidemic in the United States.

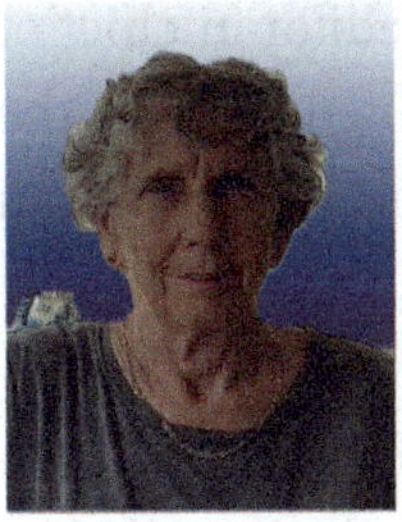

SUSIE FISHER, PHD, authored "In Search of Sol Spiegelman" in 2015 when she was an academic teaching faculty member for the MA Program in Biological Thought at The Open University of Israel. Her article "Not just 'a clever way to detect whether DNA really made RNA': The invention of DNA-RNA hybridization and its outcome" on Sol Spiegelman, based on research at the NLM, was published in October 2015 in *Studies in the History and Philosophy of Biological and Biomedical Sciences*. Today, she is retired from teaching at the Open University of Israel, engaged with a project concerning the early history of bacteriophage therapy in the USA, and applying digital humanities tools to investigate the scientific and medical networks that were involved in the rise and fall of this therapy.

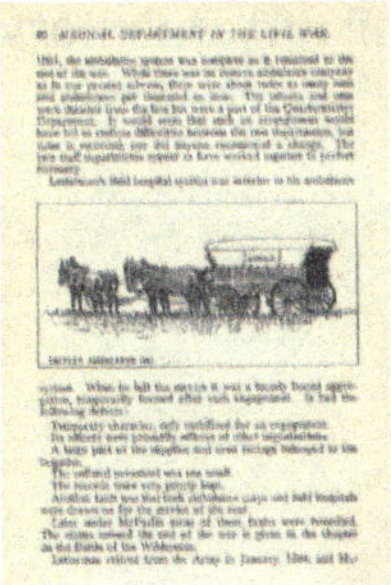

BENJAMIN FORREST authored "Following the Rear: Travails of the Union Army's Ambulance Core" in 2019 when he was a fourth-year medical student at the University of Birmingham, United Kingdom. He completed an intercalated degree program in the History of Medicine, which supported his research at the National Library of Medicine and other institutions.

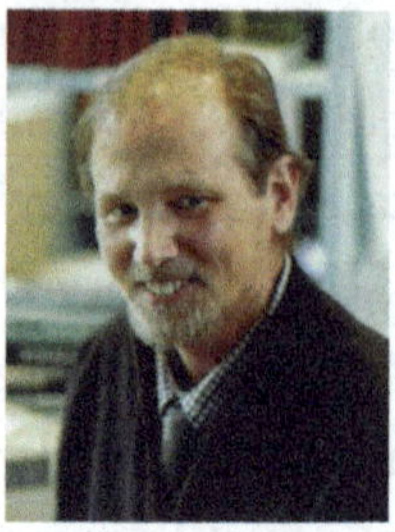

RUSSELL M. FRANKS authored "John E. Fogarty: From Providence to Profiles" in 2015 when he was Librarian for Special and Archival Collections at the Phillips Memorial Library, Providence College. Retiring in 2019, he and his wife relocated to Georgia to enjoy being near their children and three grandsons. In his spare time, Russell continues to pursue the art and craft of nineteenth-century photographic processes and researching the expansion of the western frontier during the first half of the nineteenth century.

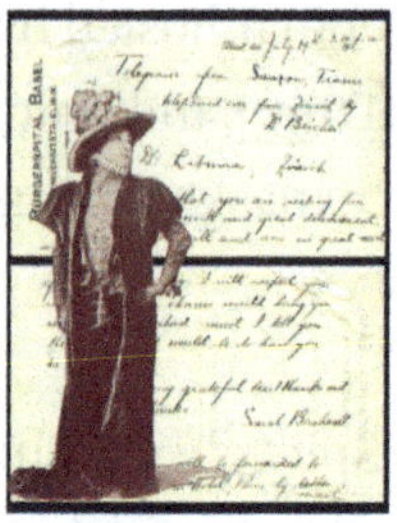

ROBERT GOTTLIEB (1931–2023) authored "The Divine Sarah and Her Divine Doctor" in 2014 based on his critically acclaimed book *Sarah: The Life of Sarah Bernhardt*. He was also author of *George Balanchine: The Ballet Maker*; *Great Expectations: The Sons and Daughters of Charles Dickens*, and most recently *Garbo*. From 1987 to 1992, he was the editor of *The New Yorker*. Before that, he served as editor-in-chief of Simon & Schuster and Alfred A. Knopf, and he edited some of the most significant books of the twentieth century, from *Catch-22* to Toni Morrison's *Beloved* to Robert Caro's *The Power Broker*.

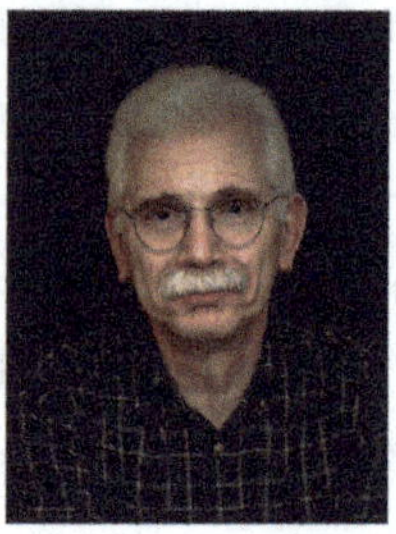

STEPHEN J. GREENBERG, MSLS, PHD, authored "A Book Unfinished: Paracelsus in Hand-Press Sheets" in 2016 when he was Coordinator of Public Services for the History of Medicine Division at the NLM. He was subsequently Head of the Rare Books and Early Manuscripts Section of the division. Dr. Greenberg retired from the NLM in 2021, but he remains active in the field, working with the Medical Library Association (MLA) and Librarians, Archivists, and Museum Professionals in the History of the Health Sciences (LAMPHHS). His personal projects are centered on work combining history, memory, poetry, and photography.

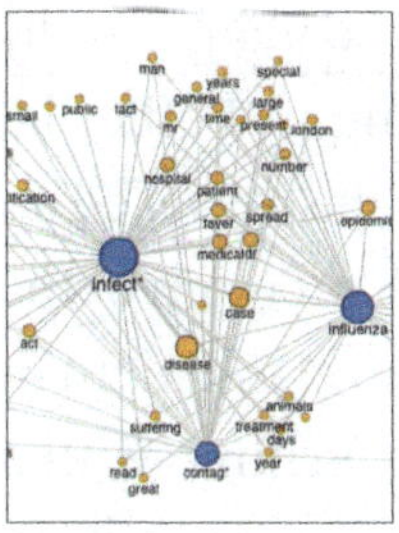

IAN HARGREAVES co-authored "Revealing Data: Measuring Mortality during an Epidemic" in 2018, with E. Thomas Ewing, Jessica King, Andrew Pregnall, and Tyler Talnagi, shortly before he graduated from Virginia Tech with degrees in foreign languages (German) and international studies and enrolled at The George Washington University Law School. Today, Ian is an associate attorney at the Federal Practice Group, having graduated from The George Washington Law School in May 2021. Ian is barred in the District of Columbia, where his practice focuses on government contracts and civil litigation.

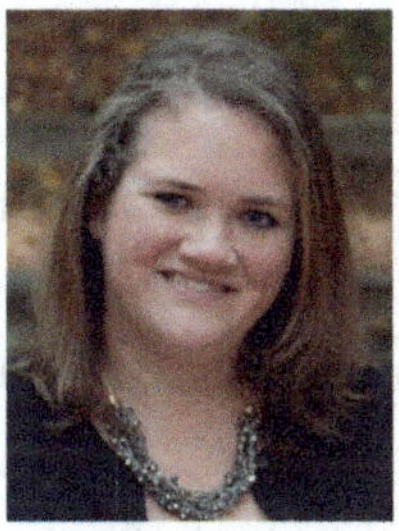

MAUREEN HARLOW, MSLS, MPA, authored "Autism and Alzheimer's on the Web" in 2014 when she was a member of the inaugural 2013 cohort of residents in the National Digital Stewardship Residency program, an initiative of the Library of Congress and the Institute of Museum and Library Services, on assignment to the National Library of Medicine. Today, she is the Director of the Media Library at PBS, overseeing the intake and preservation of over fifty years of broadcast media.

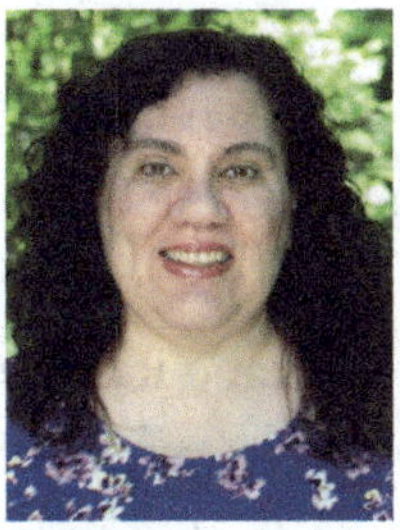

LAURA HARTMAN, MLIS, authored the introduction to chapter two when she was Acting Head of the Rare Books and Early Manuscripts Section of the NLM History of Medicine Division. She continues her public service at the NLM today, specializing in fifteenth- and sixteenth-century European imprints and remaining fascinated by investigating their provenance and tracking how they have passed from owner to owner through the centuries. Outside of work, she serves as a Girl Scout troop leader and enjoys supporting her two active teenagers in their community service projects and outdoor adventures. In quiet moments, she enjoys reading, gardening, putting together LEGOs and puzzles, and walking the C&O towpath and other local park trails.

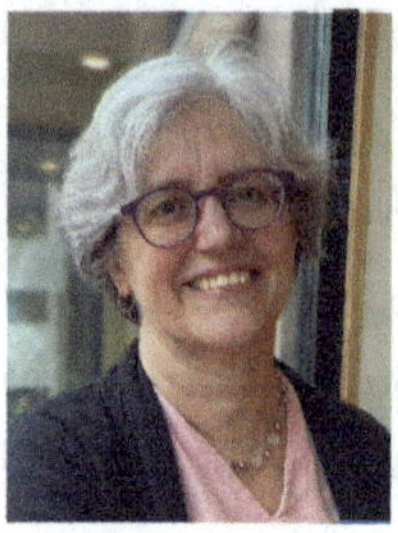

KRISTIN HEITMAN, PHD, authored "Revealing Data: London's Deadly Visitation" in 2017 as an independent scholar living in Bethesda, Maryland. It was part of the lead-up to a symposium she convened on the London Bills of Mortality under the 2017 to 2018 program of the Folger Research Institute in Washington, DC. Today, Dr. Heitman continues her independent historical research and writing, with a focus on the history of metrics and systematic records, especially in fifteenth- to seventeenth-century Europe. She now serves as Deputy Director and Senior Historian in the Office of NIH History and Stetten Museum.

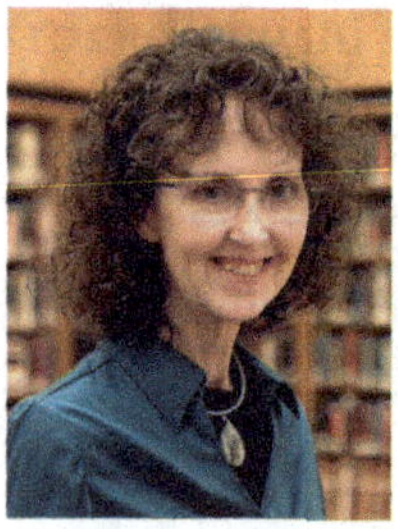

HOLLY HERRO, MLIS, co-authored "Preserving Nirenberg's Genetic Code Chart" in 2014, with Kristi Wright, when she was Conservation Librarian for the History of Medicine Division at the NLM, a position she held as Senior Conservator until her retirement in 2023. In this role, she enjoyed investigating ways data science intersects with conservation and served as a member of the Leather Discussion Group with Kristi Wright and colleagues from Pennsylvania State University and Smithsonian Libraries.

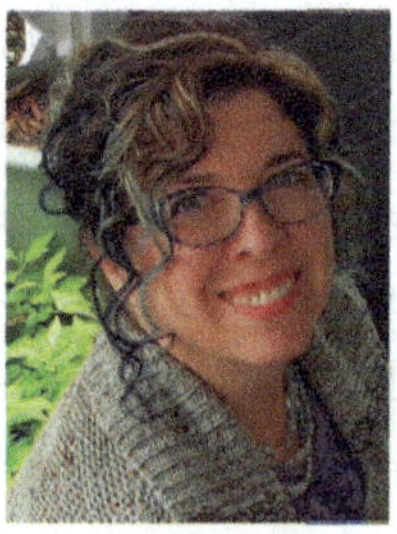

DAWN HUNTER, MFA, authored "Drawn To, Drawn From Experience" in 2017 when she was serving as the Fulbright España Senior Research Fellow at the Instituto Cajal in Madrid, Spain. Her new body of work is a suite of biographical drawings and paintings about Santiago Ramón y Cajal, the father of modern neuroscience. Her series is comprised of creative works and formal investigations of Cajal's scientific drawings that are currently on display at the John Porter Neuroscience Research Center at the National Institute of Health, Bethesda, Maryland. Her artwork about Santiago Ramón y Cajal has been well received and garnered recognition in the neuroscience community. She has been awarded fellowships and grants supporting this series, most notably a Senior Research Fellowship through the Fulbright Foundation, Washington, DC. Dawn has participated in numerous solo and multiple artist exhibitions throughout the United States and Europe, and she is an Associate Professor at the School of Visual Art and Design, University of South Carolina, Columbia, SC.

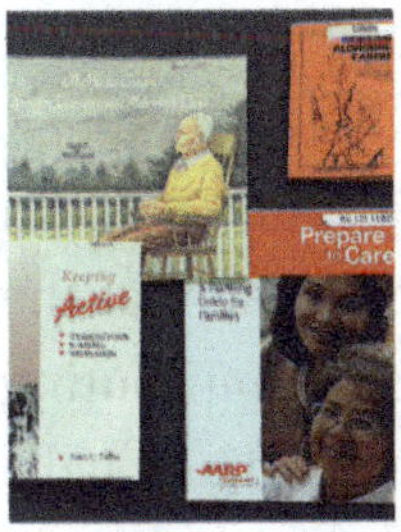

MARGARET KAISER authored "Alzheimer's Disease Collection Received" in 2013 when she was Acquisitions Librarian for the Rare Books and Early Manuscripts Section in the History of Medicine Division of the NLM.

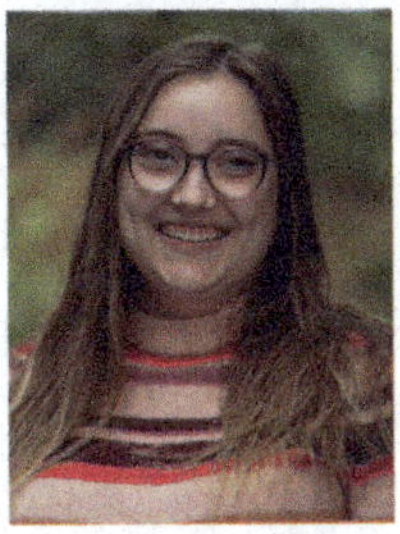

JESSICA KING, MA, co-authored "Revealing Data: Measuring Mortality during an Epidemic" in 2018, with E. Thomas Ewing, Ian Hargreaves, Andrew Pregnall, and Tyler Talnagi, shortly before she graduated from Virginia Tech with majors in communication and international studies with a minor in German and enrolled in the Virginia Tech graduate program in communication. Today, she has completed her master's degree in communication with research focused on queer representation in pop culture. She currently works in digital advertising for mission-driven organizations in Atlanta, Georgia.

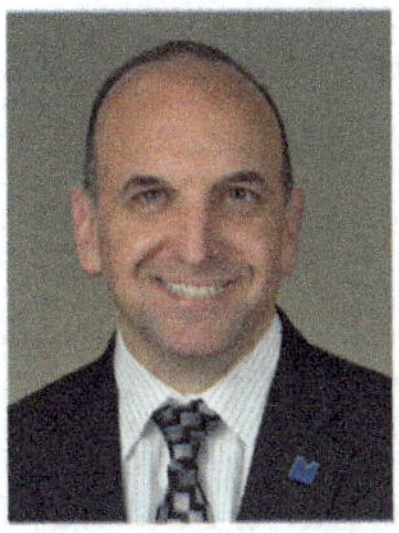

KENNETH M. KOYLE, MA, co-authored "Art on the Edge" in 2017, with Ginny A. Roth and Krista Stracka, when he was Deputy Chief of the History of Medicine Division at the NLM. He continues his public service at the NLM today, focused on supporting colleagues as they implement strategic changes to better serve current and future researchers. He continues to write blog posts for *Circulating Now* and other blogs, along with articles about history and management topics.

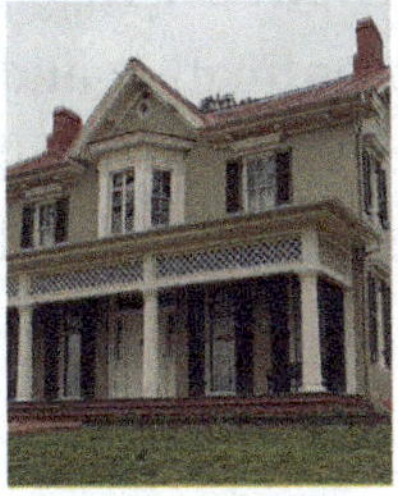

JULIE KUTRUFF co-authored "Power to the People: Washington Gives Back" in 2016 with Anne Armstrong, Jennifer Brier, Erin Carlson Mast, and Patricia Tuohy, when she was the Community Outreach and Partnership Coordinator for National Capital Parks-East (NACE), which manages the Frederick Douglass House in the Anacostia neighborhood of Washington, DC. She is currently the Special Events Manager for NACE.

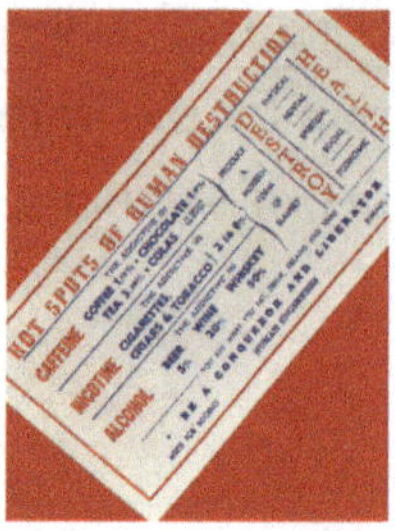

JAMES LABOSIER, MA, MLS, author of the introduction to chapter one, wrote "Hot Spots of Human Destruction: The Howard Bishop Papers" in 2019 when he was Associate Curator for the Archives and Modern Manuscripts Program in the History of Medicine Division at the NLM. He continues his public service at the NLM today, contributing his experience and expertise to management of the NLM's globally appreciated archival collections.

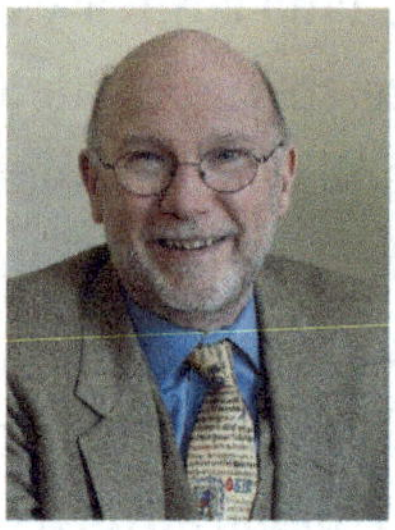

THOMAS LAWRENCE LONG, PHD, authored "Remembering & Witnessing: AIDS35 and the NLM Exhibition "Surviving and Thriving"" in 2017 when he was associate professor in residence in the UConn School of Nursing, with a joint appointment on the faculty of Women's, Gender and Sexuality Studies, and the curator of the School of Nursing's Josephine Dolan Nursing History Collection. He has published scholarly articles on cultural representations of HIV/AIDS/SIDA, including the book *AIDS and American Apocalypticism: The Cultural Semiotics of an Epidemic.* Now retired, he continues with teaching part-time and finishing back-burner scholarly manuscripts.

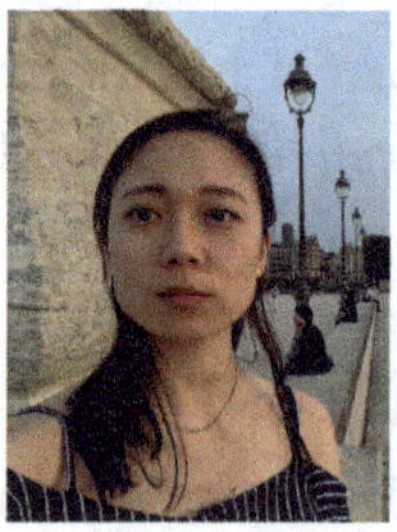

SHANNON LU authored "A Peek at Some Pamphlets" in 2014 when she was a sophomore at Wellesley College where she studied economics, computer science, and the Russian language. She was a Pathways Intern at the National Library of Medicine during summer of 2013. Today, Shannon works in San Francisco as a Lead Software Engineer, building tools to solve challenges like healthcare coordination and applying for insurance. When she's not coding, she continues to fulfill her passion for languages and international affairs through travel and civic engagement.

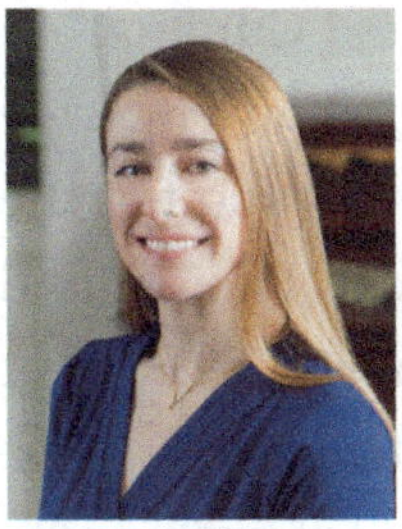

ERIN CARLSON MAST, MA, co-authored "Power to the People: Washington Gives Back" in 2016 with Anne Armstrong, Jennifer Brier, Julie Kutruff, and Patricia Tuohy, when she was CEO and Executive Director at President Lincoln's Cottage at the Soldiers' Home, a Washington, DC, historic site where Lincoln made nation-changing decisions about freedom and democracy. Today, she's based in the Chicago area and serves as President & CEO of the Lincoln Presidential Foundation. The Foundation's vision is a world where freedom and democracy flourish, inspired by the life and work of Abraham Lincoln.

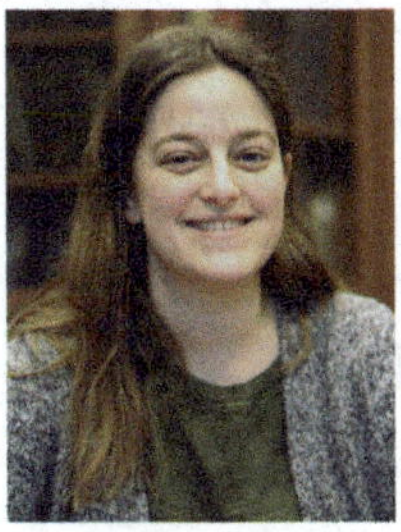

LAURA MCNULTY, MS, authored "Doctoring the Art of Medicine Series" in 2013 when she was a recent graduate of the University of Massachusetts Amherst and working as a conservation intern at the American Philosophical Society in Philadelphia, Pennsylvania following her 2012 summer internship in the conservation lab at the NLM. In 2021, Laura received her Master of Science from the Winterthur/University of Delaware Program in Art Conservation where she specialized in the conservation of archival and library materials. In addition to her internships at the American Philosophical Society and the National Library of Medicine, she has completed internships at the Colonial Williamsburg Foundation, the National Museum of American History, the Hirshhorn Museum & Sculpture Garden, the United States Holocaust Memorial Museum, and the Library of Congress, and a two-year, post-graduate fellowship at Johns Hopkins University. Today, she is a contract book conservator at the NLM.

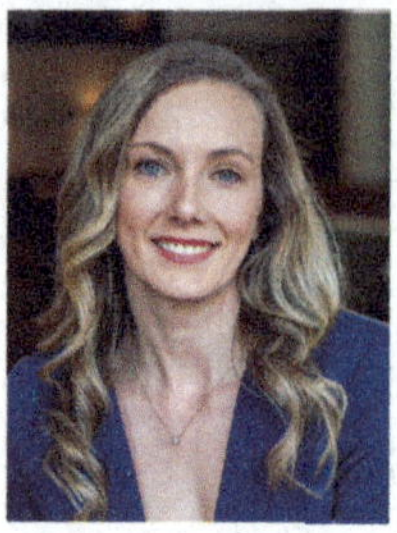

LOREN E. MILLER, PHD, authored "Collaboration and Curation" in 2017 when she was a guest curator of the NLM exhibition *Physician Assistants: Collaboration and Care* and a curatorial assistant at the Smithsonian National Museum of African American History and Culture (NMAAHC). Today, she is the senior curator at the Office of NIH History and Stetten Museum where she develops exhibitions, advances and maintains the museum's collection, and contributes to educational content. In addition to public history, her research interests include visual and material culture, women's and gender history, and African American history.

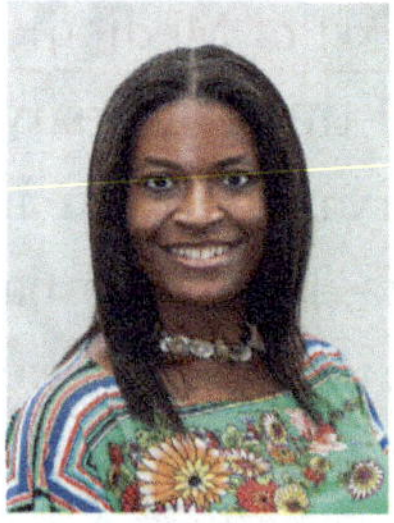

ERIKA MILLS authored "By the Teachers, For the Teachers" in 2013 and "Kick Polio Out of Nigeria" in 2014 when she was a community outreach coordinator for the Exhibition Program in the History of Medicine Division of the NLM. Today, she is an exhibit specialist for the program. She has co-curated exhibitions on a collection of images from the World Health Organization and the first history of the NLM as presented in the institution's first exhibition.

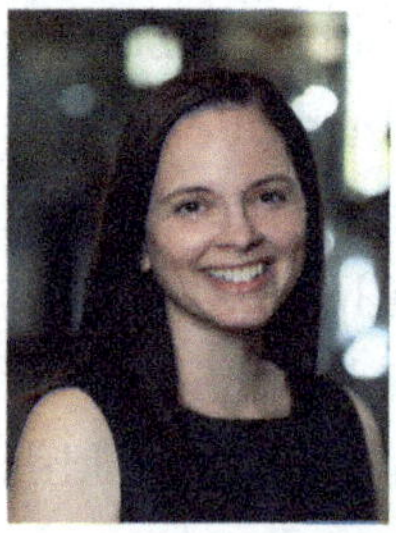

CHRISTIE MOFFATT, MLIS, authored "Smoking in America: 50 Years On" in 2014, and "Revealing Data: Explorations of Data in Collections" in 2017, when she was Manager of the Digital Manuscripts Program in the History of Medicine Division at the NLM. Today, she continues her public service at the NLM, collaborating with colleagues across the Library on digitization and access to twentieth-century historical collections in science, medicine, and public health, and web archiving on topics and events related to NLM collecting interests, including the ongoing COVID-19 pandemic, HIV/AIDS, and the opioid epidemic.

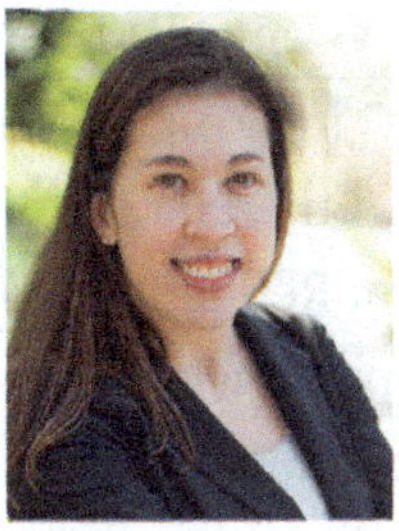

HEIDI MOREFIELD, PHD, author of the introduction to chapter five, authored "Tinkering with Profitability: DeBakey and the Affordable Blood Transfusion Instrument" in 2017 when she was a doctoral candidate in the history of medicine at Johns Hopkins University and an NLM Michael E. DeBakey Fellow. Her dissertation focused on the history of the appropriate technology movement in international health. Today, she works as a consultant, advising companies within the United States and internationally on strategy, particularly in the wake of the COVID-19 pandemic. Her book, *Developing to Scale: Technology and the Making of Global Health* is out with the University of Chicago Press.

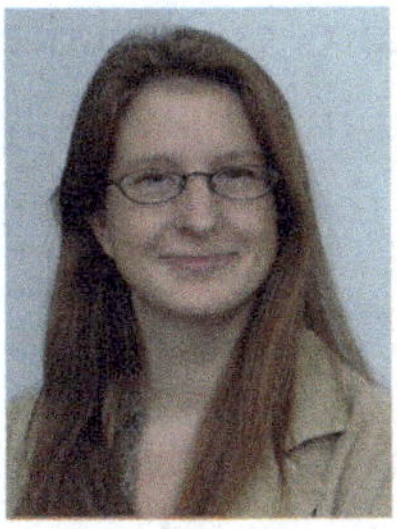

ELIZABETH A. MULLEN, MA, co-editor of this book with Jeffrey S. Reznick, and co-author with him of its introduction, wrote "MCCR Was There" in 2013 and "A Remarkable Career in Psychiatry" in 2014, when she was Manager of Web Development and Social Media in the History of Medicine Division at the NLM. As managing editor of *Circulating Now*, she has been privileged to work closely with many creative and dedicated NLM staff members who have served on the editorial board for the blog and to meet and learn from a wide range of historians, artists, curators, students, educators, and members of the public who have found meaning in the collections and shared their enthusiasm for the history of medicine.

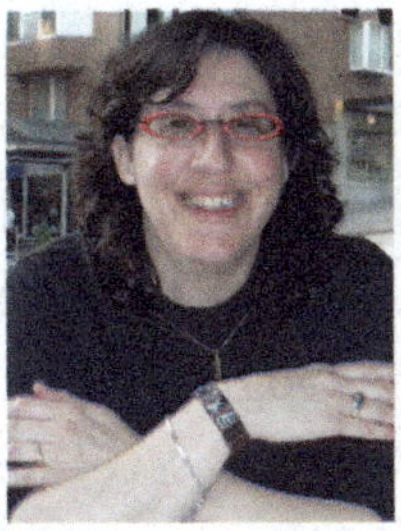

JILL L. NEWMARK, author of the introduction to chapter three, wrote "A Civil War Surgeon's Books Rediscovered" in 2014 when she was an Exhibition Specialist for the Exhibition Program in the History of Medicine Division at the NLM. Today, she is an independent historian and author of *Without Concealment, Without Compromise: The Courageous Lives of Black Civil War Surgeons*, published in 2023. She continues her research on African American medical personnel who served during the American Civil War, lecturing and presenting to the public on the subject. In her spare time, she enjoys working with dogs as a canine massage therapist.

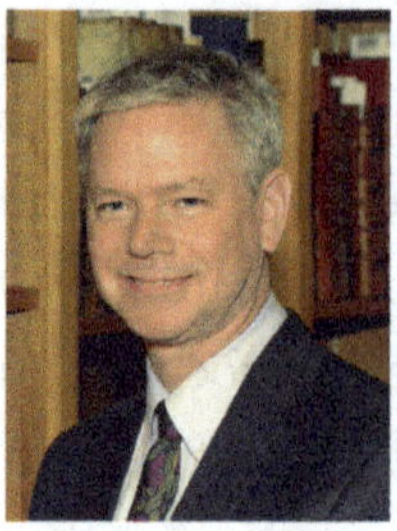

MICHAEL J. NORTH, MS, MSLS, authored "Andreas Vesalius at 500" in 2013, and "Making a Medical Heritage Milestone" in 2014, when he was Head of Rare Books and Early Manuscripts in the History of Medicine Division at the NLM. Today, he is the Head of Reference and Reader Services in the Rare Book and Special Collections Division at the Library of Congress, where he connects researchers and the public with the Library's vast rare book collections, ranging from fifteenth-century printed books to early Americana, artists' books, and popular literature.

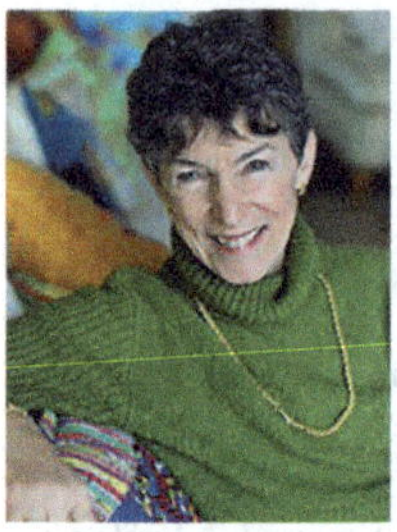

KERRY KELLY NOVICK was interviewed on *Circulating Now* in 2014, in "On Combat Fatigue Irritability: Kerry Kelly Novick Part III." She is a practicing psychoanalyst and the daughter of Gene Kelly and actress Betsy Blair. Today, she continues her active career of practice and community service. She teaches nationally and internationally and, with her husband, Jack Novick, has published three additional books since 2016.

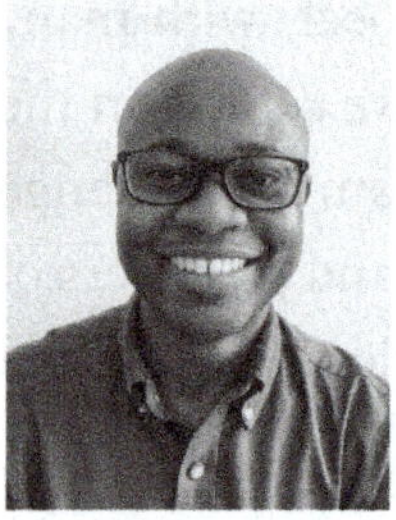

ALEXANDER NWALA, PHD, authored "Revealing Data: Why We Need Humans to Curate Web Collections" in 2018 when he was a computer science PhD student and member of the Web Science and Digital Libraries research group at Old Dominion University, Norfolk Virginia. Today, he is an assistant professor of data science at William and Mary, Williamsburg, Virginia. His research interest is interdisciplinary, encompassing social media/computational social science, web/data science, web archiving, and (local) news.

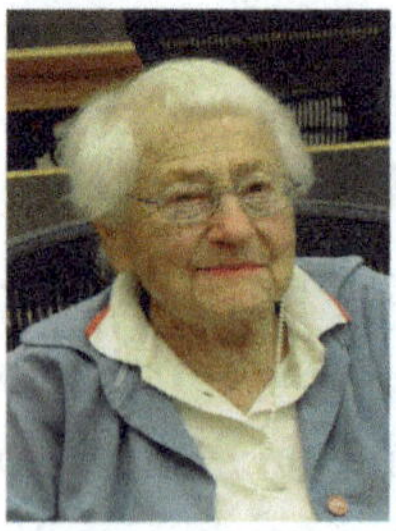

LUCY OZARIN, MD, (1914–2017) was featured in *Circulating Now* in 2014, in "A Remarkable Career in Psychiatry." She volunteered at the NLM from 2004 to 2013 researching and writing biographies of notable American psychiatrists and curating the NLM's *Diseases of the Mind* website. Before her service with us as a medical historian, Lucy earned a living as a psychiatrist. From 1943 to 1946, she served in the Navy where she earned the distinction of being one of the first women psychiatrists commissioned in the Navy (and only one of seven women Navy psychiatrists in World War II). She died on September 17, 2017, at the age of 103.

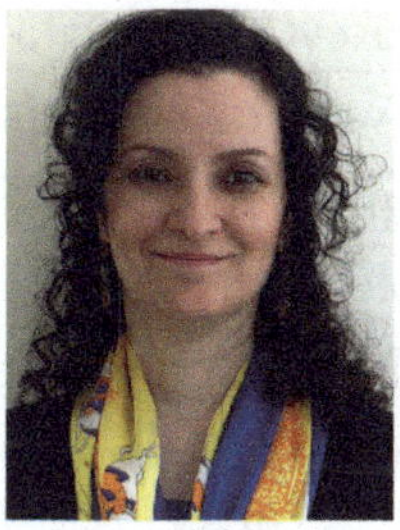

HOMIRA PASHAI, MA, authored "A Mughal Era Manuscript Curiously Illustrated" in 2016 when she was a volunteer in the History of Medicine Division of the NLM, where she updated the Library's catalog of Arabic manuscripts, identified the scribes and translated information from flyleaves and end leaves, and researched and published articles on selected manuscripts. Previously, she interned at the Library, and received her master's degree in historical research—public history in 2011, and her master's degree in education curriculum and instruction in 2018. She also worked at the Smithsonian's Freer Gallery of Art, updating descriptions of Persian and Islamic manuscripts and creating a descriptive narrative for the gallery's Islamic manuscript digitized record. She also worked in the Persian Studies Department of the University of Maryland, creating lesson plans and teacher's guides for instruction. Today, she is working on a book about 1911 Persia, with her acquaintance with manuscripts continuing to grow as it has since her childhood when she examined her grandfather's papers.

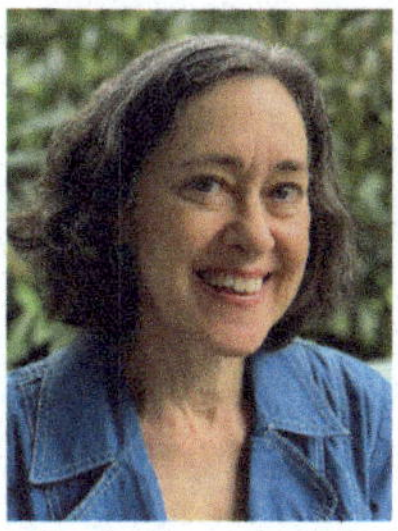

ABIGAIL PORTER authored "Leonidas H. Berry and the Fight to Desegregate Medicine" in 2018 when she was a researcher and exhibition coordinator in the History of Medicine Division's Exhibition Program at the NLM. Today, she continues her work as an exhibition writer, researcher, and project coordinator. During her career, she has worked on more than thirty historical and scientific exhibition projects for museums and libraries. Currently she is working on exhibition projects for the U.S. Capitol Visitor Center in Washington, DC. She recently completed research and script writing for *Congressional Investigations*. This temporary exhibition examines past investigations to show how Congress works, unpacks what happens during inquiries, and shows how investigations result in legislation.

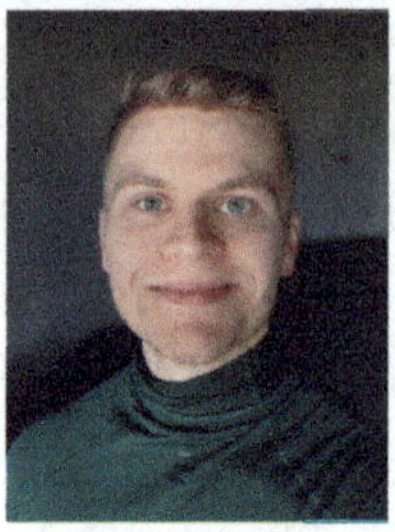

ANDREW PREGNALL, MSC, MPHIL, co-authored "Revealing Data: Measuring Mortality during an Epidemic" in 2018, with E. Thomas Ewing, Ian Hargreaves, Jessica King, and Tyler Talnagi, when he was a senior at Virginia Tech pursuing degrees in microbiology and history. After graduating, Andrew read for an MSc in health data science at UCL and an MPhil in genomic medicine at University of Cambridge on a Marshall Scholarship. Today, Andrew is starting medical school at the Penn Perelman School of Medicine, and he performs research at the intersection of data science and medicine, particularly disease subtyping and cancer genomics. In his free time, he is an avid road and gravel cyclist.

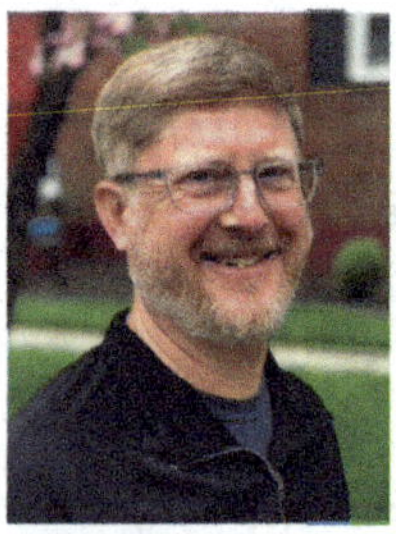

JOHN REES, MA, MLIS, author of the introduction to chapter four, wrote "A Pharmacist's Mate First Class" in 2015 when he was Archivist and Digital Resources Manager for the Archives and Modern Manuscripts Program in the History of Medicine Division at the NLM. He continues his public service at the NLM today, contributing his leadership, experience, and expertise to management of the NLM's globally appreciated archival collections.

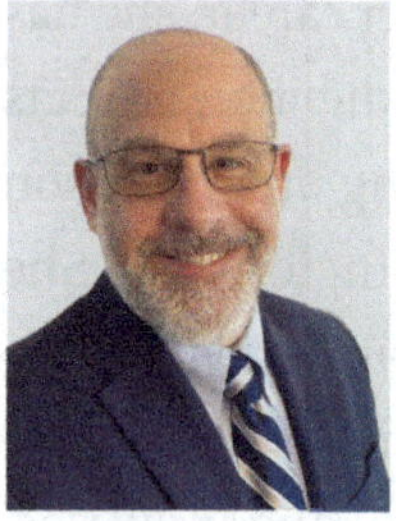

JEFFREY S. REZNICK, PHD, co-editor of this book with Elizabeth A. Mullen, and co-author with her of its introduction, co-authored "'The President Is Somewhat Restless…'" with Lenore Barbian, PhD, in 2013 when he was Chief of the NLM History of Medicine Division. He is also co-editor, with Kenneth M. Koyle, of *Images of America: U.S. National Library of Medicine* (Arcadia Publishing, 2017), and author of *War and Peace in the Worlds of Rudolf H. Sauter: A Cultural History of a Creative Life* (Anthem Press, 2022). He continues his public service at the NLM today, working strategically with teams across the Library to provide leadership and direction to advance access to the NLM's world-renowned collection, as well as its growth and preservation for future generations. He also continues to maintain a diverse, interdisciplinary, and highly collaborative historical research portfolio supported by the Library and based on its diverse collection and associated products and services.

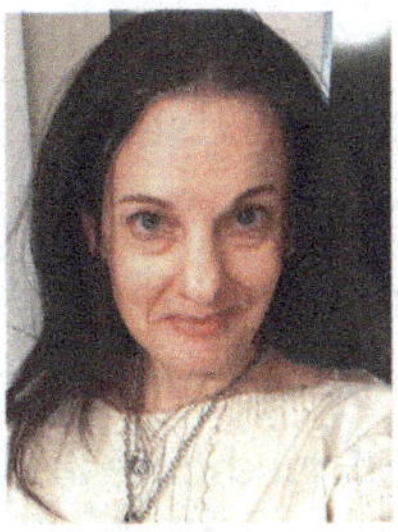

GINNY A. ROTH, MSLS, authored "Global Healing" and "Dr. Schwartz's Stamp Collection" in 2015, and co-authored "Art on the Edge" in 2017, with Kenneth M. Koyle and Krista Stracka, when she was Curator of Prints & Photographs in the History of Medicine Division at the NLM. Ginny received her MSLS at Catholic University in Washington, DC, with a focus on archives and special collections. Today, she is Assistant Section Head in the Technical Services section of the Prints and Photographs Division of the Library of Congress.

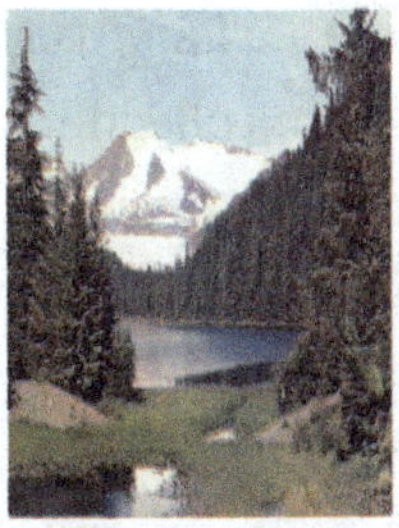

ANNE ROTHFELD, PHD, authored "America's National Parks: Preserved for Public Health" in 2016 when she was a librarian and historian in the History of Medicine Division of the NLM, a position she holds today. Currently, she's editing her dissertation manuscript for publication as well as researching and drafting her next book project on Eve Tucker, a U.S. Fine Arts Representative, and her efforts in restituting stolen cultural property in postwar Austria.

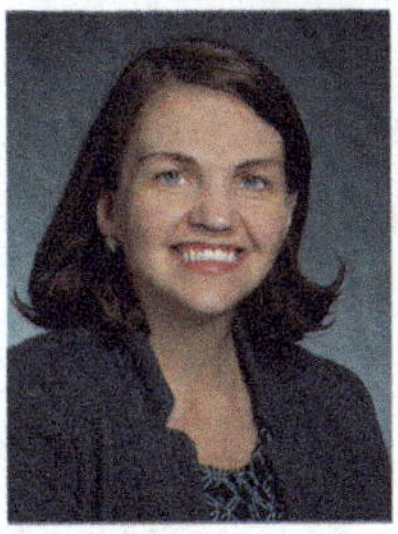

SARAH RUNCIE, PHD, was interviewed on *Circulating Now* in 2019, in "Naming, Networks, and Power in Histories of Medicine in Africa," when she was Assistant Professor of African history at the University of Louisiana at Lafayette. Today, she is Assistant Professor of history at Muhlenberg College, a position she began in fall 2020. She continues to research the history of public health in Cameroon and created a new undergraduate course at Muhlenberg called "Medicine and Power in African History."

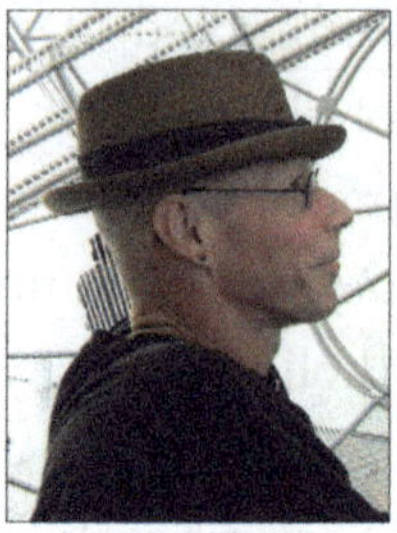

MICHAEL SAPPOL, PHD, authored "How to . . . See with the Microscope" in 2014 when he was a historian in the History of Medicine Division of the NLM. Today he lives in Stockholm, Sweden, and is a visiting researcher in the History of Science and Ideas at Uppsala University. He still loves old "how to" books and his work still focuses on the visual culture and performance of medicine and science in medical museums, illustrated publications and motion pictures. His latest book, *Queer Anatomies*, on the erotic valences of eighteenth- and nineteenth-century anatomical illustration, will be out in spring 2024. His current projects include: *Relics of Lost Medical Civilizations*, a book on the library and museum collections of Sweden's Karolinska Institute and Hagströmer Library; and "Anatomy's Photography," a history of photographic anatomy from its inception in the 1860s to the 1950s.

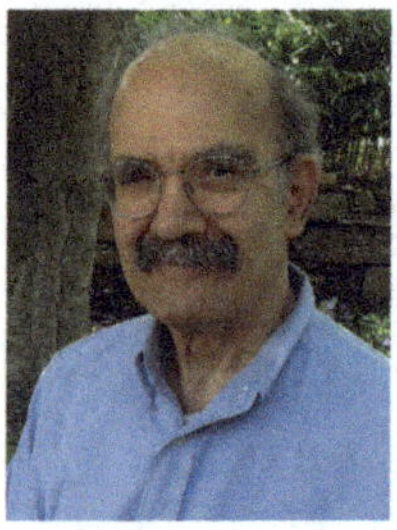

JAN SCHULTZ was interviewed on *Circulating Now* in 2019, in "The "PROMIS" of Computer-Based Medical Records." He was associated with the University of Vermont from 1969 until 1981 as a Research Associate in the College of Medicine. Today, he is semi-retired and for the past thirteen years has helped Front Porch Forum expand throughout Vermont and into parts of New York and Massachusetts. Front Porch Forum is a local social media company; see "From Bangkok to Burlington—The Public Interest Social Internet" and "How a Vermont Social Network Became a Model for Online Communities". At 79, Jan took up piano jazz.

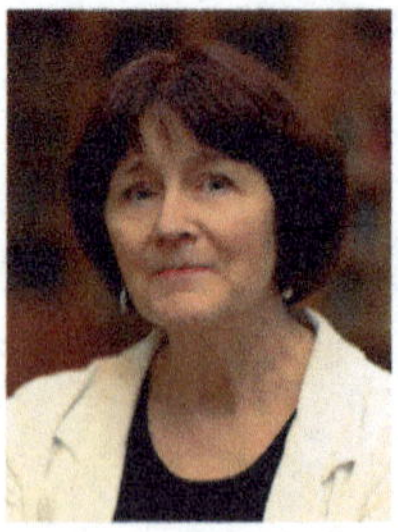

SUSAN L. SPEAKER, PHD, author of the introduction to chapter six, wrote "One Medical Officer's Armistice Day" and "Revealing Data: Collecting Data about TB, ca. 1900" in 2018 when she was Historian for the Digital Manuscripts Program of the History of Medicine Division at the NLM, working with the NLM Web Collecting and Archiving team, serving on the *Circulating Now* editorial board, and writing other blog posts and articles about the NLM and the history of medicine and public health. Susan retired in 2024.

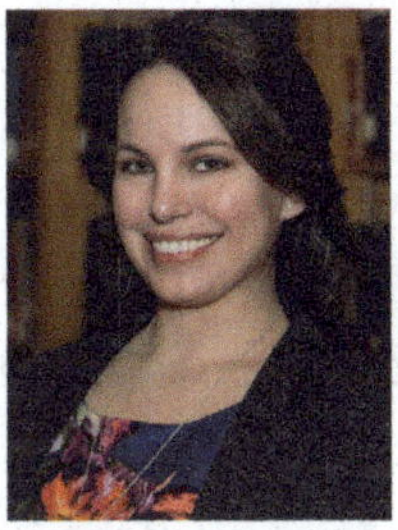

KRISTA STRACKA, MLIS, authored "Pen to Parchment: National Handwriting Day" in 2020, and co-authored "Art on the Edge" in 2017, with Kenneth M. Koyle and Ginny A. Roth, when she was a Rare Book Cataloger for the Rare Books and Early Manuscripts Section in the History of Medicine Division at the NLM. She continues her public service at the NLM today, cataloging rare and unique materials and featuring collections through social media and blog posts for *Circulating Now.*

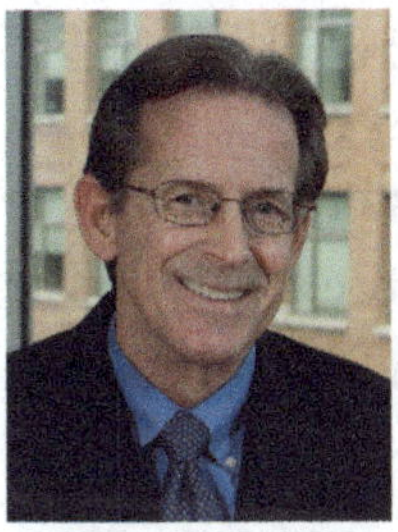

JOHN SWANN, PHD, authored "A History of the FDA Notices of Judgment" in 2015 when he was a historian at the Food and Drug Administration (FDA). He continues in this position today, researching pharmaceuticals, dietary supplements, regulation, public health, and FDA institutional history for publications, presentations, exhibitions, and social media, as well as documenting and preserving agency history for scholars and others.

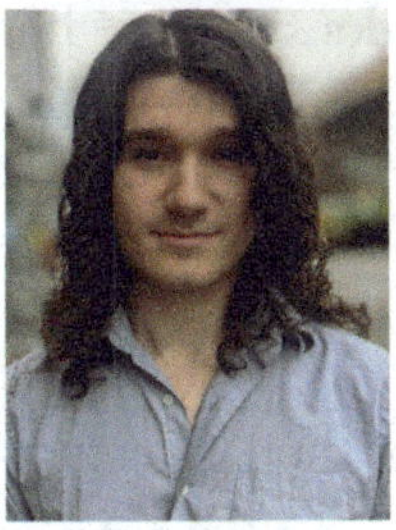

TYLER TALNAGI co-authored "Revealing Data: Measuring Mortality during an Epidemic" in 2018, with E. Thomas Ewing, Ian Hargreaves, Jessica King, and Andrew Pregnall, shortly before he graduated from Virginia Tech with degrees in German and international studies. Today, he resides in the Baltimore, Maryland, area supporting the Navy's foreign military sales programs as a consultant. He continues to utilize his passion for language and learning about different cultures, and hopes to continue traveling internationally for both business and pleasure.

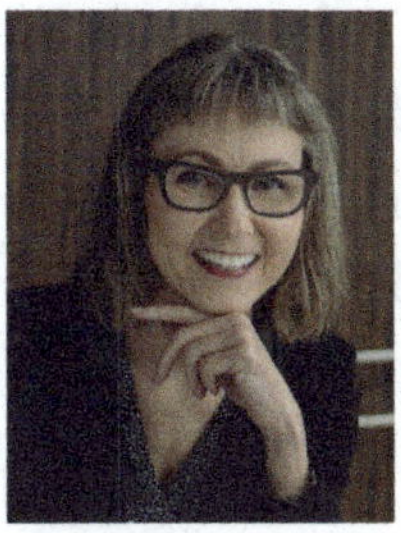

PATRICIA TUOHY co-authored "Power to the People: Washington Gives Back" in 2016 with Anne Armstrong, Jennifer Brier, and Julie Kutruff, when she was head of the Exhibition Program in the History of Medicine Division at the NLM. Patricia retired in 2022.

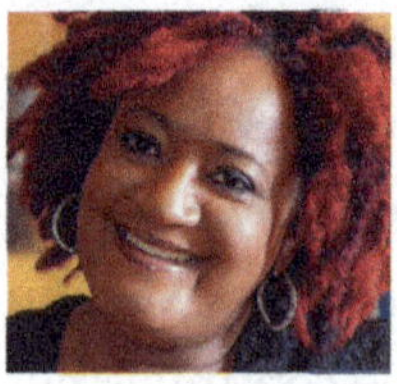

PSYCHE WILLIAMS-FORSON, PHD, authored "Sitting by the Fireside: African American History, Women's History, and Food" in 2017 when she was an associate professor and chair, Department of American Studies, University of Maryland-College Park and the guest curator of the NLM exhibition *Fire and Freedom: Food and Enslavement in Early America*. Today she is professor and still chair of the department and she has a new book *Eating While Black: Food Shaming and Race in America* (UNC Press, 2022).

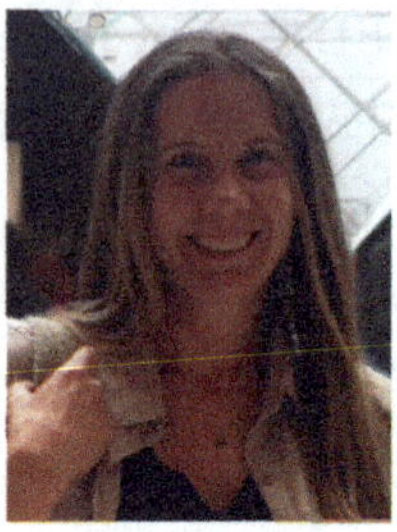

KRISTI WRIGHT, MLIS, co-authored "Preserving Nirenberg's Genetic Code Chart" in 2014, with Holly Herro, when she was a contract conservator for the Conservation Program of the History of Medicine Division at the NLM. She is principal of Wright Conservation and Framing in Front Royal, Virginia, and currently has a fascination with the effectiveness of leather as a modern conservation material and participates in the multi-institutional Leather Discussion Group. She also continues to be interested in the applications of imaging analysis in the evaluation of color shift. When she doesn't have her nose in a book, she enjoys playing music, gardening, and exploring America's wilderness areas.

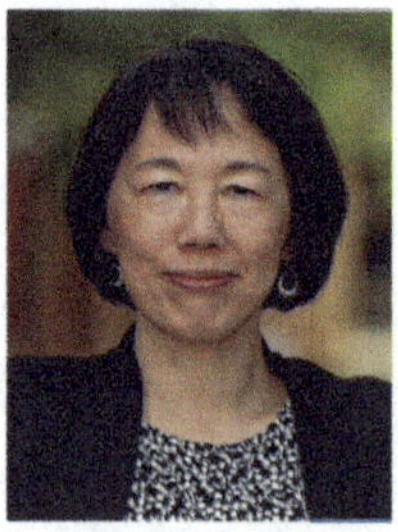

YI-LI WU, PHD, authored "'Wrapped in Flesh': Views of the Body in East Asian Medicine" when she was a Center Associate of the Lieberthal-Rogel Center for Chinese Studies at the University of Michigan, a Research Fellow of EASTmedicine, University of Westminster and an organizer of the ACLS/Chiang Ching-kuo Foundation funded workshop *Comparative perspectives on body materiality and structure in the history of Sinitic and East Asian medicines*. Today, she is an associate professor of women's and gender studies and history at the University of Michigan, where she teaches courses on gender, health, and history in East Asia. She is completing her book manuscript on the history of injury medicine.

INDEX

Page numbers followed by f denotes a figure.

Made in United States
North Haven, CT
04 November 2026

21760285R00200